Cardiac Amyloidosis

Cardiac Amyloidosis

Diagnosis and Treatment

Michele Emdin • Giuseppe Vergaro
Alberto Aimo • Marianna Fontana
Editors

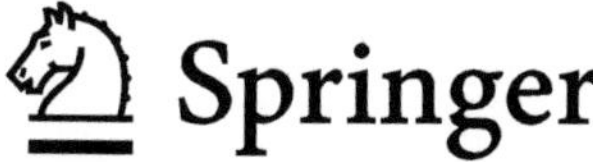
Springer

Editors
Michele Emdin
Health Science Interdisciplinary Center
Scuola Superiore Sant'Anna
Fondazione Toscana Gabriele Monasterio
Pisa, Italy

Alberto Aimo
Health Science Interdisciplinary Center
Scuola Superiore Sant'Anna
Fondazione Toscana Gabriele Monasterio
Pisa, Italy

Giuseppe Vergaro
Health Science Interdisciplinary Center
Scuola Superiore Sant'Anna
Fondazione Toscana Gabriele Monasterio
Pisa, Italy

Marianna Fontana
National Amyloidosis Centre
University College London
London, UK

ISBN 978-3-031-51759-4   ISBN 978-3-031-51757-0   (eBook)
https://doi.org/10.1007/978-3-031-51757-0

This Springer imprint is published by the registered company Springer Nature Switzerland AG
The registered company address is: Gewerbestrasse 11, 6330 Cham, Switzerland

Paper in this product is recyclable

Preface

As William Osler wrote in 1892 in his internal medicine book: "There are three phases to treatment: diagnosis, diagnosis, and diagnosis." We can then state: "There are three phases to diagnosis: knowledge, knowledge, and knowledge," and that this is particularly true for cardiac amyloidosis (CA), a once called rare disease, now increasingly recognized and treated thanks to the advances of knowledge most recently achieved by an impressive worldwide research effort.

CA is a disease caused by the accumulation of amyloid fibrils in the extracellular space of the myocardium, leading to profound changes in the heart's substrate, electrical properties, and function, which are the basis for the clinical syndrome, characterized by arrhythmias, conduction disturbances, and a progressive impairment of diastole and systole, progressively leading to overt heart failure. Until very recently, CA was almost always diagnosed very lately and after multiple hospitalizations in emergency medicine, cardiology, pulmonology, and internal medicine wards. Once the clinical suspicion was raised, the demonstration of tissue amyloid deposits was required for the final diagnosis, using highly invasive procedures such as endomyocardial biopsy. Furthermore, when the diagnosis was made, no effective therapeutic options could be offered to the patient. The perception of CA as a rare disease did not stimulate the scientific community and the pharmaceutical industry to support the research and development of new dedicated tools for either diagnosis or treatment.

Afterwards, the intuition and tireless activity of several masters, including Claudio Rapezzi in Bologna and Ferrara; Giampaolo Merlini in Pavia, Italy; Angela Dispenzieri and Martha Grogan at the Mayo Clinic School in Rochester; Mathew Maurer at the Columbia University, NYC, USA; Julian Gillmore and Philip Hawkins, joined by Marianna Fontana at the University College London, UK, and paralleled in Italy by the initiative of Gianfranco Sinagra in Trieste; and Michele Emdin and Giuseppe Vergaro in Pisa, prompted a true revolution in our current approach to CA.

The goals of a noninvasive diagnostic algorithm for transthyretin CA (ATTR-CA), and of the availability of safe, disease-modifying, and lifesaving therapies for light-chain and variant or wild-type transthyretin CA, were achieved. National and international scientific societies, such as the International Society of Amyloidosis, were born; recommendations on diagnosis and management were issued; as well as a specialty journal such as *Amyloid*, research consortia and forum, and patient support groups were formed, worldwide. In turn, this interest in CA and the increased disease awareness in the medical community, favored by several educational initiatives, prompted the identification of an increasing number of cases diagnosed and treated.

Much work is still needed: the ability to recognize and treat patients with CA should become part of the core curriculum of cardiologists as well as internal medicine specialists, general practitioners, neurologists, nephrologists, and hematologists, and both individual and collaborative research should focus on the unsolved issues regarding CA pathophysiology, epidemiology, diagnostics, and therapeutics, as well as on novel strategies for promoting screening in high-risk populations and noninvasive, comprehensive diagnostic paths including novel answers at a local, regional, and national level through the creation of clinical and research networks supported by the scientific societies, as it is the case for Italy.

Our purpose is to give to all the clinicians and researchers interested in the field the integration of the state-of-the-art knowledge with the contribution of specialists from the leading centers in Europe and the United States.

The book is dedicated first to Claudio Rapezzi, to the man who paved the way for the current clinical and research approach to CA, as well as to the clinicians working all over the world to prolong survival and improve the quality of life of patients with CA, and, finally, to our patients, whose well-being is the final goal of all our efforts.

Pisa, Italy   Michele Emdin
Pisa, Italy   Giuseppe Vergaro
Pisa, Italy   Alberto Aimo
London, UK   Marianna Fontana

Contents

Tribute to Claudio Rapezzi

Gianfranco Sinagra and Aldostefano Porcari

There may be many ways to start a tribute to Claudio Rapezzi, no one is easy in the heart of those who have spent part of their life with him. He was a unique and extremely rare concentration of human and scientific qualities that cannot be expressed only with words. If we were to choose a single characteristic to describe Claudio, we would say that he was primarily a mentor with the unique ability to ignite the minds and the hearts of friends and colleagues with his scientific passion. Many have known him as a brilliant mind, many others as a trustful and distinguished partner in research with flashes of extraordinary intelligence, and many more as a close friend with extremely sharp irony and culture.

Although he was aware of his exceptional qualities, Claudio was extremely humble and had a natural disposition in human relationships, with his eyes wide open to the world of young physician and advancing medical knowledge. Claudio dedicated his life to the study of medicine and became a master in the art of observation. During a career spanning almost 50 years, he has deeply transformed the

G. Sinagra (✉)
Centre for Diagnosis and Treatment of Cardiomyopathies, Cardiovascular Department,
Azienda Sanitaria Universitaria Giuliano-Isontina (ASUGI), University of Trieste, European
Reference Network for Rare, Low Prevalence and Complex Diseases of the Heart-ERN
GUARD-Heart, Trieste, Italy
e-mail: gianfranco.sinagra@asugi.sanita.fvg.it

A. Porcari
Centre for Diagnosis and Treatment of Cardiomyopathies, Cardiovascular Department,
Azienda Sanitaria Universitaria Giuliano-Isontina (ASUGI), University of Trieste, European
Reference Network for Rare, Low Prevalence and Complex Diseases of the Heart-ERN
GUARD-Heart, Trieste, Italy

Division of Medicine, National Amyloidosis Centre, University College London, London, UK
e-mail: aldostefano.porcari@nhs.net

M. Emdin et al. (eds.), *Cardiac Amyloidosis*,
https://doi.org/10.1007/978-3-031-51757-0_1

cardiological and the amyloidosis community worldwide. Crossing the path of Claudio marked a fundamental moment in the career of many young researchers, sometimes in unexpected ways.

Claudio approached the many congresses on heart failure and cardiomyopathies as useful opportunities to connect with young physicians and discuss the grey areas encountered in clinical practice, the limitations of the official guidelines for the treatment of heart failure and the need to follow critical thinking when approaching uncommon clinical scenarios (Fig. 1.1). As a teacher, he embodied the qualities of curiosity, critical thinking, observation, passion and creativity. He inspired and feed deep passion for medical knowledge, analysis of details and inconsistencies in clinical profiles and presentation, and for deduction as preferred methodology to deal with the many problems faced in clinical practice of medicine. He had that exceptional quality of merging scientific knowledge with his passion for the philosophy of Kant, Popper, the nosological question raised by Umberto Eco, the renewed songs from Vasco Rossi and his love for Art. His friends and colleagues will never forget his ability to use iconic paintings such as Arcimboldo' self-portrait to explain

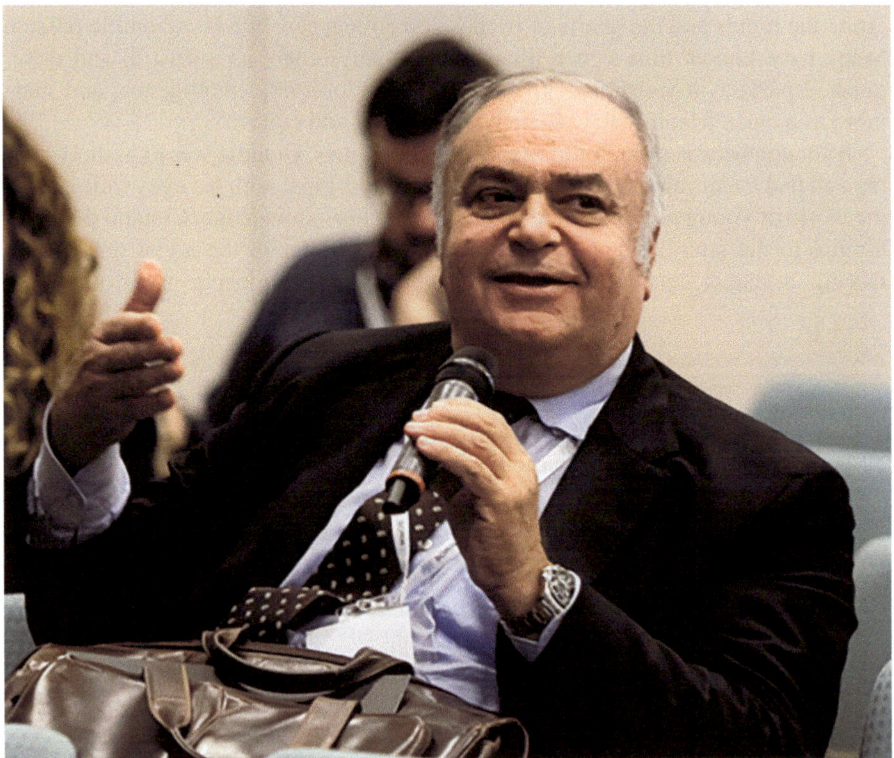

Fig. 1.1 Professor Claudio Rapezzi during a discussion at the "Advances in Heart Failure, Cardiomyopathies and Pericardial Diseases" held in Trieste (Italy)

the heterogeneous clinical phenotypes of patients presenting with systemic amyloidosis.

He was the exemplar of the physician and detective character in a contemporary version of Sherlock Holmes [1]. He shared with the cardiology community the "red flag approach" in cardiomyopathies and, particularly, in amyloidosis [2, 3]. He was among the first researchers to understand the key value of carpal tunnel syndrome as an early clinical marker of future development of cardiac amyloidosis [4, 5]. In the old days, through his expert interpretation of surface ECG, Claudio was able to characterise myocardial tissue composition and spot the presence of amyloid deposits. This is something that endomyocardial biopsy and cardiac magnetic resonance would have demonstrated many years later [6, 7]. He was very passionate on dissecting the heterogeneous clinical phenotype of ATTR amyloidosis [8, 9]. He has identified 3 main clinical phenotypes—cardiac, neurological and mixed—that have been implemented in clinical practice for diagnosing ATTR amyloidosis and for orienting therapeutic strategies worldwide. He was involved in the Transthyretin Amyloid Outcome Survey (THAOS), with the final aim of understanding and characterising the natural history of ATTR amyloidosis [10]. In seminal papers published in early 2000s, Claudio demonstrated the clinical applications of scintigraphy with bone tracers for the diagnosis of cardiac amyloidosis [11, 12]. Ten years later, that intuition paved the way for the development of a non-invasive algorithm for the diagnosis of transthyretin amyloid cardiomyopathy (ATTR-CM) in an international collaboration with the National Amyloidosis Centre (London, UK) which has deeply transformed the paradigm for diagnosing ATTR-CM [13–15].

Claudio coordinated the international phase 3 Safety and Efficacy of Tafamidis in Patients With Transthyretin Cardiomyopathy (ATTR-ACT) trial of tafamidis [16], which is the only drug ever tested in ATTR-CM with a proven impact on survival. In 2018, he presented the results of the ATTR-ACT at the European Society of Cardiology Congress held in Munich and ignited the audience with his passion and culture. Claudio considered tafamidis as the drug of the first four times:

- The first time that a drug is effective in ATTR-CM.
- The first example of precision medicine in the treatment of a cardiomyopathy.
- The first time a drug is effective in heart failure with preserved ejection fraction.
- The first time a drug without anti-neurohormonal activity is effective in heart failure.

The ATTR-ACT study has transformed the treatment of ATTR cardiomyopathy and represented a real revolution for patients and physicians worldwide (Fig. 1.2).

On top of his undisputed scientific expertise, Claudio was a great estimator of the writer Umberto Eco and the philosopher Karl Popper and was highly considered for his critical approach to the clinical methodology. A recent example is offered by the impossible interview between Sherlock Holmes and David Sackett about the fundamental question "how much can we trust the guidelines?" [17]. His pupils will never forget his positive approach to "error in medicine" as a source of thinking and a unique opportunity to overcome grey areas in medicine. In the field of classification

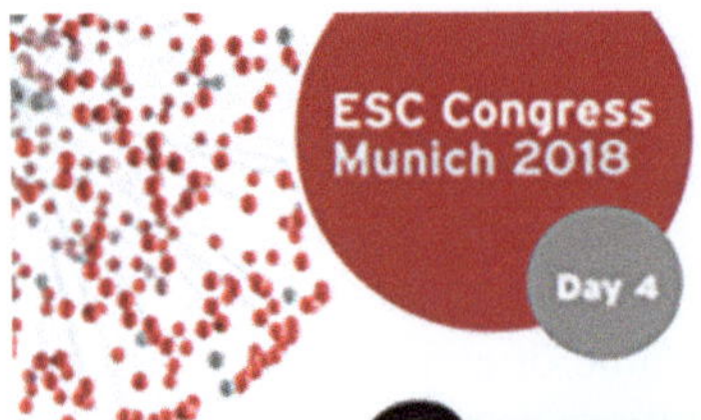

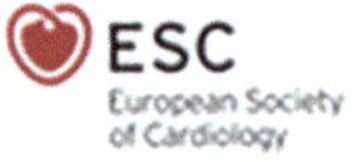

Congress News

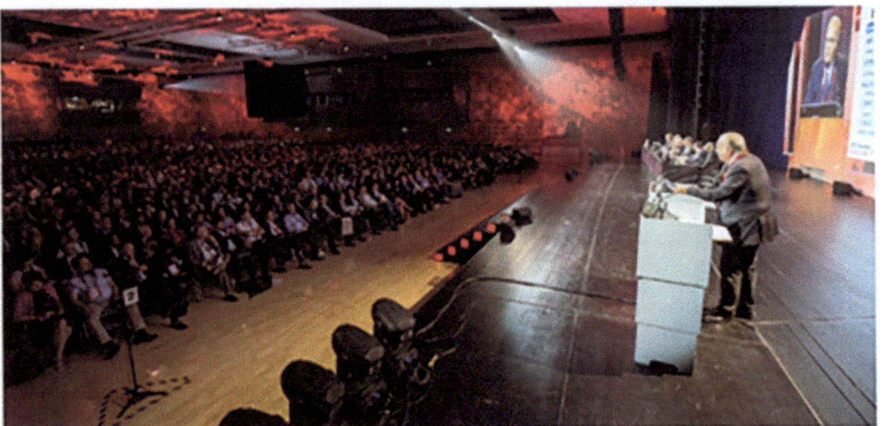

Tafamidis improves outcome in
transthyretin amyloid cardiomyopathy

Fig. 1.2 Professor Rapezzi presenting the results of the ATTR-ACT study at the European Society of Cardiology congress held in Munich

and nosology, Claudio was part of an international group of researchers that defined the criteria for classification of cardiomyopathies in 2008 [18]. More recently, he identified the limitations of that classification among patients diagnosed and managed in the real world, especially in the setting of restrictive cardiomyopathy. Therefore, he has proposed a new definition of this specific form of heart disease [19].

In the latest years, Claudio moved the centre of his activity to Ferrara where he closely collaborated with Prof. Roberto Ferrari, estimated colleague and friend. At the Ferrara University, Claudio entered in a very fruitful phase of his career characterised by multicentre collaborations. With the national and international network that he built during 50 years of clinical and scientific activity, Claudio started a number of research collaborations with friends and young physician with an interest in cardiac amyloidosis all around the world. In Ferrara, he conceived the design of the CAUSATIVE study, which is currently ongoing, with the aim of investigating the potential applications of computed tomography for the identification of cardiac amyloidosis among patients with severe aortic valve stenosis. With this project, he strenghtened the connections created with other Italian centres such as the cardiological amyloidosis community in Pisa under the leadership of Prof. Michele Emdin, close friend and partner in research, and his team of young physicians. The proposal for a re-definition of restrictive cardiomyopathy in the contemporary era was born from the intense cultural relationship between Claudio, Michele and the cardiological community in Trieste [19]. In Trieste, Claudio was used to attend the bi-annual congress "Incontri in Cardiologia" and give lectures on unmet needs in heart failure and cardiomyopathies. Young and adult cardiologists from Trieste keep a special memory of Claudio and, in particular, of the strong human and professional connection with him. With his unconventional spirit, he has inspired and encouraged, always with laughter, them and many young researchers to step into his path in the international amyloidosis community.

Claudio never forgot his old pupils from Bologna, grown in the research field of amyloidosis and disseminated in Italy and worldwide. His spirit and attitude were brighter when he met them during international congresses, he had that glimpse in his eyes when he had the opportunity of spending some time with them, a bond that time and life events could not weaken in any way.

Among the last quests of Claudio, there is definitively the foundation of the Italian Network for cardiac amyloidosis [20], that he has designed to promote collaboration among Italian centres for diagnosis and treatment of patients with suspected or confirmed cardiac amyloidosis. Sadly, Claudio has left us with many grey areas to untagle in the field of amyloidosis as well as with many ideas and research questions that awaits to be explored by his pupils disseminated worldwide. He was an extremely active part in many research projects, part of which are still ongoing such as the role of electrocardiography in the contemporary care of patients with cardiac amyloidosis [21], the cardiomyopathy-oriented interpretation of ECG findings [22, 23], the different behaviour of bone tracers validated for the diagnosis of ATTR-CM [24], the impact of tafamidis in ATTR-CM patients with NYHA class III, genotype-phenotype correlation in ATTR amyloidosis, gender differences in ATTR-CM [25–27], new treatment strategies and the possibility of combination therapy [28].

Professor Claudio Rapezzi was a giant of the amyloid field, an unattainable mentor and a unique friend.

We are close to his beloved Marinella, friends and colleagues in Ferrara, Bologna and all around the world.

He will be greatly missed and will continue being an inspiration for the next generations.

References

1. Ferrari R. A memory for Claudio Rapezzi. Eur Heart J. 2023; https://doi.org/10.1093/eurheartj/ehac773/7115482.
2. Rapezzi C, Arbustini E, Caforio ALP, Charron P, Gimeno-Blanes J, Helio T, et al. Diagnostic work-up in cardiomyopathies: bridging the gap between clinical phenotypes and final diagnosis. A position statement from the ESC Working Group on Myocardial and Pericardial Diseases. Eur Heart J. 2013;34(19):1448–58.
3. Garcia-Pavia P, Rapezzi C, Adler Y, Arad M, Basso C, Brucato A, et al. Diagnosis and treatment of cardiac amyloidosis: a position statement of the ESC Working Group on Myocardial and Pericardial Diseases. Eur Heart J. 2021;42(16):1554–68.
4. Porcari A, Pagura L, Longo F, Sfriso E, Barbati G, Murena L, et al. Prognostic significance of unexplained left ventricular hypertrophy in patients undergoing carpal tunnel surgery. ESC Hear Fail. 2022;9(1):751–60.
5. Milandri A, Farioli A, Gagliardi C, Longhi S, Salvi F, Curti S, et al. Carpal tunnel syndrome in cardiac amyloidosis: implications for early diagnosis and prognostic role across the spectrum of aetiologies. Eur J Heart Fail. 2020;22(3):507–15.
6. Rapezzi C, Merlini G, Quarta CC, Riva L, Longhi S, Leone O, et al. Systemic cardiac amyloidoses. Circulation. 2009;120(13):1203–12.
7. Maurer MS, Elliott P, Comenzo R, Semigran M, Rapezzi C. Addressing common questions encountered in the diagnosis and management of cardiac amyloidosis. Circulation. 2017;135(14):1357–77.
8. Rapezzi C, Longhi S, Milandri A, Lorenzini M, Gagliardi C, Gallelli I, et al. Cardiac involvement in hereditary-transthyretin related amyloidosis. Amyloid Int J Exp Clin Investig. 2012;19(Suppl 1):16–21.
9. Porcari A, Merlo M, Rapezzi C, Sinagra G. Transthyretin amyloid cardiomyopathy: an uncharted territory awaiting discovery. Eur J Intern Med. 2020;82:7–15.
10. Maurer MS, Hanna M, Grogan M, Dispenzieri A, Witteles R, Drachman B, et al. Genotype and phenotype of transthyretin cardiac amyloidosis: THAOS (transthyretin amyloid outcome survey). J Am Coll Cardiol. 2016;68(2):161–72.
11. Perugini E, Guidalotti PL, Salvi F, Cooke RMT, Pettinato C, Riva L, et al. Noninvasive etiologic diagnosis of cardiac amyloidosis using 99m Tc-3,3-diphosphono-1,2-propanodicarboxylic acid scintigraphy. J Am Coll Cardiol. 2005;46(6):1076–84.
12. Rapezzi C, Quarta CC, Guidalotti PL, Pettinato C, Fanti S, Leone O, et al. Role of (99m) Tc-DPD scintigraphy in diagnosis and prognosis of hereditary transthyretin-related cardiac amyloidosis. JACC Cardiovasc Imaging. 2011;4(6):659–70.
13. Rauf MU, Hawkins PN, Cappelli F, Perfetto F, Zampieri M, Argiro A, et al. Tc-99m labelled bone scintigraphy in suspected cardiac amyloidosis. Eur Heart J. 2023; https://doi.org/10.1093/eurheartj/ehad139/7083543.
14. Porcari A, Baggio C, Fabris E, Merlo M, Bussani R, Perkan A, et al. Endomyocardial biopsy in the clinical context: current indications and challenging scenarios. Heart Fail Rev. 2022;28(1):123–35.
15. Gillmore JD, Maurer MS, Falk RH, Merlini G, Damy T, Dispenzieri A, et al. Nonbiopsy diagnosis of cardiac transthyretin amyloidosis. Circulation. 2016;133(24):2404–12.
16. Maurer MS, Schwartz JH, Gundapaneni B, Elliott PM, Merlini G, Waddington-Cruz M, et al. Tafamidis treatment for patients with transthyretin amyloid cardiomyopathy. N Engl J Med. 2018;379(11):1007–16.
17. Rapezzi C, Sinagra G, Merlo M, Ferrari R. The impossible interviews-Sherlock Holmes interviews David Sackett: "how much can we trust the guidelines?". Eur Heart J Engl. 2021;42:3422–4.
18. Elliott P, Andersson B, Arbustini E, Bilinska Z, Cecchi F, Charron P, et al. Classification of the cardiomyopathies: a position statement from the European Society of Cardiology Working Group on Myocardial and Pericardial Diseases. Eur Heart J. 2008;29(2):270–6.

19. Rapezzi C, Aimo A, Barison A, Emdin M, Porcari A, Linhart A, et al. Restrictive cardiomyopathy: definition and diagnosis. Eur Heart J. 2022;43(45):4679–93.
20. Sinagra G, Emdin M, Merlo M, Vergaro G, Aimo A, Biagini E, et al. Rationale and significance of the Italian Network for Cardiac Amyloidosis. G Ital Cardiol (Rome). 2023;24(2):93–8.
21. Cipriani A, De Michieli L, Porcari A, Licchelli L, Sinigiani G, Tini G, et al. Low QRS voltages in cardiac amyloidosis. JACC CardioOncol. 2022;4(4):458–70.
22. Merlo M, Porcari A, Pagura L, Cameli M, Vergaro G, Musumeci B, et al. A national survey on prevalence of possible echocardiographic red flags of amyloid cardiomyopathy in consecutive patients undergoing routine echocardiography: study design and patients characterization — the first insight from the AC-TIVE study. Eur J Prev Cardiol. 2022;29(5):e173–7.
23. Merlo M, Pagura L, Porcari A, Cameli M, Vergaro G, Musumeci B, et al. Unmasking the prevalence of amyloid cardiomyopathy in the real world: results from phase 2 of the AC-TIVE study, an Italian nationwide survey. Eur J Heart Fail. 2022;24(8):1377–86.
24. Porcari A, Hutt DF, Grigore SF, Quigley AM, Rowczenio D, Gilbertson J, et al. Comparison of different technetium-99m-labelled bone tracers for imaging cardiac amyloidosis. Eur J Prev Cardiol. 2023;30(3):e4–6. https://doi.org/10.1093/eurjpc/zwac237/6763179.
25. Patel RK, Ioannou A, Razvi Y, Chacko L, Venneri L, Bandera F, et al. Sex differences among patients with transthyretin amyloid cardiomyopathy – from diagnosis to prognosis. Eur J Heart Fail. 2022;24(12):2355–63.
26. Aimo A, Tomasoni D, Porcari A, Vergaro G, Castiglione V, Passino C, et al. Left ventricular wall thickness and severity of cardiac disease in women and men with transthyretin amyloidosis. Eur J Heart Fail. 2023;25(4):510–4.
27. Caponetti AG, Rapezzi C, Gagliardi C, Milandri A, Dispenzieri A, Kristen AV, et al. Sex-related risk of cardiac involvement in hereditary transthyretin amyloidosis: insights from THAOS. JACC Heart Fail. 2021;9(10):736–46.
28. Porcari A, Fontana M, Gillmore JD. Transthyretin cardiac amyloidosis. Cardiovasc Res. 2023;118(18):3517–35.

Giampaolo Merlini and the Pavia School

2

Michele Emdin

The great advances in the diagnosis and treatment of cardiac amyloidosis (CA) are the result of a collective effort inspired by the pioneering work of a few masters. Among them Giampaolo Merlini (Fig. 2.1) is a giant, whose work and research contributed to advance modern clinical hematology and internal medicine. Giampaolo Merlini graduated in medicine and surgery at the University of Pavia as a student of the Ghislieri College and specialized in Hematology and Laboratory Medicine at the University of Pavia. Afterwards, he trained in clinical and laboratory investigations of monoclonal gammopathies at Malmö General Hospital, Lund University, Sweden under the supervision of Jan Waldenström. The teaching of Waldenström shaped his scientific interests, which have focused on the investigation of the molecular mechanisms of diseases, and namely on the biological activities of monoclonal proteins and related conditions. He further developed these research lines at the Institute of Cancer Research, College of Physicians & Surgeons, Columbia University, New York City, under the supervision of Elliott Osserman and together with chemist Elvin Kabat. Osserman introduced him to systemic amyloidoses and specifically to amyloidosis caused by misfolded monoclonal immunoglobulin light chains.

He was then the director of the center for the study and treatment of systemic amyloidosis and of the biotechnology research laboratories located in Pavia at the San Matteo Polyclinic Foundation, long recognized as a national referral center for the disease. This center, currently directed by Giovanni Palladini, a former student of Merlini, was founded in 1986 and employs the most advanced diagnostic tools and the most recent therapeutic resources, including experimental ones. This center

M. Emdin (✉)
Interdisciplinary Center for Health Sciences, Scuola Superiore Sant'Anna, Pisa, Italy

Cardio-thoracic Department, Fondazione Toscana Gabriele Monasterio, Pisa, Italy
e-mail: m.emdin@santannapisa.it

M. Emdin et al. (eds.), *Cardiac Amyloidosis*,
https://doi.org/10.1007/978-3-031-51757-0_2

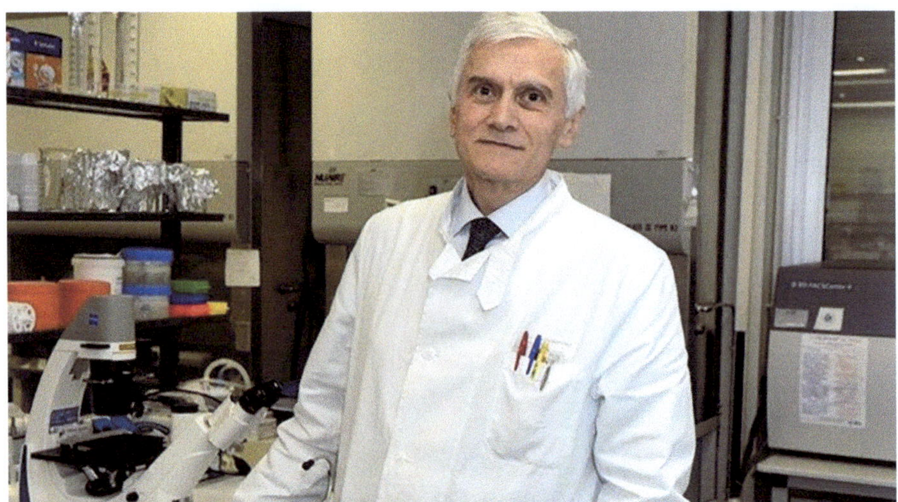

Fig. 2.1 Giampaolo Merlini

is devoted to the care of patients with amyloidosis, has been instrumental in the introduction of new tools for diagnosis, risk prediction, and management, and has been one of the leading centers in the world in terms of scientific output [1]. He was full Professor (now *Emeritus*) of Clinical Biochemistry at the University of Pavia and President of the Postgraduate Course in Medical Biotechnology. Further, he directed the International Society of Amyloidosis and the Italian Society for Amyloidosis and was the Chairman of the Committee on Plasma Proteins of the International Federation of Clinical Chemistry and Laboratory Medicine.

Prof. Merlini's research interests included the pathogenesis, natural history, diagnosis, and treatment of monoclonal gammopathies, namely of immunoglobulin light chain amyloidosis. His research focused on the study of the molecular mechanisms of cardiac damage, the investigation of biomarkers for the assessment of prognosis and response to therapy, and on the development of new therapeutic agents and treatments. He was principal investigator of several research projects funded by the European Community and by national and international research agencies, and received several international awards: the Ham-Wasserman Lecture 2017 at the American Society of Hematology Congress, the Robert Kyle Award at the International Workshop on Waldenström's Macroglobulinemia in 2018, the Jan G. Waldenström Award of the International Myeloma Society in 2019, the Giampaolo Merlini Prize by the International Society of Amyloidosis in 2020, dedicated to his person, the "Standing on the Shoulders of the Giants" Award by the International Academy of Clinical Hematology in 2022.

His scientific output is extraordinary, with an H index of 102 (Scopus, June 2023) and over 650 publications; he is a highly cited researcher for the years 2021 and 2022. His most notable scientific achievements include a novel system to stage multiple myeloma [2]; the proposal of biphosphonates as effective drugs in multiple myeloma [3]; the identification of 4′-iodo-4′-deoxy doxorubicin as a possible treatment for amyloidosis [4]; N-terminal pro-B-type natriuretic peptide as a possible biomarker for this condition [5]; the proposal of the melphalan-dexamethasone combination as an effective and safe treatment regimen for AL amyloidosis [6]; and the most recent evidence of the efficacy of birtamimab (a novel humanized monoclonal antibody designed to neutralize light chain aggregates and deplete organ-deposited amyloid via macrophage-induced phagocytosis) plus standard of care in Mayo stage IV light chain amyloidosis patients [7].

On a personal note, he was, and still is, always there, when I asked for an advice either on a difficult patient or on the research strategy and clinical governance: His words were always, and still are, enlightening. We share our faith in man and our commitment to the patient.

Curiositas felix, great culture and deep humanity, ability to organize and educate are some of the unique qualities of the man. Finally, Dante Alighieri's words *"Facesti come quei che va di notte, che porta il lume dietro e sé non giova, ma dopo sè fa le persone dotte"* (*"You acted like who goes at night carrying a light behind him, and does not help himself but makes people learned"*) [8] best describe Giampaolo Merlini's attitude toward his disciples and his lesson to scholars, physicians, and researchers.

References

1. http://www.amiloidosi.it/index.php/it/
2. Merlini G, Waldenström JG, Jayakar SD. A new improved clinical staging system for multiple myeloma based on analysis of 123 treated patients. Blood. 1980;55:1011–9.
3. Attardo-Parrinello G, Merlini G, Pavesi F, Crema F, Fiorentini ML, Ascari E. Effects of a new aminodiphosphonate (aminohydroxybutylidene diphosphonate) in patients with osteolytic lesions from metastases and myelomatosis. Comparison with dichloromethylene diphosphonate. Arch Intern Med. 1987;147:1629–33.
4. Merlini G, Ascari E, Amboldi N, Bellotti V, Arbustini E, Perfetti V, Ferrari M, Zorzoli I, Marinone MG, Garini P, et al. Interaction of the anthracycline 4′-iodo-4′-deoxydoxorubicin with amyloid fibrils: inhibition of amyloidogenesis. Proc Natl Acad Sci U S A. 1995;92:2959–63.
5. Palladini G, Campana C, Klersy C, Balduini A, Vadacca G, Perfetti V, Perlini S, Obici L, Ascari E, d'Eril GM, Moratti R, Merlini G. Serum N-terminal pro-brain natriuretic peptide is a sensitive marker of myocardial dysfunction in AL amyloidosis. Circulation. 2003;107:2440–5.
6. Palladini G, Perfetti V, Obici L, Caccialanza R, Semino A, Adami F, Cavallero G, Rustichelli R, Virga G, Merlini G. Association of melphalan and high-dose dexamethasone is effective and well tolerated in patients with AL (primary) amyloidosis who are ineligible for stem cell transplantation. Blood. 2004;103:2936–8.
7. Gertz MA, Cohen AD, Comenzo RL, Kastritis E, Landau HJ, Libby EN, Liedtke M, Sanchorawala V, Schönland S, Wechalekar AD, Zonder JA, Palladini G, Walling J, Guthrie S, Nie C, Karp C, Jin Y, Kinney GG, Merlini G. Birtamimab plus standard of care in light chain amyloidosis: the phase 3 randomized placebo-controlled VITAL trial. Blood. 2023;142:1208–18. https://doi.org/10.1182/blood.2022019406. Epub ahead of print. PMID: 37366170.
8. Alighieri D. Divina Commedia. Purgatorio, Canto XXII, 67–69.

A Brief History of Amyloidosis

3

Assuero Giorgetti, Angela Pucci, and Alberto Aimo

Abbreviations

AL	Amyloid light chain amyloidosis
ATTR	Amyloid transthyretin amyloidosis (v, variant; wt, wild-type)
ATTR-ACT	Tafamidis in transthyretin cardiomyopathy clinical trial
CA	Cardiac amyloidosis
PET	Positron emission tomography

Amyloidoses are considered rare diseases resulting from the extracellular deposition of amyloid, a fibrillar material derived from various precursor proteins that self-assemble with highly ordered abnormal cross β-sheet conformation. Deposition of amyloid can occur in the presence of an abnormal protein (e.g., variant transthyretin amyloidosis [ATTRv] and immunoglobulin light-chain [AL] amyloidosis), in association with prolonged and excessive secretion of a normal protein (e.g., reactive systemic amyloidosis and β2-microglobulin dialysis-related amyloidosis), or, in ageing process with unknown mechanisms (e.g., wild-type ATTR [ATTRwt] and atrial natriuretic peptide in isolated atrial amyloidosis) [1].

A. Giorgetti (✉)
Fondazione Toscana Gabriele Monasterio, Pisa, Italy
e-mail: asso@ftgm.it

A. Pucci
University Hospital of Pisa, Pisa, Italy
e-mail: a.pucci@ao-pisa.toscana.it

A. Aimo
Fondazione Toscana Gabriele Monasterio, Pisa, Italy

Scuola Superiore Sant'Anna, Pisa, Italy
e-mail: aimoalb@ftgm.it

© The Author(s), under exclusive license to Springer Nature
Switzerland AG 2024
M. Emdin et al. (eds.), *Cardiac Amyloidosis*,
https://doi.org/10.1007/978-3-031-51757-0_3

The term "amyloid" was introduced in the scientific literature by the German botanist Matthias Schleiden (1804–1881), who first applied the iodine-sulfuric acid test for starch in plants [2]. Schleiden demonstrated the presence of a starch-like substance, which he defined as "amyloid" in his book *Grundzige der wissenschaftlichen Botanik* ("Principles of Scientific Botany"), published in 1842–1843 [3]. The term derives from the Greek ἄμυλον and Latin "amylum", meaning "starch" [2].

Lesions attributable to amyloid deposits had already been described in the liver and spleen, already in 1639 [2]. The first use of the term "amyloid" in human disease is attributed to the physician and physiologist Rudolf Virchow (1821–1902) in his publication *Über eine in Gehirn und Rückenmark des Menschen aufgefundene Substanz mit der chemischen Reaction der Cellulose* ("About a substance found in the human brain and spinal cord with the chemical reaction for cellulose"), dating to 1854 [4]. In this text, Virchow described small roundish deposits in the gray matter of individuals with dementia, stating that those structures showed the same color reaction with iodine and sulfuric acid, i.e., a change from brown to blue, as starch. Virchow then proposed that these lesions had the same composition of starch, and defined them as "corpora amylacea." Over the following years, Virchow used the staining method with iodine and sulfuric acid on other amyloid-laden tissues [2].

In 1859, the German chemist August Kekulé (1829–1896) reported that organs infiltrated by amyloid had a high nitrogen content. Kekulé then proposed that the amyloid substance was composed mainly of protein, rather than carbohydrate, compounds [2]. Virchow did disagree with this conclusion, that he deemed wrong because whole tissue specimens were analyzed, rather than the lesions alone [5]. Virchow also did not agree with the use of methyl violet stain to detect amyloid, which was proposed independently by three scientists in 1875. Already in 1876, Soyka reported having found amyloid in the cardiac tissue with the use of this new method. Ackroyd and Ehrlich described methyl violet stain as "metachromatic" in 1878. Metachromatic stains challenged Virchow's iodine sulfuric acid test for decades, but were eventually replaced by Congo red [2, 5].

The Congo red dye was invented by the German chemist Paul Böttiger in 1884 as the first dye that did not require additional substances for fixation to the textile fibers [6]. In 1922, the German chemist Herman Bennhold discovered the Congo red ability to bind amyloid [7]. Reactivity with Congo red stain or "Congophilia with apple green birefringence" became the first diagnostic criterion for amyloid, introduced by the Belgian physician Paul Divry in 1927 [8]. The Puchtler's modification of Congo red staining, developed in 1962, is currently used to detect amyloid in histological specimens [9]. For histology, the samples are mostly formalin-fixed and paraffin-embedded, then 8–10 μm thick sections (such thickness increasing the staining sensibility) are stained with Congo red, and viewed in a light microscope under polarized light where amyloid is shown as green birefringent homogeneous material (red staining without light polarization is not specific of amyloid) [2]. Congo red is a symmetrical molecule with a hydrophobic center composed of two phenyl rings and two charged terminal naphthalene moieties; the terminal parts of Congo red contain sulphonic acid and amine groups. Although the interaction mechanisms between Congo red and amyloid fibrils have been intensively

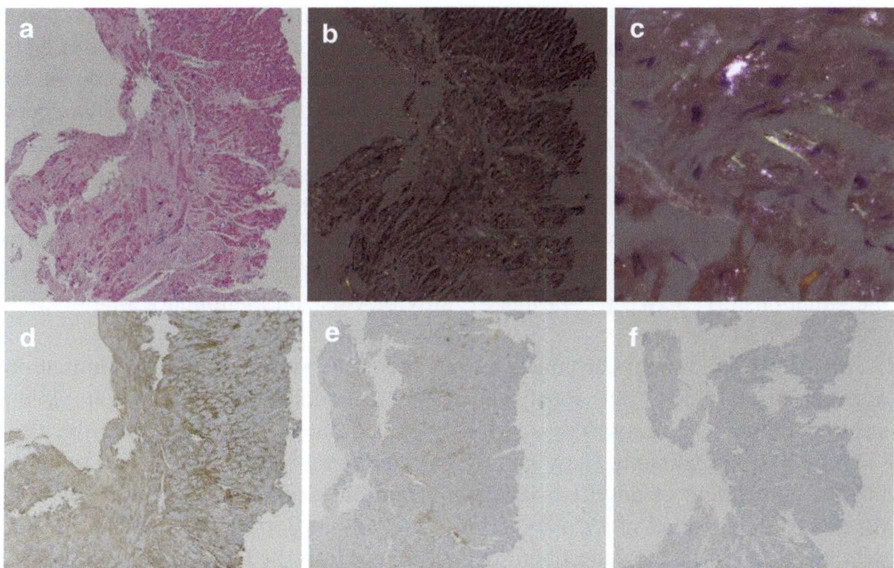

Fig. 3.1 Histology findings on an endomyocardial biopsy specimen. Routine histology showing enlarged interstitial spaces with amorphous and eosinophilic deposits (**a**). Amyloid deposits are demonstrated by green birefringence on the Congo red staining under polarized light (**b**), highlighting also very thin amyloid deposits surrounding single myocytes (**c**). Immunohistochemistry shows immunoglobulin light-chain Lambda immunoreactivity (**d**) with negative light-chain λ (**e**) and transthyretin (TTR) immunostaining (**f**). (**a**) Hematoxylin and eosin staining; (**b, c**): Congo red staining; (**d–f**): Immunoperoxidase staining and hematoxylin counterstaining. Original magnification: **a, b** and **d–f**: 4×; **c**: 40×

investigated, the process is not completely clarified. Congo red binding has been assumed to depend on the secondary, β-pleated configuration of the fibril, possibly mediated by hydrophobic interactions of the benzidine centers as well as the electrostatically charged terminal groups. The binding of Congo red to amyloid induces a characteristic shift in the maximal optical absorbance of the molecule from 490 nm to 540 nm, which causes the characteristic apple green birefringence under polarized light [2, 10] (Fig. 3.1).

3.1 Characterization of the Structure and Biochemical Composition of Amyloid Deposits

Besides the identification of amyloid in the brain of a patient with dementia by Alzheimer, in 1907 [11], no major breakthroughs in the research on amyloid came before the late 50 s. American researchers Alan S Cohen and Evan Calkins described the first extraction method that consisted of gentle physical separation and homogenization of the material in saline, followed by low-speed centrifugation [12]. Alternative methods involving the use of an alkaline solution of sodium glycinate

[13] and, most importantly, the "water extraction method" of Pras were proposed [14]. This last method has been widely used to extract almost all amyloid types except for Aβ and prion protein amyloid and enabled the identification of the β-pleated sheet configuration of amyloid proteins and the discovery of the biochemical structure of those proteins [2].

The secondary structure of amyloid consists of the polypeptide backbone, mostly in the β-pleated sheet conformation, oriented perpendicular to the fibril axis. This β-pleated sheet structure was revealed by X-ray diffraction analysis of isolated amyloid protein fibrils starting from 1968 [15, 16]. Glenner and coworkers also reported the relationship between "primary" amyloidosis and immunoglobulin light chains [17].

During the following years, many amyloid proteins were identified. Inflammation-associated amyloidosis, previously called the "secondary" and today AA amyloidosis, was shown to be caused by amyloid protein A, an acute phase protein in 1971 [18]. In 1978, prealbumin (now known as transthyretin, TTR) was found to be the protein constituent of amyloid deposits in familial amyloid polyneuropathy [19], the disorder described in 1951 by Corino Andrade in Portugal [20]. Similar disorders were found in the subsequent decades especially in Japan and Sweden. The Finnish type of familial amyloidosis, today known as AGel amyloidosis, was described in 1969 [21]. In 1980, TTR was characterized as the amyloid protein also in "senile cardiac amyloidosis" [22], later renamed as senile systemic amyloidosis, and now as ATTR. Over the following years, more than 30 circulating proteins were identified in tissue deposits in patients with amyloidotic disorders, including the Aβ peptide in Alzheimer disease and β2-microglobulin in dialysis-related arthropathy [2]. The development of molecular biology techniques allowed also to identify a growing number of mutations associated with hereditary forms and to establish some correlations between the genotype and clinical phenotype.

The identification of the amyloid precursors led to the development of the modern nomenclature of amyloidosis. The first official nomenclature committee was established in 1979 [2], and the latest nomenclature update was published in 2022 [23].

3.2 Novel Diagnostic Techniques

Thioflavin stain allows amyloid visualization using the fluorescence microscope. Thioflavin-T (Basic Yellow 1 or CI 49005) is a benzothiazole salt. When the dye binds to β sheets, it undergoes a 120 nm red shift of its excitation spectrum that may selectively be excited at 450 nm, resulting in a fluorescence signal at 482 nm. Thioflavin-S is a mixture of compounds resulting from the methylation of dehydro-thiotoluidine with sulfonic acid. The fluorescence method is specific for amyloid similarly to Congo red and very sensitive [24]. Thioflavin stains are possible alternatives to Congo red staining. In both cases, the identification of the amyloid protein requires immunohistochemistry techniques, and then the use of antibodies targets the amyloid precursors. A definite diagnosis requires amyloid typing by immunohistochemistry, immunoelectron microscopy, or mass spectrometry-based proteomic analysis, the latter one preferably after isolation of amyloid plaques by laser microdissection [25].

A major breakthrough in the field of diagnosis was the finding that technetium-based bone tracers bind ATTR deposits in the heart [26] (Fig. 3.2). In a multicenter center study on 1217 patients referred with suspected cardiac amyloidosis, an abnormal bone scintigraphy scan combined with a negative evaluation for a monoclonal gammopathy was shown to have a positive predictive value of 100% for ATTR cardiac amyloidosis (CA) [27]. An algorithm for the noninvasive diagnosis of ATTR-CA was then developed, in 2016 [27], and is now recommended by all the international documents to diagnose this condition [28].

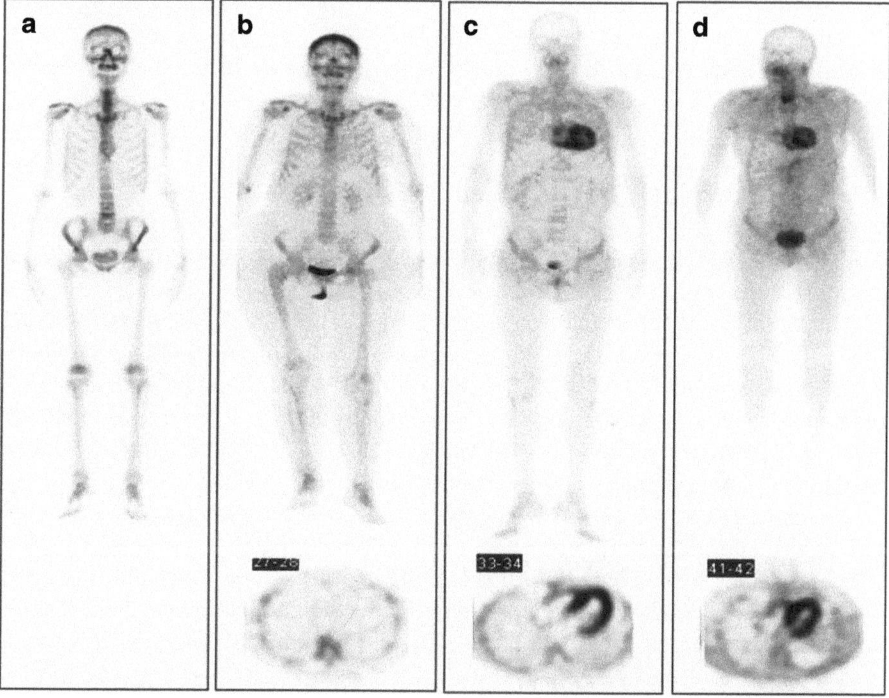

Fig. 3.2 Proposal of the Perugini scoring system. Representative examples illustrating the spectrum of ^{99m}Tc-3,3-diphosphono-1,2-propanodicarboxylic acid (^{99m}Tc-DPD) uptake among patients with transthyretin (TTR)-related or monoclonal immunoglobulin light-chain (AL) cardiac amyloidosis and unaffected controls (top row = whole-body scans, anterior view; bottom row = cross-sectional views of cardiac single-photon emission computed tomography in the same patients). A: Unaffected control subject without visually detectable uptake. B: Patient with AL amyloidosis and echocardiographic documentation of cardiac involvement without any visually detectable sign of myocardial ^{99m}Tc-DPD uptake; mild uptake of the tracer is visible only at the soft tissue level. C and D: Two patients with TTR-related amyloidosis and echocardiographic documentation of cardiac involvement, both showing strong myocardial ^{99m}Tc-DPD uptake (with absent bone uptake); in one of the patients (D), splanchnic uptake is also visible. Reprinted with permission from: Perugini et al. JACC [26]

In 1988, Hawkins described the use of antibodies targeting the amyloid serum P component (a protein found in all types of amyloid deposits) and labelled with ^{123}I, in a murine model of amyloidosis [29]; two years later, the same technique was employed successfully in human patients [30]. Another novel development was the discovery of Pittsburgh compound B, a positron emission tomography (PET) tracer labelled with ^{11}C and able to bind selectively the Aβ peptide. This tracer allowed to detect noninvasively the amyloid deposits in patients with suspected Alzheimer disease [31]. ^{18}F-labelled tracers, including ^{18}F-flutemetamol, ^{18}F-florbetapir, and ^{18}F-florbetaben are increasingly investigated in view of their longer half-time that avoids the need for on-site cyclotrons. Contrary to bone tracers, positron emission tomography amyloid-binding tracers demonstrate higher affinity for light-chain fibrils and may accurately distinguish patients with different types of CA. Specifically, patients with AL-CA display a persistent tracer uptake, while there is a rapid decrease in the signal in patients with ATTR-CA or those without CA [32]. Assessment of the diagnostic yield of PET imaging versus histological analysis is pending.

3.3 Therapeutic Approaches

AL and ATTR amyloidosis account for the vast majority of cases of CA. Their treatment will be analyzed in detail in dedicated chapters.

The therapy of AL amyloidosis has evolved in parallel with the therapy of multiple myeloma. The main stages of this process were the identification of melphalan as an effective therapy (in the 1970s and 1980s) [33], autologous stem cell transplantation (beginning of the 1990s) [34], the introduction of immunomodulatory agents and proteasome inhibitors (beginning of the 2000s) [35], and the recent identification of daratumumab as a possible first-line therapy [36].

As for ATTR amyloidosis, the attention was focused for a long time on hereditary forms, and particularly on patients with polyneuropathy. Liver transplantation was introduced at the beginning of the 1990s and was soon restricted to patients with early-onset, Val30Met-related disease (in whom cardiac involvement is much less common than polyneuropathy) [37]. The TTR tetramer stabilizer tafamidis was first characterized as an effective drug for patients with polyneuropathy [38]. In 2018, the phase 3 study tafamidis in Transthyretin Cardiomyopathy Clinical Trial (ATTR-ACT) demonstrated that tafamidis (a drug that stabilizes the TTR tetramer) improves the prognosis of patients with ATTR amyloidosis (either wild-type or variant) and cardiac involvement [39]. Following this study, tafamidis became the first approved drug for ATTR-related cardiomyopathy in May 2019. At present, tafamidis is the only therapeutic option for patients with ATTRwt-CA or ATTRv with isolated cardiac involvement, while those with cardiomyopathy and polyneuropathy may receive either tafamidis or patisiran (a blocker of TTR translation in the liver) [40]. Many therapies are under investigation, including gene editing [41] or the removal of tissue amyloid deposits through specific antibodies [42].

3.4   Conclusions

Our knowledge of amyloidosis has dramatically improved from the description by Virchow, but the term "amyloid" is still used to identify the abnormal substance whose tissue accumulation causes heterogeneous disease manifestations. Except for the noninvasive diagnosis of ATTR-CA by means of bone scintigraphy and the exclusion of a monoclonal protein, amyloidosis is always diagnosed by demonstrating tissue amyloid deposits and identifying the amyloidogenic protein. Major challenges are the need to perform often highly invasive biopsies (such as endomyocardial or renal biopsy), and the availability of immunohistochemistry, immunoelectron microscopy, or proteomics. An intriguing perspective is the introduction of an algorithm for the noninvasive diagnosis of AL-CA through PET tracers. While the mechanisms, whereby these tracers bind amyloid fibers, are still incompletely understood, the in-depth characterization of the amyloidogenic cascade has allowed the development of targeted therapeutic strategies such as TTR tetramer stabilizers, gene editing, or antibodies targeting tissue fibers.

References

1. Wechalekar AD, Gillmore JD, Hawkins PN. Systemic amyloidosis. Lancet. 2016;387:2641–54.
2. Tanskanen M. "Amyloid"—historical aspects. In: Feng D, editor. Amyloidosis [Internet]. London: IntechOpen; 2013. [cited 2022 Dec 27]. https://www.intechopen.com/chapters/44870. https://doi.org/10.5772/53423.
3. Scleiden MJ, Schwann T, Schulze M. Klassische Schriften zur Zellenlehre. In: Ostwalds klassiker der exakten Wissenschaften, band 275: Verlag Harri Deutsch. http://ww.books.google/fi/books/about/Klassische_Schriften_zur_Zellenlehre.html?=h9_WFhLD8uYC&redir_esc=y.
4. Virchow R. Über eine im Gehirn und Rückenmark des Menschen aufgefundene Substanz mit der chemischen Reaction der Cellulose. Virchows Archiv Pathol Anat Klinische Med Berlin. 1854;6:135–8.
5. Kyle RA. Amyloidosis: a convoluted story. Br J Haematol. 2001;114:529–38.
6. SteensmaDP. "Congo" red: out of Africa? Arch Pathol Lab Med. 2001;125:250–2.
7. Bennhold H. Eine spezifische Amyloidfärbung mit Kongorot. Münchener Medizinische Wochenschrift (November) 1922:1537–1538.
8. Divry P. Etude histo-chimique des plaques seniles. J de Neurologie et de Psychiatrie. 1927;27:643–57.
9. Puchtler H, Sweat F, Levine M. On the binding of Congo red by amyloid. J Histochem Cytochem. 1962;10:355–64.
10. Yakupova EI, Bobyleva LG, Vikhlyantsev IM, Bobylev AG. Congo red and amyloids: history and relationship. Biosci Rep. 2019;39:BSR20181415.
11. Alzheimer A. Über eine eigenartige Erkrankung der Hirnrinde. Allg Zeitschr Psychtiatr Psych Gerichtl Med. 1907;64:146–8.
12. Cohen AS, Calcins E. Electron microscopic observations on a fibrous component in amyloid of diverse origins. Nature. 1959;183:1202–3.
13. Glenner GG, Bladen HA. Purification and reconstitution of the periodic fibril and unit structure of human amyloid. Science. 1966;154:271–2.
14. Pras M, Schubert M, Zucker-Franklin D, Rimon A, Franklin EC. The characterization of soluble amyloid prepared in water. J Clin Invest. 1968;47:924–33.
15. Eanes ED, Glenner GG. X-ray diffraction studies on amyloid filaments. J Histochem Cytochem. 1968;16(11):673–7.

16. Bonar L, Cohen AS, Skinner MM. Characterization of the amyloid fibril as a crossbeta protein. Proc Soc Exp Biol Med. 1969;131:1373–5.

17. Glenner GG, Terry W, Harada M, Isersky C, Page D. Amyloid fibril proteins: proof of homology with immunoglobulin light chains by sequence analyses. Science. 1971;172:1150–1.

18. Bendit EP, Eriksen N. Chemical similarity among amyloid substances associated with long standing inflammation. Lab Investig. 1971;26:615–25.

19. Costa PP, Figueira AS, Bravo FR. Amyloid fibril protein related to prealbumin in familial amyloidotic polyneuropathy. Proc Natl Acad Sci U S A. 1978;75:4499–503.

20. Corino de Andrade M. Preliminary note on an unusual form of peripheral neuropathy. Rev Neurol. 1951;85:302–6.

21. Meretoja J. Familial systemic paramyloidosis with lattice dystrophy of the cornea, progressive cranial neuropathy, skin changes and various internal symptoms. A previously unrecognized heritable syndrome. Ann Clin Res. 1969;1:314–24.

22. Sletten K, Westermark P, Natvig JB. Senile cardiac amyloid is related to prealbumin. Scand J Immunol. 1980;12:503–6.

23. Buxbaum JN, Dispenzieri A, Eisenberg DS, Fändrich M, Merlini G, Saraiva MJM, Sekijima Y, Westermark P. Amyloid nomenclature 2022: update, novel proteins, and recommendations by the International Society of Amyloidosis (ISA) Nomenclature Committee. Amyloid. 2022, 29:213–9.

24. Biancalana M, Koide S. Molecular mechanism of Thioflavin-T binding to amyloid fibrils. Biochim Biophys Acta. 2010;1804:1405–12.

25. Wisniowski B, Wechalekar A. Confirming the diagnosis of amyloidosis. Acta Haematol. 2020;143:312–21.

26. Perugini E, Guidalotti PL, Salvi F, Cooke RM, Pettinato C, Riva L, Leone O, Farsad M, Ciliberti P, Bacchi-Reggiani L, Fallani F, Branzi A, Rapezzi C. Noninvasive etiologic diagnosis of cardiac amyloidosis using 99mTc-3,3-diphosphono-1,2-propanodicarboxylic acid scintigraphy. J Am Coll Cardiol. 2005;46:1076–84.

27. Gillmore JD, Maurer MS, Falk RH, Merlini G, Damy T, Dispenzieri A, Wechalekar AD, Berk JL, Quarta CC, Grogan M, Lachmann HJ, Bokhari S, Castano A, Dorbala S, Johnson GB, Glaudemans AW, Rezk T, Fontana M, Palladini G, Milani P, Guidalotti PL, Flatman K, Lane T, Vonberg FW, Whelan CJ, Moon JC, Ruberg FL, Miller EJ, Hutt DF, Hazenberg BP, Rapezzi C, Hawkins PN. Nonbiopsy diagnosis of cardiac transthyretin amyloidosis. Circulation. 2016;133:2404–12.

28. Rapezzi C, Aimo A, Serenelli M, Barison A, Vergaro G, Passino C, Panichella G, Sinagra G, Merlo M, Fontana M, Gillmore J, Quarta CC, Maurer MS, Kittleson MM, Garcia-Pavia P, Emdin M. Critical comparison of documents from scientific societies on cardiac amyloidosis: JACC state-of-the-art review. J Am Coll Cardiol. 2022;79:1288–303.

29. Hawkins PN, Myers MJ, Lavender JP, Pepys MB. Diagnostic radionuclide imaging of amyloid: biological targeting by circulating human serum amyloid P component. Lancet. 1988;1:1413–8.

30. Hawkins PN, Lavender JP, Pepys MB. Evaluation of systemic amyloidosis by scintigraphy with 123I-labeled serum amyloid P component. N Engl J Med. 1990;323:508–13.

31. Klunk WE, Wang Y, Huang GF, Debnath ML, Holt DP, Mathis CA. Uncharged thioflavin-T derivatives bind to amyloid-beta protein with high affinity and readily enter the brain. Life Sci. 2001;69:1471–84.

32. Genovesi D, Vergaro G, Giorgetti A, Marzullo P, Scipioni M, Santarelli MF, Pucci A, Buda G, Volpi E, Emdin M. [18F]-Florbetaben PET/CT for differential diagnosis among cardiac immunoglobulin light chain, transthyretin amyloidosis, and mimicking conditions. JACC Cardiovasc Imaging. 2021;14:246–55.

33. Kyle RA, Wagoner RD, Holley KE. Primary systemic amyloidosis: resolution of the nephrotic syndrome with melphalan and prednisone. Arch Intern Med. 1982;142:1445–7.

34. Majolino I, Marcenò R, Pecoraro G, et al. High-dose therapy and autologous transplantation in amyloidosis-AL. Haematologica. 1993;78:68–71.

35. Kumar SK, Rajkumar SV, Dispenzieri A, et al. Improved survival in multiple myeloma and the impact of novel therapies. Blood. 2008;111:2516–20.
36. Kastritis E, Palladini G, Minnema MC, Wechalekar AD, Jaccard A, Lee HC, Sanchorawala V, Gibbs S, Mollee P, Venner CP, Lu J, Schönland S, Gatt ME, Suzuki K, Kim K, Cibeira MT, Beksac M, Libby E, Valent J, Hungria V, Wong SW, Rosenzweig M, Bumma N, Huart A, Dimopoulos MA, Bhutani D, Waxman AJ, Goodman SA, Zonder JA, Lam S, Song K, Hansen T, Manier S, Roeloffzen W, Jamroziak K, Kwok F, Shimazaki C, Kim JS, Crusoe E, Ahmadi T, Tran N, Qin X, Vasey SY, Tromp B, Schecter JM, Weiss BM, Zhuang SH, Vermeulen J, Merlini G, Comenzo RL, ANDROMEDA Trial Investigators. Daratumumab-based treatment for immunoglobulin light-chain amyloidosis. N Engl J Med. 2021;385:46–58.
37. Ericzon BG, Wilczek HE, Larsson M, Wijayatunga P, Stangou A, Pena JR, Furtado E, Barroso E, Daniel J, Samuel D, Adam R, Karam V, Poterucha J, Lewis D, Ferraz-Neto BH, Cruz MW, Munar-Ques M, Fabregat J, Ikeda S, Ando Y, Heaton N, Otto G, Suhr O. Liver transplantation for hereditary transthyretin amyloidosis: after 20 years still the best therapeutic alternative? Transplantation. 2015;99:1847–54.
38. Coelho T, Maia LF, Martins da Silva A, Waddington Cruz M, Planté-Bordeneuve V, Lozeron P, Suhr OB, Campistol JM, Conceição IM, Schmidt HH, Trigo P, Kelly JW, Labaudinière R, Chan J, Packman J, Wilson A, Grogan DR. Tafamidis for transthyretin familial amyloid polyneuropathy: a randomized, controlled trial. Neurology. 2012;79:785–92.
39. Maurer MS, Schwartz JH, Gundapaneni B, et al. Tafamidis treatment for patients with transthyretin amyloid cardiomyopathy. N Engl J Med. 2018;379:1007–16.
40. Garcia-Pavia P, Rapezzi C, Adler Y, Arad M, Basso C, Brucato A, Burazor I, Caforio ALP, Damy T, Eriksson U, Fontana M, Gillmore JD, Gonzalez-Lopez E, Grogan M, Heymans S, Imazio M, Kindermann I, Kristen AV, Maurer MS, Merlini G, Pantazis A, Pankuweit S, Rigopoulos AG, Linhart A. Diagnosis and treatment of cardiac amyloidosis: a position statement of the ESC Working Group on Myocardial and Pericardial Diseases. Eur Heart J. 2021;42:1554–68.
41. Gillmore JD, Gane E, Taubel J, Kao J, Fontana M, Maitland ML, Seitzer J, O'Connell D, Walsh KR, Wood K, Phillips J, Xu Y, Amaral A, Boyd AP, Cehelsky JE, McKee MD, Schiermeier A, Harari O, Murphy A, Kyratsous CA, Zambrowicz B, Soltys R, Gutstein DE, Leonard J, Sepp-Lorenzino L, Lebwohl D. CRISPR-Cas9 in vivo gene editing for transthyretin amyloidosis. N Engl J Med. 2021;385:493–502.
42. Griffin JM, Rosenblum H, Maurer MS. Pathophysiology and therapeutic approaches to cardiac amyloidosis. Circ Res. 2021;128:1554–75.

Alberto Giannoni, Chiara Arzilli, and Alberto Aimo

Abbreviations

AL	Amyloid light chain amyloidosis
ATTR	Amyloid transthyretin amyloidosis (vATTR, variant form; wtATTR, wild-type form)
ISA	International Society of Amyloidosis
SAA	Serum amyloid A protein
SAP	Serum amyloid P component
TTR	Transthyretin

4.1 Definition and Nomenclature

The definition of "amyloidosis" encompasses a group of disorders caused by tissue deposition, mainly extracellular, of misfolded proteins, which aggregate into insoluble fibrils that compose the amyloid substance [1]. Immunohistochemistry or proteomic analyses allow classifying the different types of amyloidosis based on the

A. Giannoni (✉) · A. Aimo
Interdisciplinary Center for Health Sciences, Scuola Superiore Sant'Anna, Pisa, Italy

Cardiology Division, Fondazione Toscana Gabriele Monasterio, Pisa, Italy
e-mail: alberto.giannoni@santannapisa.it; aimoalb@ftgm.it

C. Arzilli
Cardiology Division, Fondazione Toscana Gabriele Monasterio, Pisa, Italy
e-mail: carzilli@monasterio.it

specific proteins that form the amyloid fibrils. The International Society of Amyloidosis (ISA) currently recognizes 42 different amyloidogenic proteins in humans. According to the nomenclature established by ISA, the amyloid protein is defined by the letter "A," followed by a suffix indicating the specific protein. This notation is also used to designate the different pathologies. The term amyloid refers to the specific protein involved, while amyloidosis refers to the disease caused by the amyloid protein. For example, when amyloid deposits are composed of immunoglobulin light chains, the amyloid protein is designated as AL and the disease is AL amyloidosis [1].

4.2 Amyloid Fibers

All forms of amyloidosis are characterized by tissue accumulation of insoluble fibrils composed of misfolded proteins. Amyloid fibrils have a 7–13 nm diameter and are composed by of 2–8 protofilaments, each having a 2–7 nm diameter, either intertwined or arranged side by side. Protofilaments are composed of β-sheet structures with hydrogen bonds between amino and carboxyl terminals of the amino acid chain [2]. The extremely regular structure of amyloid fibrils explains the characteristic apple green birefringence that can be seen on polarized light after Congo red staining [2].

The mechanisms underlying the formation of amyloid fibrils have not been completely characterized, but it is thought to depend on the intrinsic characteristics and local concentration of the amyloidogenic protein, its interaction with cell membranes and the extracellular matrix, and the insufficient removal of misfolded proteins by proteasomes (before protein release into the circulation) and macrophages [3–5]. The amyloidogenic potential of a protein is related to at least three factors, not mutually exclusive: (1) the intrinsic propensity of a protein to form amyloid deposits, (2) proteolytic changes, and (3) changes in the amino acid sequence. Some proteins are defined as "intrinsically misfolded" as they have at least a region without a fixed secondary or tertiary structure and can then change their conformation to better interact with their ligands [6]. Some examples are apolipoproteins AI, AII and the serum amyloid A protein (SAA) [7, 8]. The propensity to form amyloid deposits can be increased in some conditions, for example, when circulating concentration increases, as in the case of β2-microglobulin amyloidosis [9]. Alternatively, a normal protein can undergo proteolytic changes within the cell or in the extracellular spaces, and this process can increase its propensity to form amyloid deposits: this process occurs in many forms of amyloidosis [3] and has been well characterized in Alzheimer's disease [10]. Furthermore, a gene mutation can reduce protein stability, as in the familial forms of amyloidosis [11] or in mutations in the variable regions of immunoglobulin light chains [12–14] (Fig. 4.1).

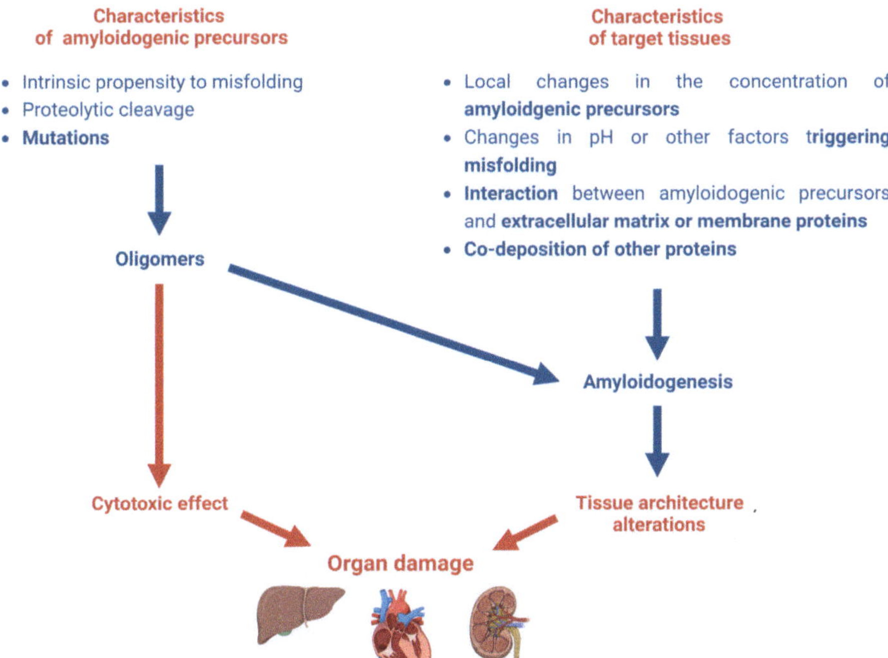

Fig. 4.1 Main characteristics of the amyloidogenic process and the resulting organ damage. The formation of amyloid deposits in tissues is attributed both to intrinsic characteristics of the amyloidogenic protein and to specific aspects of target tissues. Organ damage is caused by structural changes caused by amyloid deposition, and possibly also by a direct cytotoxic effect of protein oligomers

The process of amyloidogenesis is characterized by at least two phases. Indeed, all the interactions and conformational changes needed to form an initial amyloid deposit require a very long time to occur. After the so-called nucleation phase, the velocity of protein deposition increases markedly ("elongation phase" or "phase of sigmoidal growth"). During this phase, new nucleation processes can occur at the surface of fibrils or as a result of fibril fragmentation [3, 6].

In addition to amyloid fibrils, amyloid deposits include other protein components such as collagen [4], glycosaminoglycans, and proteoglycans (particularly dermatan sulfate and heparan sulfate), which form a scaffold promoting amyloid deposition [15] and may concur to cause organ tropism of amyloidogenic precursors [3]. Another protein very frequently encountered in deposits is serum amyloid P component (SAP), a pentraxin that has a high affinity for amyloid fibrils and protects them from proteolytic degradation and phagocytosis [16].

4.3 Pathophysiology of Organ Damage

Organ damage in amyloidosis is partially related to changes in tissue architecture caused by amyloid deposits. This, for example, explains diastolic dysfunction and the restrictive phenotype of amyloid cardiomyopathy [17]. On the other hand, several studies in AL amyloidosis have reported that renal and cardiac function and neuropathy improve after chemotherapy has blocked the production of light chains, despite the persistence of tissue amyloid deposits [18]. Organ dysfunction seems then to derive, at least in some cases, from a direct cytopathic effect of soluble oligomer species. Several observations stand in agreement with this proposed mechanism: Aβ oligomers have a neurotoxic effect [19]; in patients with ATTR amyloidosis related to *TTR* gene mutations, small protein aggregates interact with cell receptors inducing oxidative stress and neuronal damage [20]; in AL amyloidosis, light chains cause oxidative stress and mitochondrial damage in cardiomyocytes by altering intracellular calcium dynamics and reducing the contractile and relaxation properties of cardiomyocytes [21, 22]. It has also been postulated that oligomers, thanks to their antiparallel β-sheet conformation, are able to directly damage the integrity of plasma membrane by inducing the formation of structures similar to pores [5] (Fig. 4.1).

The different amyloidogenic proteins show a particular organ tropism. For example, β2-microglobulin deposits mostly in the joints while mutated TTR molecules in the peripheral nervous system and the heart. This tropism seems to depend on local factors such as higher protein concentration in different tissues or pH variations that promote protein misfolding as well as specific interactions with extracellular matrix proteins [23] or cell receptors [24]. Furthermore, in AL amyloidosis, it has been demonstrated that different mutations in genes coding for the variable region of immunoglobulin light chain contribute to determine the sites of deposition [25].

Table 4.1 Characteristics of the main forms of systemic amyloidosis

	Acquired/hereditary	Cause	Abnormal protein	Heart	Kidneys	Liver	Neuropathy	Other organs	Therapy
AL	Acquired	Plasma cell dyscrasia	Immunoglobulin light chains	+++	+++	++	+	GI tract, soft tissues	Chemotherapy, ASCT
ATTR	Acquired Hereditary	*TTR* gene mutations	TTR *wild type* Mutated TTR	+++ ++	– –	– –	– +++	Carpal tunnel syndrome	Supportive therapy, tetramer stabilizers Supportive therapy, organ transplant, tetramer stabilizers, inhibitors of TTR synthesis
AA	Acquired	Chronic inflammation	SAA	–/+	+++	+ (late)	–		Anti-inflammatory therapies
ALECT2	Acquired	Uncertain	LECT2	–	+++	++	–		Supportive therapy
Aβ2M	Acquired Hereditary	Chronic hemodialysis β2-microglobulin gene mutations	β2-microglobulin	–	–	–	–/+	Carpal tunnel syndrome, joints	Supportive therapy, organ transplant
AFib	Hereditary		Fibrinogen	–	+++	–/+	–		Supportive therapy, organ transplant
AApoAI	Hereditary	Mutations in the apolipoprotein A1 gene	Altered ApoA1	+	++	++	+/–	Testes	Supportive therapy, organ transplant
ALys	Hereditary	Lysozyme gene mutations	Mutated lysozyme	–	+	++	–	GI tract, skin	Supportive therapy
AGel	Hereditary	Gelsolin gene mutations	Mutated gelsolin	–	–/+	–	++		Supportive therapy

Adapted from Buxbaun et al. [1]

AA inflammatory/reactive amyloidosis, *AApoAI* apolipoprotein AI amyloidosis, *Aβ2M* β2-microglobulin amyloidosis, *AFib* amyloidosis with deposition of the α chain of fibrinogen A, *AGel* gelsolin amyloidosis, *AL* amyloid light chain amyloidosis, *ALECT2* LECT2 amyloidosis, *ALys* lysozyme amyloidosis, *ASCT* autologous stem cell transplantation, *ATTR* amyloid transthyretin amyloidosis, *LECT2* leukocyte cell-derived chemotaxin-2, *SAA* serum amyloid A, *TTR* transthyretin. +++ very common, ++ common, + uncommon, –/+ rars, – not applicable or not occurring in this condition

4.4   Classification and Epidemiology

Forty-two proteins have been classified as potentially amyloidogenic in humans. From a clinical perspective, amyloidosis can be classified into familial (related to inherited mutations) or acquired, and into systemic or localized forms [1]. Table 4.1 summarizes the characteristics of some of the most common forms of systemic amyloidosis [1].

Amyloidosis is still considered a rare disease, which, by definition, means a condition affecting <5 people in 10,000 [26]. However, several recent studies based on novel diagnostic algorithms and tools have highlighted that amyloidosis and particularly ATTR is more common than expected (Fig. 4.2) and, presumably, still partly under-recognized [27].

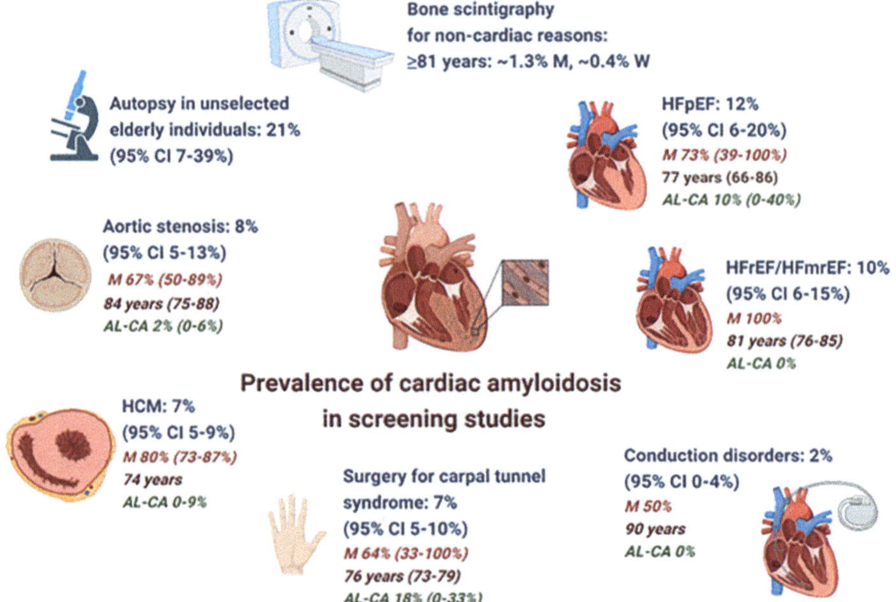

Fig. 4.2 Prevalence of cardiac amyloidosis (CA) in different settings. Except for two specific settings (bone scintigraphy for non-cardiac reasons and autopsy in unselected elderly individuals), the mean and 95% confidence interval (CI) or the range of prevalence of CA across studies (blue), the percentage of males out of all patients with CA (average and range; red), the mean/median age of patients with CA (brown), and the percentage of patients with amyloid light chain (AL) CA out of all patients with CA (green) are reported. *HCM* hypertrophic cardiomyopathy, *HFmrEF* heart failure with mildly reduced ejection fraction, *HFpEF* heart failure with preserved ejection fraction, *HFrEF* heart failure with reduced ejection fraction, *M* men. (Reprinted with permission from Aimo et al. [27])

4.4.1 Acquired Forms

Acquired forms of amyloidosis include some of the most encountered forms of systemic amyloidosis, such as AL, ATTR (wild-type), serum amyloid A (AA), and leukocyte chemotactic factor-2 (ALECT2) amyloidosis.

AL amyloidosis is characterized by the deposition of misfolded light chains from monoclonal immunoglobulins. In 10–15% of cases, it is associated with multiple myeloma, but it more commonly develops from an indolent plasma cell clone (*smouldering myeloma*, Waldenström macroglobulinemia, or monoclonal gammopathy of uncertain significance). AL amyloidosis has been long considered the most common form of systemic amyloidosis, even though the rising prevalence of ATTR amyloidosis is currently challenging this assumption. The main organ targets are the heart, kidneys, liver, and peripheral nervous system (particularly the autonomic fibers) [28].

Two large epidemiological studies have clarified the incidence and prevalence of AL amyloidosis in two areas of the US (Olmsted County, Minesota) and Europe (Limoges, France). A first report from the Mayo clinic and its affiliated hospitals (year range 1950–1989) found an overall age- and sex-adjusted annual rate per million-person years of 8.9 (corresponding to an estimated 2225 new cases per year over a population of 250 million US citizen in 1989) [29]. Another report from the same area was then updated (year range covered 1990–2015) with an overall age- and sex-adjusted annual rate per million-person years of 12 (corresponding to an estimated 3852 new cases over a population of 321 million US citizen in 2015) [30]. Incidence rises with age and is usually higher in males than females [31]. In a study by Quock et al. based on US claim data, AL amyloidosis incidence seems to remain stable across the time window included in the study (2007–2015), ranging from 9.7 to 14.0 cases per million-person, while prevalence increase significantly (annual percentage change of 12%) from 15.5 cases per million in 2007 to 40.5 in 2015 [32]. Differences in incidence and prevalence rates have been described among different countries, with lowest rates observed in Brazil and highest in Japan [31]. A recent systematic review has tried to redefine the epidemiology of cardiac amyloidosis (CA) in specific subset of patients and found a prevalence of AL-CA in up to 13% of cases (in patients with heart failure and preserved ejection fraction—HFpEF, ≥65 years and no coronary artery disease) [27].

Wild-type ATTR amyloidosis (ATTRwt), previously known as senile amyloidosis, typically involves elderly men. It is caused by the accumulation of TTR amyloid fibrils, particularly in the heart and tendons. ATTR epidemiology is rapidly evolving due to the increased use of cardiac scintigraphy as a noninvasive diagnostic tool. By using national health registries in Denmark, Finland, Norway, and Sweden, a mean prevalence of ATTR-CM of 33 cases per million was found in 2018, with a progressive increase in prevalence from 2008 to 2018 across the different countries. While no differentiation was made between wild-type and hereditary forms, the mean age at diagnosis (73.1 years) suggests a higher proportion of ATTRwt among the diagnosed cases.

The prevalence of ATTRwt is higher in specific patient subsets with red flags commonly associated with amyloidosis. Indeed, Castaño et al. found that around 13% of patients hospitalized for HFpEF and with a wall thickness >12 mm may have ATTRwt, and approximately 16% of patients with severe calcific aortic stenosis undergoing percutaneous transcatheter aortic valve implantation actually have ATTR-CA [33]. Similar series have confirmed those findings [27]. Likewise, the prevalence of ATTR-CA was found to be ranging from 2% to 7% in patients undergoing surgery for carpal tunnel syndrome over a certain age (≥50 years in men and ≥60 years in women) [34]. Despite being more recognized than in the past, ATTR amyloidosis prevalence is likely still underestimated, as autoptic studies report a prevalence of ATTR fibrils in around 25% of subjects over 80 years [35]. Indeed, wild-type ATTR amyloidosis, also known as senile systemic amyloidosis, seems the most common form of systemic amyloidosis in older adults, particularly in men.

AA amyloidosis is also known as inflammatory or reactive amyloidosis and develops as a complication of chronic inflammatory disorders, such as autoimmune disorders, infections, or neoplasms. In this form of amyloidosis, there is a deposition of fibrils of serum amyloid A protein (SAA), an acute phase protein synthetized by the liver. SAA is an apolipoprotein part of high-density lipoprotein, synthesized by hepatocytes under the transcriptional regulation of proinflammatory cytokines. The median plasma concentration of SAA may increase from 3 mg/L (in a healthy subject) to >2000 mg/L during acute inflammation [36]. A sustained increase in SAA should be present to then develop AA amyloidosis, although for reasons unknown, amyloidosis only occurs in a minority of patients with chronic inflammatory disorders [36]. In facts, this variety of amyloidosis is becoming less frequent in western countries and constitutes <10% of all amyloidosis subtypes [37]. The kidney is involved in virtually all patients, with proteinuria and worsening renal function, progressing to end-stage renal failure. Beyond renal involvement, SAA may affect also the spleen and liver, while cardiac involvement or neuropathy are usually later manifestations [38]. Targeted anti-inflammatory treatment promotes normalization of circulating SAA levels preventing amyloid deposition and renal damage. Novel therapies aimed at promoting clearance of existing amyloid deposits soon may be an effective treatment approach.

Amyloidosis can also be caused by accumulation of leukocyte cell-derived chemotaxin-2 (*LECT2*). Besides its soluble functioning as a cytokine or hepatokine, LECT2 may cause a specific form of amyloidosis (ALECT2) [39]. Previously considered a rare condition, ALECT2 has emerged as a common form of renal amyloidosis (after AL and AA amyloidosis) and liver amyloidosis, with a quite slow progression. It is particularly frequent in some ethnic groups such as Hispanic individuals [40]. ALECT2 should be suspected when all markers for AL and AA are negative. ALECT2 can be found in association with other types of amyloidosis as well as malignancies or autoimmune diseases [39].

Beta-2 microglobulin amyloidosis is an important complication of chronic intermittent hemodialysis and is due to the accumulation of β2-microglobulin, mostly in the joints and heart. The prevalence and incidence of dialysis-related cardiac β2-microglobulin amyloidosis are unclear [41]. Currently, the condition is uncommon and typically associated with prior dialysis schemes with low-flow membranes. Today, specific techniques of β-2 microglobulin removal, such as hemodiafiltration or an adsorbent column, may prove advantageous, but randomized controlled studies are needed [42].

4.4.2 Forms of Amyloidosis Related to Gene Mutations

These conditions are due to gene mutation that cause the synthesis of unstable proteins, with a propensity to form fibrils. These are systemic disorders often characterized by peripheral neuropathy, cardiac and renal involvement. ATTRv amyloidosis is the most common form. Other forms are due to mutations in the fibrinogen α chain, apolipoprotein A I, lysozyme, or gelsolin (Table 4.1).

The *TTR* gene is located on chromosome 18 and consists of four exons, each one coding for a single monomer. Point mutations occurring in the *TTR* gene sequence can destabilize the encoded protein leading to amyloid fibrils formation. *Variant ATTR amyloidosis (ATTRv)* is inherited in a dominant autosomic fashion with incomplete penetrance. Over 120 mutations in the *TTR* gene have been described, but not all of them have been associated with ATTRv. Each disease-causing mutation has a specific geographical distribution. The specific mutation influences the pattern of organ involvement, but the phenotype can vary even within families carrying the same mutations. V122I, T60A, V30M, I68L, and L111M are most commonly associated with predominant cardiac involvement [17]. ATTRv has a global distribution, but some geographic regions are more affected than others. For instance, the prevalence of ATTRv is high in certain areas of Portugal, Sweden, and Japan, where some of the most common mutations occur [43–45]. The age of onset and severity of ATTRv can vary depending on the specific mutation and may range from early-onset, rapidly progressive disease to late-onset disease with slow progression [43–45].

Together with specific pathogenetic mutations, it is likely than many gene variants are associated with a different likelihood of developing amyloidosis. A prominent example is represented by AA amyloidosis, which develops only a minority of patients with chronic inflammatory conditions. To date, the only established predisposing factor is *SAA* genotype, particularly some *SAA1* alleles, which significantly increase the risk of AA amyloidosis in different populations (*SAA1.1* in Caucasian and *SAA1.3* in Japanese subjects) [38].

4.5 Prognostic Significance of Different Types of Amyloidosis

Amyloidosis is a progressively debilitating disease with a poor prognosis and a poor quality of life. The natural history of amyloidosis is mainly determined by the extent of cardiac involvement and secondarily of renal involvement. Amyloid infiltration of the heart causes a progressive atrial and ventricular wall thickening, resulting in diastolic dysfunction and further progression to heart failure, usually with preserved ejection fraction. Systolic dysfunction usually occurs in later stages of the disease. Cardiac symptoms (e.g., fatigue, shortness of breath, syncope) and conduction abnormalities (e.g., atrioventricular block or tachi-arrhythmias) also become increasingly clinically apparent with severe progression over time. Increased disease awareness coupled with earlier and improved diagnosis due to the use of disease-modifying therapies aimed at reducing or stopping amyloid deposition (though not reversing cardiac damage) has led to progressive improvements in outcomes. This is exemplified by a study conducted by Westin et al. on two cohorts of patients with cardiac amyloidosis in Denmark. The 1-year mortality rate was 74% for patients diagnosed in 1998–2002, decreasing to 39% for patients diagnosed in 2013–2017 [46].

4.5.1 AL Amyloidosis

Systemic AL amyloidosis was historically considered as an inevitably fatal disease. The natural history of AL amyloidosis is determined by cardiac and renal involvement. Early diagnosis is vital to prevent irreversible organ damage and improve overall survival: diagnosis at a late stage, when cardiac and renal damages are very advanced, is associated with a poor survival measured in weeks; instead, early diagnosis, when cardiac and renal damages are absent or minimal, is associated with a better survival, measured in several years [28]. Before the introduction of treatments against the underlying plasma cell dyscrasia, prognosis was indeed poor with an expected average survival of 12–13 months and, among those with symptomatic heart involvement, of only 6 months [47, 48].

AL amyloidosis survival rate has improved over the years due to a new standard of care. In the 1990s, the introduction of high-dose melphalan and autologous stem cell transplantation (HDM/SCT) significantly improved the prognosis for carefully selected AL patients [49]. HDM/SCT treatment was associated with a longer-term survival of 15–20 years in ~30% of patients treated [50]. Unfortunately, 65–75% of newly diagnosed patients with AL amyloidosis were ineligible for HDM/SCT. Recently, new therapeutic treatments have emerged, including cyclophosphamide-bortezomib-dexamethasone regimens, novel proteasome inhibitors, next-generation immunomodulatory drugs, and anti-CD38 monoclonal antibodies [51]. They are associated with high clonal response rates and prolonged progression-free survival.

In 2000s, standardized risk stratification and treatment response assessment, thanks to the advent of the serum-free light chain assay and cardiac biomarkers [52], have helped to develop risk-adapted therapies and to further improve survival. The current staging system of AL amyloidosis was originally defined by the Mayo Clinic in 2012 and was based on cardiac biomarkers, for evaluating the cardiac damage and immunoglobulin light chain levels and for evaluating the clonal plasma cells activity. Threshold value of cTnT ≥ 0.025 ng/mL (or cTnI 0.1 ng/mL, or hs-cTnT 40 ng/L), NT-proBNP ≥ 1800 ng/L and difference between involved and uninvolved light chain (FLC-diff) ≥18 mg/dL allow to classify AL amyloidosis into four stages with different clinical risk and consequent survival. In stage I, all markers are below the cutoffs; in stage II, one marker is above the cutoffs; in stage III, two markers are above the cutoffs; in stage IV, all markers are above the cutoffs [53]. This staging system has been revised by European study group in 2013 for a better classification of stage III amyloidosis: patients in stage III with NT-proBNP <8500 ng/L and systolic blood pressure (SBP) >100 mmHg show a very good hematologic response to chemotherapy (stage IIIa), while patients with NT-proBNP >8500 ng/L and SBP <100 mmHg have a poor prognosis with a median survival of only 3 months (stage IIIb) [54].

Today, long-term survival is becoming more common: one of five patients now lives 10 years after diagnosis [55]. Data from the United Kingdom National Amyloidosis Centre database showed that AL amyloidosis patients have experienced a significant improvement in survival from a median of 1.5 years for patients diagnosed in late 1990s to more than 5 years in contemporary cohorts [56]. Staron and colleagues showed that the overall survival increased steadily since 1980s onwards, with median values of 1.4 years for AL patients diagnosed in 1980–1989 increasing to 4.6 years for AL patients diagnosed in 2010–2019 at the Boston University Amyloidosis Center. However, patients with age at diagnosis ≥70 years only showed marginal improvements in survival over time. On the other hand, AL amyloidosis-unrelated mortality increased over time (from 3% of deaths in 1980s to 16% in 2010s) and with longer survival (29% of deaths occurring >10 years after diagnosis): the causes were infections unrelated to treatment, major vascular events, and solid tumor malignancies [57].

4.5.2 ATTR Amyloidosis

The natural history of ATTR amyloidosis is not well-defined, and risk stratification remains a challenge. Outcomes in ATTR amyloidosis depend on cardiac, renal, and neurological damage. In the past, delineating the prognosis in ATTR was difficult due to underdiagnosis or late diagnosis and the lack of effective treatments. Therefore, most studies on the outcomes of ATTR amyloidosis essentially track the natural history of the condition. Today, however, diagnosis is made earlier, and there are more effective risk stratification systems available, making the natural history of the disease clearer [58].

Overall, survival rates in ATTR patients are higher than in AL patients. Among ATTR subjects, the survival rate is lower in those with a cardiac or cardiac/neurological phenotype and ATTRwt [59]. The median survival of patients with ATTRwt is 47 months, with 78% of deaths due to cardiac involvement [60]. The median survival of untreated patients with ATTRv is between 10 and 15 years [59]. Quality of life is low for both variant and wild-type ATTR [58].

In ATTR amyloidosis, the incidence of heart failure increases during the evolution of the disease, but remains higher in patients with ATTRwt than in those with ATTRv [61]. In ATTR cardiomyopathy, life expectancy ranges from 69.2 to

24.1 months based on the severity of cardiac and renal involvement. Even after adjusting for age, the prognosis is worse in patients with more severe cardiomyopathy and renal failure, defined by a level of NT-proBNP greater than 3000 ng/L and an eGFR less than 45 mL/min [62]. Cardiac biomarkers (high-sensitivity troponin T or I, NT-proBNP, or BNP) and estimated glomerular filtration rate (eGFR), alone or in combination, are useful for predicting the prognosis in ATTR patients [63]. Martyn et al. have recently shown that the intensity of ^{99m}Tc-PYP uptake (heart-to-contralateral lung ratio) does not offer incremental prognostic discrimination in patients with ATTR-CM [64]. Circulating transthyretin (TTR) levels parallel TTR kinetic stability, correlate with disease severity, and may serve as indirect markers of ATTR-CM disease activity and response to targeted treatment [65]. Other biomarkers, such as retinol-binding protein 4, transthyretin kinetic stability, non-native transthyretin, peptide probes, and neurofilament light chain, are potential risk stratification markers in patients with transthyretin cardiac amyloidosis [65].

Tafamidis, a TTR stabilizer that attenuates TTR dissociation and slows amyloid fibril formation, was recently shown to reduce mortality and cardiac hospitalizations in patients with symptomatic heart failure due to ATTR-CM [66]. Additional studies evaluating other stabilizers or TTR gene-silencing agents are still ongoing, but again these studies include only patients with ATTR-CM and overt HF [67]. On the other hand, Gonzalez-Lopez et al. have reported that asymptomatic patients with ATTRv amyloidosis benefits of an early initiation of transthyretin (TTR) stabilizers were associated with improved prognosis [61].

β-2 Microglobulin amyloidosis remains a clinically important complication of intermittent dialysis with low-flow membranes. Today, hemodiafiltration or an adsorbent column has greatly decreased the prevalence of this amyloidosis: in a European and Japanese register, hospitalizations caused by β-2 microglobulin amyloidosis have decreased over tenfold from 1998 to 2018, but β-2 microglobulin amyloidosis nonetheless remains associated with mortality, even in the current high-flux era [68].

4.6   Conclusions

Amyloidosis encompasses a group of disorders, referred to as amyloidoses, which are heterogeneous in nature. Amyloidoses can be systemic or localized, acquired or hereditary, but always involve amyloid deposits with different misfolded proteins that stabilize and promote further deposition and a various degree of direct cell toxicity. Amyloidosis is now recognized to be prevalent, depending on the amyloid precursors, age ranges, or clinical settings, with AL and ATTR amyloidosis being the most frequently observed clinical entities. AL amyloidosis, caused by clonal plasma cells, seems to have worse outcome than ATTR amyloidosis, since the heart and kidney are often involved, with light chain related toxicity causing a more rapid progression and organ damage. In ATTR amyloidosis, the subtype and location of amyloid deposits determine the natural disease history, with cardiac involvement (more frequent in ATTRwt and some ATTRv subtypes) causing worse outcomes.

References

1. Buxbaum JN, Dispenzieri A, Eisenberg DS, Fändrich M, Merlini G, Saraiva MJM, et al. Amyloid nomenclature 2022: update, novel proteins, and recommendations by the International Society of Amyloidosis (ISA) Nomenclature Committee. Amyloid. 2022;29(4):213–9.
2. Chiti F, Dobson CM. Protein misfolding, amyloid formation, and human disease: a summary of progress over the last decade. Annu Rev Biochem. 2017;86:27–68.
3. Merlini G, Bellotti V. Molecular mechanisms of amyloidosis. N Engl J Med. 2003;349(6):583–96.
4. Merlini G, Seldin DC, Gertz MA. Amyloidosis: pathogenesis and new therapeutic options. J Clin Oncol. 2011;29(14):1924–33.
5. Berthelot K, Cullin C, Lecomte S. What does make an amyloid toxic: morphology, structure or interaction with membrane? Biochimie. 2013;95(1):12–9.
6. Karamanos TK, Kalverda AP, Thompson GS, Radford SE. Mechanisms of amyloid formation revealed by solution NMR. Prog Nucl Magn Reson Spectrosc. 2015;88–89:86–104.
7. Yakar S, Livneh A, Kaplan B, Pras M. The molecular basis of reactive amyloidosis. Semin Arthritis Rheum. 1995;24(4):255–61.
8. Andreola A, Bellotti V, Giorgetti S, Mangione P, Obici L, Stoppini M, et al. Conformational switching and fibrillogenesis in the amyloidogenic fragment of apolipoprotein a-I. J Biol Chem. 2003;278(4):2444–51.
9. Verdone G, Corazza A, Viglino P, Pettirossi F, Giorgetti S, Mangione P, et al. The solution structure of human beta2-microglobulin reveals the prodromes of its amyloid transition. Protein Sci. 2002;11(3):487–99.
10. Hardy J, Selkoe DJ. The amyloid hypothesis of Alzheimer's disease: progress and problems on the road to therapeutics. Science (New York, NY). 2002;297(5580):353–6.
11. Buxbaum JN, Tagoe CE. The genetics of the amyloidoses. Annu Rev Med. 2000;51:543–69.
12. Hurle MR, Helms LR, Li L, Chan W, Wetzel R. A role for destabilizing amino acid replacements in light-chain amyloidosis. Proc Natl Acad Sci U S A. 1994;91(12):5446–50.
13. Ozaki S, Abe M, Wolfenbarger D, Weiss DT, Solomon A. Preferential expression of human lambda-light-chain variable-region subgroups in multiple myeloma, AL amyloidosis, and Waldenström's macroglobulinemia. Clin Immunol Immunopathol. 1994;71(2):183–9.
14. Dobson CM. Protein misfolding, evolution and disease. Trends Biochem Sci. 1999;24(9):329–32.
15. McLaurin J, Yang D, Yip CM, Fraser PE. Review: Modulating factors in amyloid-beta fibril formation. J Struct Biol. 2000;130(2–3):259–70.
16. Tennent GA, Lovat LB, Pepys MB. Serum amyloid P component prevents proteolysis of the amyloid fibrils of Alzheimer disease and systemic amyloidosis. Proc Natl Acad Sci U S A. 1995;92(10):4299–303.
17. Maurer MS, Bokhari S, Damy T, Dorbala S, Drachman BM, Fontana M, et al. Expert Consensus Recommendations for the suspicion and diagnosis of transthyretin cardiac amyloidosis. Circ Heart Fail. 2019;12(9):e006075.
18. Dember LM, Sanchorawala V, Seldin DC, Wright DG, LaValley M, Berk JL, et al. Effect of dose-intensive intravenous melphalan and autologous blood stem-cell transplantation on al amyloidosis-associated renal disease. Ann Intern Med. 2001;134(9 Pt 1):746–53.
19. Lambert MP, Barlow AK, Chromy BA, Edwards C, Freed R, Liosatos M, et al. Diffusible, nonfibrillar ligands derived from Abeta1–42 are potent central nervous system neurotoxins. Proc Natl Acad Sci U S A. 1998;95(11):6448–53.
20. Sousa MM, Du Yan S, Fernandes R, Guimaraes A, Stern D, Saraiva MJ. Familial amyloid polyneuropathy: receptor for advanced glycation end products-dependent triggering of neuronal inflammatory and apoptotic pathways. J Neurosci. 2001;21(19):7576–86.
21. Brenner DA, Jain M, Pimentel DR, Wang B, Connors LH, Skinner M, et al. Human amyloidogenic light chains directly impair cardiomyocyte function through an increase in cellular oxidant stress. Circ Res. 2004;94(8):1008–10.

22. Guan J, Mishra S, Qiu Y, Shi J, Trudeau K, Las G, et al. Lysosomal dysfunction and impaired autophagy underlie the pathogenesis of amyloidogenic light chain-mediated cardiotoxicity. EMBO Mol Med. 2015;7(5):688.
23. Stevens FJ, Kisilevsky R. Immunoglobulin light chains, glycosaminoglycans, and amyloid. Cell Mol Life Sci. 2000;57(3):441–9.
24. Yan SD, Zhu H, Zhu A, Golabek A, Du H, Roher A, et al. Receptor-dependent cell stress and amyloid accumulation in systemic amyloidosis. Nat Med. 2000;6(6):643–51.
25. Comenzo RL, Zhang Y, Martinez C, Osman K, Herrera GA. The tropism of organ involvement in primary systemic amyloidosis: contributions of Ig V(L) germ line gene use and clonal plasma cell burden. Blood. 2001;98(3):714–20.
26. Moliner AM, Waligora J. The European Union Policy in the field of rare diseases. Adv Exp Med Biol. 2017;1031:561–87.
27. Aimo A, Merlo M, Porcari A, Georgiopoulos G, Pagura L, Vergaro G, et al. Redefining the epidemiology of cardiac amyloidosis. A systematic review and meta-analysis of screening studies. Eur J Heart Fail. 2022;24(12):2342–51.
28. Merlini G, Dispenzieri A, Sanchorawala V, Schönland SO, Palladini G, Hawkins PN, et al. Systemic immunoglobulin light chain amyloidosis. Nat Rev Dis Primers. 2018;4(1):38.
29. Kyle RA, Linos A, Beard CM, Linke RP, Gertz MA, O'Fallon WM, et al. Incidence and natural history of primary systemic amyloidosis in Olmsted County, Minnesota, 1950 through 1989. Blood. 1992;79(7):1817–22.
30. Kyle RA, Larson DR, Kurtin PJ, Kumar S, Cerhan JR, Therneau TM, et al. Incidence of AL amyloidosis in Olmsted County, Minnesota, 1990 through 2015. Mayo Clin Proc. 2019;94(3):465–71.
31. Kumar N, Zhang NJ, Cherepanov D, Romanus D, Hughes M, Faller DV. Global epidemiology of amyloid light-chain amyloidosis. Orphanet J Rare Dis. 2022;17(1):278.
32. Quock TP, Yan T, Chang E, Guthrie S, Broder MS. Epidemiology of AL amyloidosis: a real-world study using US claims data. Blood Adv. 2018;2(10):1046–53.
33. Castaño A, Narotsky DL, Hamid N, Khalique OK, Morgenstern R, DeLuca A, et al. Unveiling transthyretin cardiac amyloidosis and its predictors among elderly patients with severe aortic stenosis undergoing transcatheter aortic valve replacement. Eur Heart J. 2017;38(38):2879–87.
34. Sperry BW, Reyes BA, Ikram A, Donnelly JP, Phelan D, Jaber WA, et al. Tenosynovial and cardiac amyloidosis in patients undergoing carpal tunnel release. J Am Coll Cardiol. 2018;72(17):2040–50.
35. Tanskanen M, Peuralinna T, Polvikoski T, Notkola IL, Sulkava R, Hardy J, et al. Senile systemic amyloidosis affects 25% of the very aged and associates with genetic variation in alpha2-macroglobulin and tau: a population-based autopsy study. Ann Med. 2008;40(3):232–9.
36. Ledue TB, Weiner DL, Sipe JD, Poulin SE, Collins MF, Rifai N. Analytical evaluation of particle-enhanced immunonephelometric assays for C-reactive protein, serum amyloid A and mannose-binding protein in human serum. Ann Clin Biochem. 1998;35(Pt 6):745–53.
37. Georgin-Lavialle S, Savey L, Buob D, Bastard JP, Fellahi S, Karras A, et al. French practical guidelines for the diagnosis and management of AA amyloidosis. La Revue de Medecine Interne. 2023;44(2):62–71.
38. Obici L, Merlini G. AA amyloidosis: basic knowledge, unmet needs and future treatments. Swiss Med Wkly. 2012;142:w13580.
39. Zhu MH, Liu YJ, Li CY, Tao F, Yang GJ, Chen J. The emerging roles of leukocyte cell-derived chemotaxin-2 in immune diseases: from mechanisms to therapeutic potential. Front Immunol. 2023;14:1158083.
40. Dogan A. Amyloidosis: insights from proteomics. Annu Rev Pathol. 2017;12:277–304.
41. Morris AD, Smith RN, Stone JR. The pathology and changing epidemiology of dialysis-related cardiac beta-2 microglobulin amyloidosis. Cardiovasc Pathol. 2019;42:30–5.
42. Kikuchi K, Hamano T, Wada A, Nakai S, Masakane I. Predilution online hemodiafiltration is associated with improved survival compared with hemodialysis. Kidney Int. 2019;95(4):929–38.

43. Goyal A, Lahan S, Dalia T, Ranka S, Bhattad VB, Patel RR, et al. Clinical comparison of V122I genotypic variant of transthyretin amyloid cardiomyopathy with wild-type and other hereditary variants: a systematic review. Heart Fail Rev. 2022;27(3):849–56.
44. Mejia Baranda J, Ljungberg J, Wixner J, Anan I, Oskarsson V. Epidemiology of hereditary transthyretin amyloidosis in the northernmost region of Sweden: a retrospective cohort study. Amyloid. 2022;29(2):120–7.
45. Schmidt HH, Waddington-Cruz M, Botteman MF, Carter JA, Chopra AS, Hopps M, et al. Estimating the global prevalence of transthyretin familial amyloid polyneuropathy. Muscle Nerve. 2018;57(5):829–37.
46. Westin O, Butt JH, Gustafsson F, Schou M, Salomo M, Køber L, et al. Two decades of cardiac amyloidosis: a Danish nationwide study. JACC Cardio Oncol. 2021;3(4):522–33.
47. Kyle RA, Greipp PR. Amyloidosis (AL). Clinical and laboratory features in 229 cases. Mayo Clin Proc. 1983;58(10):665–83.
48. Dubrey SW, Cha K, Anderson J, Chamarthi B, Reisinger J, Skinner M, et al. The clinical features of immunoglobulin light-chain (AL) amyloidosis with heart involvement. QJM. 1998;91(2):141–57.
49. Sanchorawala V, Sun F, Quillen K, Sloan JM, Berk JL, Seldin DC. Long-term outcome of patients with AL amyloidosis treated with high-dose melphalan and stem cell transplantation: 20-year experience. Blood. 2015;126(20):2345–7.
50. Sidana S, Sidiqi MH, Dispenzieri A, Buadi FK, Lacy MQ, Muchtar E, et al. Fifteen year overall survival rates after autologous stem cell transplantation for AL amyloidosis. Am J Hematol. 2019;94(9):1020–6.
51. Griffin JM, Rosenblum H, Maurer MS. Pathophysiology and therapeutic approaches to cardiac amyloidosis. Circ Res. 2021;128(10):1554–75.
52. Palladini G, Dispenzieri A, Gertz MA, Kumar S, Wechalekar A, Hawkins PN, et al. New criteria for response to treatment in immunoglobulin light chain amyloidosis based on free light chain measurement and cardiac biomarkers: impact on survival outcomes. J Clin Oncol. 2012;30(36):4541–9.
53. Kumar S, Dispenzieri A, Lacy MQ, Hayman SR, Buadi FK, Colby C, et al. Revised prognostic staging system for light chain amyloidosis incorporating cardiac biomarkers and serum free light chain measurements. J Clin Oncol. 2012;30(9):989–95.
54. Wechalekar AD, Schonland SO, Kastritis E, Gillmore JD, Dimopoulos MA, Lane T, et al. A European collaborative study of treatment outcomes in 346 patients with cardiac stage III AL amyloidosis. Blood. 2013;121(17):3420–7.
55. Muchtar E, Gertz MA, Lacy MQ, Go RS, Buadi FK, Dingli D, et al. Ten-year survivors in AL amyloidosis: characteristics and treatment pattern. Br J Haematol. 2019;187(5):588–94.
56. Ravichandran S, Lachmann HJ, Wechalekar AD. Epidemiologic and survival trends in amyloidosis, 1987–2019. N Engl J Med. 2020;382(16):1567–8.
57. Staron A, Zheng L, Doros G, Connors LH, Mendelson LM, Joshi T, et al. Marked progress in AL amyloidosis survival: a 40-year longitudinal natural history study. Blood Cancer J. 2021;11(8):139.
58. Lane T, Fontana M, Martinez-Naharro A, Quarta CC, Whelan CJ, Petrie A, et al. Natural history, quality of life, and outcome in cardiac transthyretin amyloidosis. Circulation. 2019;140(1):16–26.
59. Damy T, Kristen AV, Suhr OB, Maurer MS, Planté-Bordeneuve V, Yu CR, et al. Transthyretin cardiac amyloidosis in continental Western Europe: an insight through the Transthyretin Amyloidosis Outcomes Survey (THAOS). Eur Heart J. 2019;43(5):391–400.
60. Grogan M, Scott CG, Kyle RA, Zeldenrust SR, Gertz MA, Lin G, et al. Natural history of wild-type transthyretin cardiac amyloidosis and risk stratification using a novel staging system. J Am Coll Cardiol. 2016;68(10):1014–20.
61. Gonzalez-Lopez E, Escobar-Lopez L, Obici L, Saturi G, Bezard M, Saith SE, et al. Prognosis of transthyretin cardiac amyloidosis without heart failure symptoms. JACC Cardio Oncol. 2022;4(4):442–54.

62. Gillmore JD, Damy T, Fontana M, Hutchinson M, Lachmann HJ, Martinez-Naharro A, et al. A new staging system for cardiac transthyretin amyloidosis. Eur Heart J. 2018;39(30):2799–806.
63. Nakashima N, Takashio S, Morioka M, Nishi M, Yamada T, Hirakawa K, et al. A simple staging system using biomarkers for wild-type transthyretin amyloid cardiomyopathy in Japan. ESC Heart Failure. 2022;9(3):1731–9.
64. Martyn T, Saef J, Hussain M, Ives L, Kiang A, Estep JD, et al. The association of cardiac biomarkers, the intensity of Tc99 pyrophosphate uptake, and survival in patients evaluated for transthyretin cardiac amyloidosis in the early therapeutics era. J Card Fail. 2022;28(10):1509–18.
65. Hood CJ, Hendren NS, Pedretti R, Roth LR, Saelices L, Grodin JL. Update on disease-specific biomarkers in transthyretin cardiac amyloidosis. Curr Heart Failure Rep. 2022;19(5):356–63.
66. Maurer MS, Schwartz JH, Gundapaneni B, Elliott PM, Merlini G, Waddington-Cruz M, et al. Tafamidis treatment for patients with transthyretin amyloid cardiomyopathy. N Engl J Med. 2018;379(11):1007–16.
67. Garcia-Pavia P, Domínguez F, Gonzalez-Lopez E. Transthyretin amyloid cardiomyopathy. Med Clin. 2021;156(3):126–34.
68. Kanda E, Muenz D, Bieber B, Cases A, Locatelli F, Port FK, et al. Beta-2 microglobulin and all-cause mortality in the era of high-flux hemodialysis: results from the Dialysis Outcomes and Practice Patterns Study. Clin Kidney J. 2021;14(5):1436–42.

Amyloid Light Chain (AL) Amyloidosis

5

Ashutosh D. Wechalekar

Abbreviations

AL	Amyloid light chain
ATTR	Amyloid transthyretin
CCND1	Cyclin D1 gene
FLC	Free light chain
hs-TnT	High-sensitivity troponin T
Ig	Immunoglobulin
IGLV	Variable region of immunoglobulin light chains
MGUS	Monoclonal gammopathy of undetermined significance
NT-proBNP	N-Terminal fraction of pro-B-type natriuretic peptide
PCD	Plasma cell dyscrasia
SAP	Serum amyloid P component
SNP	Single nucleotide polymorphism
SPIE	Serum protein electrophoresis with immunofixation
UPIE	Urine protein electrophoresis with immunofixation

Amyloid light chain (AL) amyloidosis is one of the most common forms of systemic amyloidosis. The etiology of AL amyloidosis occurs due to a clonal plasma cell expansion and the subsequent production of amyloidogenic immunoglobulin (Ig) light chains, which assume an unstable misfolded conformation and are prone to aggregate into amyloid fibril precursors. These last can cause a direct tissue

A. D. Wechalekar (✉)
National Amyloidosis Centre, University College London, London, UK

University College London Hospitals, London, UK
e-mail: a.wechalekar@ucl.ac.uk

© The Author(s), under exclusive license to Springer Nature
Switzerland AG 2024
M. Emdin et al. (eds.), *Cardiac Amyloidosis*,
https://doi.org/10.1007/978-3-031-51757-0_5

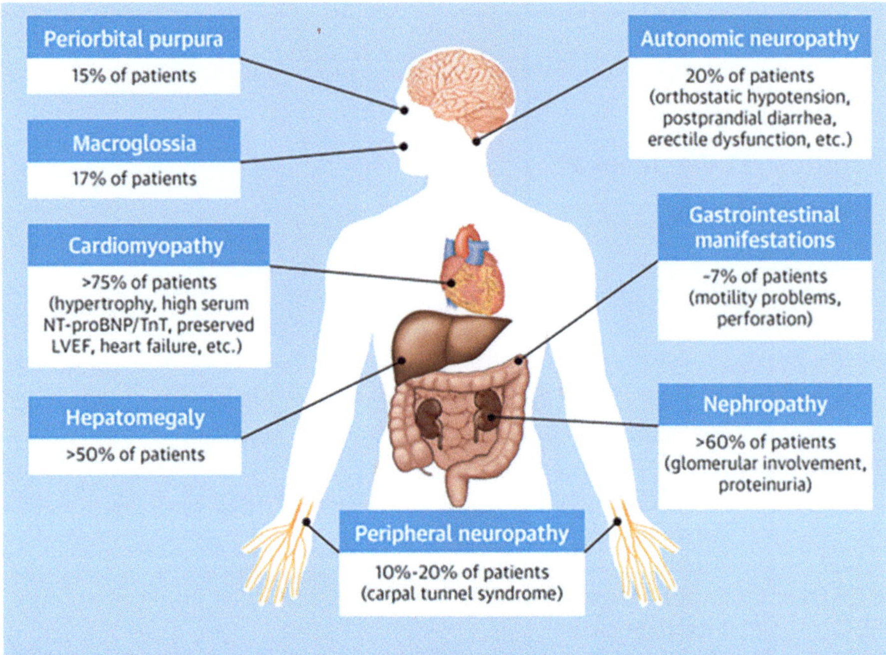

Fig. 5.1 Common clinical manifestations among patients with amyloid light chain amyloidosis. This figure summarizes the systemic manifestation of amyloid light chain amyloidosis, the number of organs and tissues that are affected, the percentage of patients in whom these organs are affected at diagnosis, and some commonly observed symptoms for the affected organ or system. *LVEF* left ventricular ejection fraction, *NT-proBNP* N-terminal pro-brain natriuretic peptide, *TnT* troponin T. (Reprinted with permission from Wechalekar et al. [3])

damage through their proteotoxicity, usually in the heart, or form stable fibrils, with organ damage related to an interstitial accumulation causing an impairment of tissue structure [1]. The most commonly affected organs are the heart and kidneys, followed by the liver, gastrointestinal tract, soft tissues, and peripheral nervous system. More than 75% of patients diagnosed with AL amyloidosis display symptoms of cardiac involvement [2]. Clinical manifestations reflect the topographic distribution reported in Fig. 5.1.

5.1 Epidemiology and Risk Factors

The epidemiology of AL amyloidosis is poorly defined, given the absence of data from large samples. A study based on the Olmsted County Project reported an incidence normalized for sex and age of 8.9 cases per million subjects per year during the period 1950–1989. An update in the interval 1990–2015 reported an incidence of 12 per million per year [4]. Another population study performed in the French Limousin region from 2012 to 2016 reported similar results than those in the

Olmsted County cohort [2]. Further estimates from population-based studies revealed a crude incidence of 3 cases per million population in England in 2008, 11 cases per million in Argentina in 2006–2014, and 9.7–14.0 cases per million-person in the US during 2007–2015 [5]. In 2018, approximately 74,000 AL amyloidosis cases worldwide were diagnosed during the preceding 20 years, revealing an estimated incidence and 20-year prevalence rates of 10 and 51 cases per million-person, respectively [5]. Interestingly, the prevalence of AL amyloidosis is increasingly growing, as suggested by the elevation from 15.5 cases per million in 2007 to 40.5 in 2015 in the US, with the incidence showing a similar trend to elevation [5, 6] but may also be due to impacts of treatment which have marked prolonged the patient survival. The incidence also increases with age, doubling after 65 years, with a mean age of approximately 63 years at diagnosis and a slight predominance in the male sex (55%) [1, 5]. Indeed, less than 5% of affected patients are under the age of 40 [7].

Two important risk factors for AL amyloidosis are the pre-existence of monoclonal gammopathies and some single nucleotide polymorphisms (SNPs). In patients with monoclonal gammopathy of uncertain significance (MGUS), the risk of developing AL amyloidosis is 8.8-fold higher than in the general population, particularly in cases with production of IgM [8]. In patients with a diagnosis of multiple myeloma, around 10–15% had overt amyloidosis, while 30–40% may have amyloid deposits on a biopsy without a clear clinical syndrome of amyloidosis deposition (asymptomatic amyloidosis) [9]. AL amyloidosis is considered to be five to ten times less frequent than multiple myeloma, but it represents the most common type of systemic amyloidosis in developed countries [4]. As for SNPs, a genome wide association study on a cohort of 1229 patients with AL amyloidosis identified ten loci associated with this condition [10]. Most notably, the rs9344 variant in a gene coding for a protein involved in chromatin remodeling promotes a translocation from the chromosome 11 to the chromosome 14 in a site near the gene coding for cyclin D1 (CCND1), a regulator of cell cycle involved in several neoplasms. This SNP is associated with an odds ratio of 1.35 of developing AL amyloidosis. AL patients harboring t(11;14) also reported a higher risk of death [11]. Another SNP increasing the risk of disease is rs79419269, which is near the SMARCD3 gene, also involved in chromatin remodeling [10].

5.2 Pathophysiology

Although all plasma cell dyscrasias (PCDs) may cause AL amyloidosis, this condition is usually caused by a clone of indolent B cells that produces monoclonal and abnormal λ light chains (in 70–80% of cases) or κ (in 20–30%) [1, 12, 13] (Fig. 5.2). A translocation from the chromosome 11 to the chromosome 14 brings the locus coding for the heavy chains near the CCND1 oncogene [15]. Furthermore, somatic mutations in the gene coding for the variable region of immunoglobulin light chains (IGLV) may reduce protein stability, thus increasing the degradation of immunoglobulins within the cells and circulating concentrations of free light chains [16].

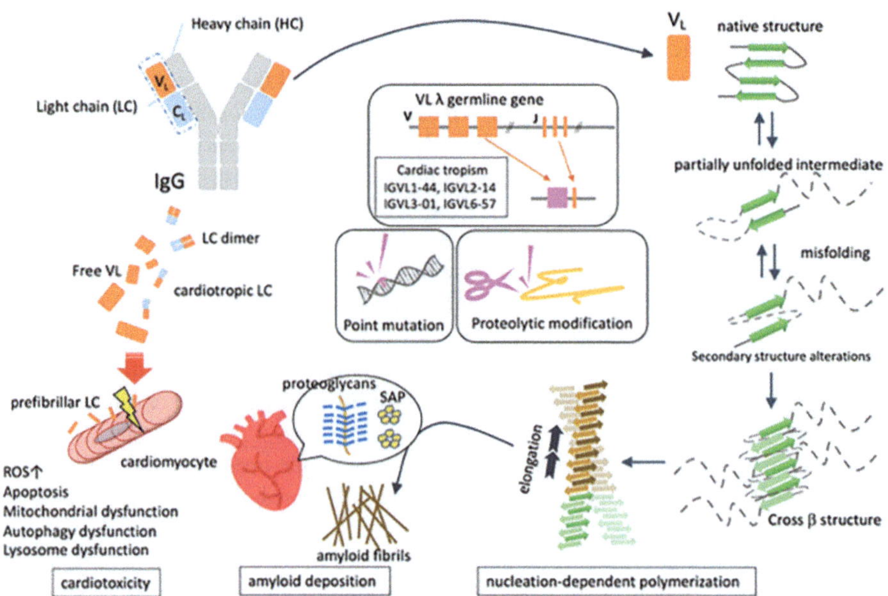

Fig. 5.2 Pathophysiology of cardiac amyloid light chain amyloidosis. A plasma cell clone produces monoclonal immunoglobulins that are structurally instable. Light chains are then released into the circulation. Because of their structural characteristics, altered equilibrium between protein synthesis and degradation, and their chemical and physical properties, they undergo misfolding and formation of protofibrils, then amyloid fibrils. The resulting organ damage derives from the precipitation of fibrils, leading to altered tissue architecture or a direct toxic damage by free light chains or protofibrils. (Reprinted with permission from Ikura et al. [14])

The fact that in AL the λ family is overrepresented also suggests that there is a gene sequence closely related to amyloid formation in the λ IGVL [17]. Light chain fibrils can infiltrate throughout the body, except for the brain, but they mainly show affinity for heart and kidney. The molecular mechanisms behind the amyloid tropism remain largely unknown, but some structural features or genetic mutations may guide amyloid deposition [1, 17].

Additionally, there appears to be post-translational modification in the light chain in form of N-glycosylation. Higher rates of N-glycosylation among clonal κ light chains (LCs) from patients with AL amyloidosis compared to other monoclonal gammopathies indicate that this post-translational modification is associated with a higher risk of developing AL amyloidosis. The group from University of Pavia reported peculiar sequence and spatial pattern of N-glycosylation in amyloidogenic κ LCs. They found that most of the N-glycosylation sites lie in the framework region 3, particularly within the E strand, and consisting mainly of the NFT sequon, setting them apart with respect to non-amyloidogenic clonal LCs. The data raises important questions about the role of this phenomenon in amyloidosis and supports that N-glycosylation may determine the pathogenic behavior of a subset of amyloidogenic LCs. Larger studies and details phenotyping may help refine current

N-glycosylation-based prognostic assessments for patients with monoclonal gammopathies.

Since immunoglobulins normally recognize a wide variety of antigens, each chain is produced with a unique amino acid sequence and three-dimensional structure. Therefore, the morphology of precursor light chains in each patient is unique and highly variable, resulting in a very diverse clinical presentation. In addition to the qualitative abnormality resulting in destabilization of the native structure, a quantitative overproduction of light chains by plasma cells occurs. Although the plasma cell clone proliferation stimulates the synthesis of light chains, amyloidogenic plasma cell clones are not abundant and overly proliferative—often akin to MGUS. The typical median bone marrow plasma cell infiltration is ~9%, and most patients do not fulfil the CRAB criteria for diagnosis of multiple myeloma [14].

The critical step in amyloidogenesis is the turning of soluble proteins into insoluble amyloid fibrils that deposit in organs. Amyloidogenesis is a multistep process requiring the unfolding and misfolding of precursor proteins, with the subsequent nucleation and fibril elongation. The initial nucleation phase can be a slow process but once the nucleation has initiated, the fibril elongation is rapid and exponential. When there is an equilibrium between protein synthesis and degradation (proteostasis), extracellular chaperone proteins promote the correct folding of these chains and prevent their aggregation [14]. When there is an excessive synthesis of light chains, for example, due to mutations or because the efficiency of proteostasis declines with age, the formation and precipitation of amyloid fibrils become more likely. In some cases, even specific interactions with the microenvironment (such as components of the extracellular matrix, proteases, or metal ions) can promote fibril formation in an organ or tissue [1]. When light chain oligomers have formed, the process of aggregation into organized and stable structures is started, also because these structures bind serum amyloid P (SAP) component, which seems to protect protein aggregates from degradation [1].

The formation of amyloid aggregates starts with the native protein in a monomeric, partially misfolded form. When these proteins reach a critical concentration, a fibrillar nucleus forms and catalyzes fibril elongation. This concentration is variable and depends on the stability or instability of the specific light chains. The less stable light chains have lower critical concentrations, while the most stable chains have higher concentrations. When this threshold is reached, the velocity of fibril formation increases exponentially [1].

Organ damage in amyloidosis is generally considered to be related with fibrils that accumulate in large amount within the tissue interstitium between the parenchymal cells, impairing the coordination and the physical characteristics of the tissue. Amyloid fibrils are also capable to interact with biological membranes and promote inflammatory response [18]. Cardiac involvement is a main determinant of survival, and heart dysfunction can result from both amyloid deposits causing disruption of tissue architecture and from proteotoxicity of the light chains [1]. In *C. elegans* model, infusion of light chains from a cardiac amyloid patient results in proteome remodeling, associated with apoptosis activation and oxidative stress. The proteome alterations affect proteins involved in cytoskeletal organization, protein synthesis and quality control, mitochondrial activity and metabolism, signal transduction, and molecular trafficking. Interestingly, the amount of amyloid infiltration in an AL heart is lower than that in patients with transthyretin amyloidosis (ATTR), but AL patients show higher cardiac damage and lower survival rates. Therefore, clinical and experimental evidence suggest that the primary mechanism of injury is likely related to direct cellular toxicity from amyloid precursors or the rate of accumulation of amyloid fibrils [19]. A rapid build up reduces the time for any potential myocyte adaptation to injury initiating a positive back loop that can only end once the production of amyloidogenic precursors ends.

Misfolded proteins have well-documented toxic effects and promote oxidative stress even before fibril formation, causing mitochondrial damage and cell death (Fig. 5.2). These are challenging to capture in clinical practice especially as the basis of proteotoxicity has not been completely clarified. Amyloidogenic light chains are internalized by cardiac myocytes, possibly leading to activation of the p38 mitogen-activated protein kinase pathway, increased reactive oxygen species, altered calcium dynamics, abnormal cell functioning, and apoptosis [20, 21]. However, there is still little evidence for in vivo analysis, and further research may elucidate the molecular mechanisms of cardiac damage in AL.

5.3 Clinical Manifestations

The clinical features of AL amyloidosis depend on the organs and tissues involved [1]. This can be influenced also by the structure of light chains or the genetic abnormality at the basis of protein instability. For example, the IGLV6-57 variant often displays renal involvement, while the IGLV1-44 variant provides a fivefold increase in the risk of dominant heart involvement. Even mutation in κ chains with involvement of IGKV may be associated with different patterns of organ involvement; for example, IGKV1-33 is often associated with liver disease [1, 16, 22]. The heart disease is the most frequent presentation in AL amyloidosis, followed by nephropathy (>60%), hepatic involvement (>50%), neuropathy (10–20%), macroglossia (17%), and periorbital purpura (15%) [3]. Certain features such as marked macroglossia are almost pathognomonic of AL amyloidosis. In patients with cardiac amyloidosis, the simple presence of monoclonal protein in the serum is not adequate to distinguish the presence of AL from ATTR amyloidosis. A pathway with imaging and a tissue biopsy need to be carefully followed to arrive the accurate diagnosis.

The typical phenotype of cardiac amyloidosis is heart failure with preserved ejection fraction but in the advanced case, patients will have a profound low output state with ejection fraction, blood pressure, cardiorenal manifestations, and fatigue [23]. The amyloidotic heart shows a symmetrical increase in biventricular wall thickness (pseudohypertrophy) with markedly increase in the LV stiffness and filling pressures in the presence of nondilated or small ventricles. Of indeed both mechanisms, the cause of rapid clinical progression in AL amyloidosis remains unclear and can be either due to rapid accumulation because of high levels of an unstable precursor or from a direct toxic damage by light chains or protofibrils. Additionally, most patients with amyloidosis have significant perfusion abnormalities in AL amyloidosis which may also contribute to the clinical phenotype. This rapid progression drives the greater clinical and prognostic severity of AL cardiac amyloidosis [24]. Overall, symptoms of cardiac disease can be attributed to diastolic or systolic heart failure. The patient presents with exertional dyspnea, orthopnea, or paroxysmal nocturnal dyspnea, and symptoms related to right heart involvement with severe fluid retention, hepatomegaly, and ascites. Most patients also have less specific symptoms such as anorexia, profound fatigue, and asthenia. Patients may have pleural and pericardial effusions, and ascites.

Renal involvement manifests with a nephrotic syndrome, with hypoalbuminemia-related peripheral edema. Patients will have gradual but progressive loss of renal excretory function. Cardiorenal syndrome also contributes to renal impairment in many patients with AL amyloidosis. Soft tissues deposits occur in 15–20% of patients and, when present, are pathognomonic signs of AL. As these may not occur or only present in the advanced patient, they are not reliable markers for the diagnosis of AL amyloidosis (Fig. 5.1).

Gastrointestinal involvement can present with early satiety, weight loss, constipation, or profound diarrhea (or alternating constipation/diarrhea). These symptoms often overlap with symptoms of autonomic GI involvement. Liver involvement presented as initially asymptomatic hepatomegaly with a slow increase in the alkaline phosphatase followed later by increase in transaminases. Bilirubin increase is a late and ominous feature followed by rapid decline and death in many patients.

About a fifth of all patients have significant peripheral or autonomic neuropathy. The neuropathy is typically a mixed axonal-demyelinating neuropathy. Small fire involvement is common and often an early feature which may not be detected on standard nerve conduction studies. Patients with autonomic neuropathy present with postural hypotension, gut symptoms (overlapping those described for GI involvement) but can progress to difficulty in micturition, blurring of vision, and repeated syncopal episodes. These patients can present with bleeding or thrombosis. Factor deficiency is seen in patients with significant amyloid deposits due to adsorption of factor X on the amyloid fibrils. Patients additionally have marked increase in capillary fragility which can contribute to bleeding in the skin or gut. Patients with marked nephrotic syndrome can be markedly prothrombotic due to loss of anticoagulant factors and, conversely, may need prophylactic anticoagulation.

5.4 Diagnosis

AL amyloidosis is considered as a great "mimic." The initial and even later clinical features of AL amyloidosis are very nonspecific sign and symptoms. There is no single diagnostic test for amyloidosis. Therefore, the diagnosis requires a complex multistep process with key, and often missed, initial step of suspicion of amyloidosis. Once AL is suspected, the next steps are to identify amyloid deposits on histology on a tissue biopsy, type these deposits for confirmation of the fibril type, and then define the organs involved (Fig. 5.3). The presentation of heart failure combined with different and unexplained extracardiac symptoms should trigger the supposition of cardiac amyloidosis. The suspicion may also rise in case of hypotension or absence of hypertension co-existing with elevation of left ventricular mass or wall thickness, especially when associated with enhanced right ventricular mass [26].

Fig. 5.3 Presenting features and diagnostic algorithm for AL amyloidosis. Amyloidosis can be suspected if elevated biomarkers of organ involvement are detected during follow-up of patients with MGUS or if suggestive symptoms arise. The first scenario is ideal and enables early presymptomatic diagnosis. Based on relative rates of progression, appropriate screening programs should detect one patient with MGUS progressing to AL amyloidosis for every seven to ten who develop multiple myeloma. In patients with MGUS in whom elevated NT-proBNP or BNP is found, cardiac magnetic resonance imaging can be used as a higher specificity confirmatory test. If symptoms of systemic amyloidosis arise in a patient in whom a pre-existing monoclonal gammopathy is not known, the first step should be searching for a monoclonal component, particularly if heart involvement is suspected, so as not to delay diagnosis. Only the combination of immunofixation of both serum and urine and FLC measurement grants adequate diagnostic sensitivity to detect amyloidogenic monoclonal proteins. MS-based methods are under investigation. Patients with suspected cardiac amyloidosis without monoclonal components can have an attempted nonbiopsy diagnosis of ATTR amyloidosis with cardiac scintigraphy with bone tracers. Validated tracers are 99mTc-diphosphono-propanodicarboxylic acid, 99mTcpyrophosphate, and 99mTc-hydroxymethylene diphosphonate. DNA analysis is necessary to differentiate between hereditary and wild-type ATTR amyloidosis and to rule out other rarer hereditary forms. All other patients require a tissue diagnosis. Amyloid deposits can be found in abdominal fat, minor salivary glands, and bone marrow, and most patients can be spared biopsy of the involved organ. However, if amyloidosis is deemed probable, for a prompt start of treatment, organ biopsy should not be deferred. Amyloid deposits are recognized as nonbranching fibrils of 7–10 nm in width, detected by light microscopy with green birefringence under polarized light after staining with Congo red or by electron microscopy. The diagnostic sensitivity of abdominal fat aspirate combined with bone marrow or minor salivary gland biopsy is approximately 90% at referral centers, but the recognition of amyloid deposits is affected by the experience of the pathologist. With a few exceptions (e.g., patients with a monoclonal component and periorbital purpura and/or macroglossia, or combination of amyloid heart and renal involvement with albuminuria), the clinical presentation of AL amyloidosis cannot reliably be differentiated from that of other types of systemic amyloidosis. Thus, amyloid tissue typing with adequate technology is mandatory. Standard light microscopy immunohistochemistry does perform satisfactorily, and patients should be referred to specialized centers for typing with adequate technology (immunohistochemistry with custom-made antibodies, IEM, or MS). Accurate clonal studies, biomarker-based staging, and assessment of comorbidities are necessary to design the therapeutic strategy. *ATTR* transthyretin amyloidosis, *FLC* free light chain, *IEM* immunoelectron microscopy, *MGUS* monoclonal gammopathy of undetermined significance, *MRI* magnetic resonance imaging, *MS* mass spectrometry, *NT-proBNP* N-terminal fraction of pro-B-type natriuretic peptide. (Reprinted with permission from Palladini et al. [25])

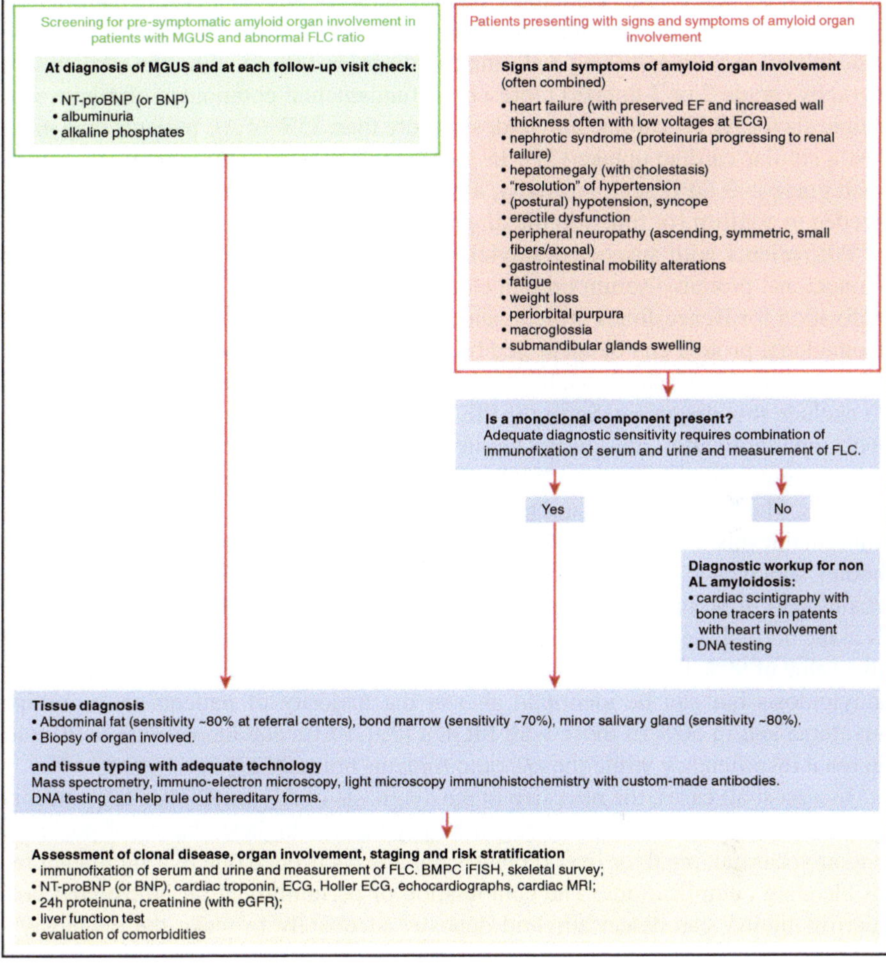
Screening for pre-symptomatic amyloid organ involvement in patients with MGUS and abnormal FLC ratio
At diagnosis of MGUS and at each follow-up visit check:
• NT-proBNP (or BNP)
• albuminuria
• alkaline phosphates
Patients presenting with signs and symptoms of amyloid organ involvement
Signs and symptoms of amyloid organ Involvement (often combined)
• heart failure (with preserved EF and increased wall thickness often with low voltages at ECG)
• nephrotic syndrome (proteinuria progressing to renal failure)
• hepatomegaly (with cholestasis)
• "resolution" of hypertension
• (postural) hypotension, syncope
• erectile dysfunction
• peripheral neuropathy (ascending, symmetric, small fibers/axonal)
• gastrointestinal mobility alterations
• fatigue
• weight loss
• periorbital purpura
• macroglossia
• submandibular glands swelling
Is a monoclonal component present?
Adequate diagnostic sensitivity requires combination of immunofixation of serum and urine and measurement of FLC.
Yes
No
Diagnostic workup for non AL amyloidosis:
• cardiac scintigraphy with bone tracers in patents with heart involvement
• DNA testing
Tissue diagnosis
• Abdominal fat (sensitivity ~80% at referral centers), bond marrow (sensitivity ~70%), minor salivary gland (sensitivity ~80%).
• Biopsy of organ involved.
and tissue typing with adequate technology
Mass spectrometry, immuno-electron microscopy, light microscopy immunohistochemistry with custom-made antibodies. DNA testing can help rule out hereditary forms.
Assessment of clonal disease, organ involvement, staging and risk stratification
• immunofixation of serum and urine and measurement of FLC. BMPC iFISH, skeletal survey;
• NT-proBNP (or BNP), cardiac troponin, ECG, Holler ECG, echocardiographs, cardiac MRI;
• 24h proteinuna, creatinine (with eGFR);
• liver function test
• evaluation of comorbidities

A number of recent guidelines have elucidated the diagnostic pathway for patients with systemic amyloidosis. This always starts with the identification of a monoclonal protein assessing a plasma cell disorder. Indeed, although cardiac scintigraphy (grade 2 or 3 uptake) represents a fundamental component of noninvasive diagnosis for ATTR cardiac amyloidosis, more than 25% of AL patients may manifest a similar cardiac uptake [27]. In presence of monoclonal protein, in a patient with grade 2–3 DPD scan positivity, a biopsy (often an endomyocardial biopsy) is needed to confirm (or rule out) the diagnosis of cardiac amyloidosis.

All patients with suspected amyloidosis need a full panel for assessment of a monoclonal protein—serum protein electrophoresis, immunofixation, urine immunofixation for Bence Jones protein, and measurement of serum free light chains. A monoclonal protein can be identified by standard electrophoresis in around 50% of patients with AL amyloidosis, but a negative electrophoretic tracing does not allow to exclude this diagnosis. Serum (SPIE) and urine (UPIE) protein electrophoreses with immunofixation are always required, and there are rare cases in which only urine examination is positive [28]. Immunofixation can be negative in around 20% of cases. The key test is measurement of free light chain (FLC) assay which detects abnormal levels of immunoglobulin light chains in serum. The assay relies on antibodies which bind epitopes of light chains normally masked by binding to heavy chains [29]. If no monoclonal protein is identified by SPIE/UPIE and the FLC ratio is in the normal range, then AL amyloidosis can be excluded with a negative predictive value of 99% [30, 31]. Presence of abnormally elevated FLCs is not specific of amyloidosis but can be identified also in the majority of patients with multiple myeloma and in 50% of those with MGUS [29]. FLCs can increase up to 20 folds in renal insufficiency while the κ/λ ratio remains normal [29].

In almost all cases, the next step in the diagnosis of AL amyloidosis is confirmatory biopsy. While the involved organ biopsy has the highest chance of positivity, endomyocardial, renal, or liver biopsy is not always needed due to a significant risk of bleeding complications. The combination of periumbilical fat biopsy and bone marrow biopsy can detect amyloid deposits adequately to make the diagnosis in around 85% of cases of AL amyloidosis [1].

Accurately documenting organ involvement is critical. Detecting cardiac involvement is nonetheless crucial as survival of patients with AL amyloidosis depends on the presence and severity of cardiac disease [1, 23]. Echocardiography with demonstration of LV wall thickness >12 mm in absence of another cause is the key step one. Impairment of longitudinal strain is characteristic of amyloidosis and helps to differentiate from other causes of heart thick-walled cardiomyopathies. Cardiac MRI scan is the most sensitive and specific test for diagnosis of cardiac amyloidosis and is indicated in cases where the diagnosis is not clear on echocardiography. Abnormal echocardiography together with N-terminal pro-B-type natriuretic peptide (NT-proBNP) >332 ng/L (in the absence of atrial fibrillation and kidney disease) and low voltage on 12-lead electrocardiography suggests the presence of cardiac disease [32, 33]. Conversely, normal NT-proBNP allows to reliably exclude cardiac disease [34]. Other useful biomarkers are high-sensitivity troponins (I or T). Patients with AL amyloidosis show a chronic release of troponin, and negative troponin values make unlikely (but do not rule out) the diagnosis of cardiac disease. On the contrary, elevated troponin levels increase the likelihood of cardiac disease, as well as stratifying patient risk, as in the case of natriuretic peptides [21, 35]. Findings from electrocardiogram and imaging techniques are relevant for the diagnosis of AL amyloidosis [36–39], as discussed in detail in the following chapters.

5.5 Prognosis

The prognosis of patients with cardiac amyloidosis has markedly improved over the last decades. The major determinant of outcome in amyloidosis still remains the extent of cardiac involvement. An early diagnosis is essential as median survival is only 3–6 months in the absence of hematological treatments [40]. In the decade following the turn of the millennium, the median survival of patients with AL amyloidosis was about 2.5 years which remained unchanged for rest of the decade. The survival improved with access to more effective anti-plasma cell therapies. Bortezomib-based regimes were introduced in the treatment paradigm by 2009–2010 which was a significant step change in the prognosis of AL amyloidosis. The survival for patients diagnosed in mid-2000s was a median of approx. 3 years which has increased to over 6 years in the contemporary cohorts. Introduction of daratumumab-based regimes, which achieve even deeper responses, is expected to significantly improve outcomes even further. However, 20% of the patients are present with advanced cardiac disease. There is still a significant unmet medical need in this patient population where 50–60% may succumb to the disease within a few months of diagnosis irrespective of treatment. Patients with significant renal involvement (even without cardiac involvement) remain at risk of renal progression (two-thirds of renal stage III patient need dialysis within 2 years of presentation). While this does not directly, in absence of cardiac involvement, impact overall survival, the marked morbidity and impact on quality of life of an individual patient are very substantial.

Risk stratification is also essential to modulate the therapeutic approach based on the risk/benefit ratio of each patient, considering the likelihood of response and individual frailty. The current staging system is based on the use of biomarkers, which reflect both organ damage and the degree of activation of the plasma cell clone. The Mayo Clinic 2004 model classified patients into three stages based on the dosing of NT-proBNP and troponin T [41]. The 2015 European modification of the Mayo Clinic 2004 model added a fourth category for patients with NT-proBNP greater than 8500 pg/mL. The Mayo 2012 model classifies patients based on the troponin T or high-sensitivity troponin T, NT-proBNP additionally incorporating the difference between the involved and the uninvolved FLC value [42]. All models had a similar predictive value for survival, even if the 2004 model better predicts for early death and the 2012 model provides a better prediction for long-term survival [2]. Global longitudinal strain is an independent prognostic marker in AL and addition of LS% to the European modification of the Mayo staging provided further refinement in outcome prediction. A staging system of renal involvement to predict the progression toward the need for dialysis has been developed and validated [43]. Although not predictive of mortality, this score estimates the risk of progression of renal disease and information on patient life quality and the possibility to prescribe some cancer therapies. Interestingly, because of the changing standards of care and the increased knowledge of the disease, survival improved and early mortality declined over the last 40 years. Indeed, during the last four decades, the 6-month mortality of AL decreased over from 23% to 13%, and overall survival increased [44].

5.6 Conclusions

AL amyloidosis is a plasma cell disorder characterized by indolent cell clones within the bone marrow that secrete abnormal monoclonal light chains, which then aggregate into amyloid fibrils and deposit in tissues, resulting in devastating organ injury and dysfunction. AL amyloidosis is a debilitating disease with still high and early mortality. Cardiac involvement is common in and represents the most adverse prognostic feature. However, the variable or nonspecific presentation and the perceived rarity often led to delay or missing in suspecting AL amyloidosis as a cause of heart failure. A high index of suspicion as well as the collaboration between different specialists is imperative to diagnose AL amyloidosis. In addition, late diagnosis and therapy are associated with poor prognosis and survival. Hence, the critical need to increase awareness, and understanding of AL amyloidosis.

References

1. Merlini G, Dispenzieri A, Sanchorawala V, et al. Systemic immunoglobulin light chain amyloidosis. Nat Rev Dis Primers. 2018;4(1):38. https://doi.org/10.1038/s41572-018-0034-3.
2. Gertz MA, Dispenzieri A. Systemic amyloidosis recognition, prognosis, and therapy: a systematic review. JAMA. 2020;324(1):79–89. https://doi.org/10.1001/jama.2020.5493.
3. Wechalekar AD, Fontana M, Quarta CC, Liedtke M. AL amyloidosis for cardiologists: awareness, diagnosis, and future prospects: JACC: CardioOncology state-of-the-art review. JACC CardioOncol. 2022;4(4):427–41. https://doi.org/10.1016/j.jaccao.2022.08.009.
4. Kyle RA, Linos A, Beard CM, et al. Incidence and natural history of primary systemic amyloidosis in Olmsted County, Minnesota, 1950 through 1989. Blood. 1992;79(7):1817–22.
5. Kumar N, Zhang NJ, Cherepanov D, Romanus D, Hughes M, Faller DV. Global epidemiology of amyloid light-chain amyloidosis. Orphanet J Rare Dis. 2022;17(1):278. https://doi.org/10.1186/s13023-022-02414-6.
6. Quock TP, Yan T, Chang E, Guthrie S, Broder MS. Epidemiology of AL amyloidosis: a real-world study using US claims data. Blood Adv. 2018;2(10):1046–53. https://doi.org/10.1182/bloodadvances.2018016402.
7. Baker KR. Light chain amyloidosis: epidemiology, staging, and prognostication. Methodist Debakey Cardiovasc J. 2022;18(2):27–35. https://doi.org/10.14797/mdcvj.1070.
8. Kyle RA, Larson DR, Therneau TM, et al. Long-term follow-up of monoclonal gammopathy of undetermined significance. N Engl J Med. 2018;378(3):241–9. https://doi.org/10.1056/NEJMoa1709974.
9. Desikan KR, Dhodapkar MV, Hough A, et al. Incidence and impact of light chain associated (AL) amyloidosis on the prognosis of patients with multiple myeloma treated

with autologous transplantation. Leuk Lymphoma. 1997;27(3–4):315–9. https://doi.org/10.3109/10428199709059685.

10. da Silva Filho MI, Forsti A, Weinhold N, et al. Genome-wide association study of immunoglobulin light chain amyloidosis in three patient cohorts: comparison with myeloma. Leukemia. 2017;31(8):1735–42. https://doi.org/10.1038/leu.2016.387.

11. Xu L, Su Y. Genetic pathogenesis of immunoglobulin light chain amyloidosis: basic characteristics and clinical applications. Exp Hematol Oncol. 2021;10(1):43. https://doi.org/10.1186/s40164-021-00236-z.

12. Merlini G, Bellotti V. Molecular mechanisms of amyloidosis. N Engl J Med. 2003;349(6):583–96. https://doi.org/10.1056/NEJMra023144.

13. Merlini G, Stone MJ. Dangerous small B-cell clones. Blood. 2006;108(8):2520–30. https://doi.org/10.1182/blood-2006-03-001164.

14. Ikura H, Endo J, Kitakata H, Moriyama H, Sano M, Fukuda K. Molecular mechanism of pathogenesis and treatment strategies for AL amyloidosis. Int J Mol Sci. 2022;23(11):6336. https://doi.org/10.3390/ijms23116336.

15. Bochtler T, Hegenbart U, Heiss C, et al. Hyperdiploidy is less frequent in AL amyloidosis compared with monoclonal gammopathy of undetermined significance and inversely associated with translocation t(11;14). Blood. 2011;117(14):3809–15. https://doi.org/10.1182/blood-2010-02-268987.

16. Morgan GJ, Kelly JW. The kinetic stability of a full-length antibody light chain dimer determines whether endoproteolysis can release amyloidogenic variable domains. J Mol Biol. 2016;428(21):4280–97. https://doi.org/10.1016/j.jmb.2016.08.021.

17. Kourelis TV, Dasari S, Theis JD, et al. Clarifying immunoglobulin gene usage in systemic and localized immunoglobulin light-chain amyloidosis by mass spectrometry. Blood. 2017;129(3):299–306. https://doi.org/10.1182/blood-2016-10-743997.

18. Cecchi C, Stefani M. The amyloid-cell membrane system. The interplay between the biophysical features of oligomers/fibrils and cell membrane defines amyloid toxicity. Biophys Chem. 2013;182:30–43. https://doi.org/10.1016/j.bpc.2013.06.003.

19. Merlini G, Lousada I, Ando Y, et al. Rationale, application and clinical qualification for NT-proBNP as a surrogate end point in pivotal clinical trials in patients with AL amyloidosis. Leukemia. 2016;30(10):1979–86. https://doi.org/10.1038/leu.2016.191.

20. Marin-Argany M, Lin Y, Misra P, et al. Cell damage in light chain amyloidosis: fibril internalization, toxicity and cell-mediated seeding. J Biol Chem. 2016;291(38):19813–25. https://doi.org/10.1074/jbc.M116.736736.

21. Mishra S, Guan J, Plovie E, et al. Human amyloidogenic light chain proteins result in cardiac dysfunction, cell death, and early mortality in zebrafish. Am J Physiol Heart Circ Physiol. 2013;305(1):H95–103. https://doi.org/10.1152/ajpheart.00186.2013.

22. Perfetti V, Palladini G, Casarini S, et al. The repertoire of lambda light chains causing predominant amyloid heart involvement and identification of a preferentially involved germline gene, IGLV1-44. Blood. 2012;119(1):144–50. https://doi.org/10.1182/blood-2011-05-355784.

23. Selvanayagam JB, Hawkins PN, Paul B, Myerson SG, Neubauer S. Evaluation and management of the cardiac amyloidosis. J Am Coll Cardiol. 2007;50(22):2101–10. https://doi.org/10.1016/j.jacc.2007.08.028.

24. Falk RH, Alexander KM, Liao R, Dorbala S. AL (light-chain) cardiac amyloidosis: a review of diagnosis and therapy. J Am Coll Cardiol. 2016;68(12):1323–41. https://doi.org/10.1016/j.jacc.2016.06.053.

25. Palladini G, Milani P, Merlini G. Management of AL amyloidosis in 2020. Blood. 2020;136(23):2620–7. https://doi.org/10.1182/blood.2020006913.

26. Griffin JM, Rosenblum H, Maurer MS. Pathophysiology and therapeutic approaches to cardiac amyloidosis. Circ Res. 2021;128(10):1554–75. https://doi.org/10.1161/CIRCRESAHA.121.318187.

27. Quarta CC, Zheng J, Hutt D, et al. 99mTc-DPD scintigraphy in immunoglobulin light chain (AL) cardiac amyloidosis. Eur Heart J Cardiovasc Imaging. 2021;22(11):1304–11. https://doi.org/10.1093/ehjci/jeab095.

28. Gillmore JD, Wechalekar A, Bird J, et al. Guidelines on the diagnosis and investigation of AL amyloidosis. Br J Haematol. 2015;168(2):207–18. https://doi.org/10.1111/bjh.13156.
29. Dispenzieri A, Kyle R, Merlini G, et al. International Myeloma Working Group guidelines for serum-free light chain analysis in multiple myeloma and related disorders. Leukemia. 2009;23(2):215–24. https://doi.org/10.1038/leu.2008.307.
30. Writing C, Kittleson MM, Ruberg FL, et al. ACC expert consensus decision pathway on comprehensive multidisciplinary care for the patient with cardiac amyloidosis: a report of the American College of Cardiology Solution Set Oversight Committee. J Am Coll Cardiol. 2023; https://doi.org/10.1016/j.jacc.2022.11.022.
31. Garcia-Pavia P, Rapezzi C, Adler Y, et al. Diagnosis and treatment of cardiac amyloidosis: a position statement of the ESC Working Group on Myocardial and Pericardial Diseases. Eur Heart J. 2021;42(16):1554–68. https://doi.org/10.1093/eurheartj/ehab072.
32. Kumar SK, Callander NS, Adekola K, et al. Systemic light chain amyloidosis, version 2.2023, NCCN clinical practice guidelines in oncology. J Natl Compr Cancer Netw. 2023;21(1):67–81. https://doi.org/10.6004/jnccn.2023.0001.
33. Hwa YL, Fogaren T, Sams A, et al. Immunoglobulin light-chain amyloidosis: clinical presentations and diagnostic approach. J Adv Pract Oncol. 2019;10(5):470–81. https://doi.org/10.6004/jadpro.2019.10.5.5.
34. Palladini G, Campana C, Klersy C, et al. Serum N-terminal pro-brain natriuretic peptide is a sensitive marker of myocardial dysfunction in AL amyloidosis. Circulation. 2003;107(19):2440–5. https://doi.org/10.1161/01.Cir.0000068314.02595.B2.
35. Kristen AV, Giannitsis E, Lehrke S, et al. Assessment of disease severity and outcome in patients with systemic light-chain amyloidosis by the high-sensitivity troponin T assay. Blood. 2010;116(14):2455–61. https://doi.org/10.1182/blood-2010-02-267708.
36. Murtagh B, Hammill SC, Gertz MA, Kyle RA, Tajik AJ, Grogan M. Electrocardiographic findings in primary systemic amyloidosis and biopsy-proven cardiac involvement. Am J Cardiol. 2005;95(4):535–7. https://doi.org/10.1016/j.amjcard.2004.10.028.
37. Phelan D, Collier P, Thavendiranathan P, et al. Relative apical sparing of longitudinal strain using two-dimensional speckle-tracking echocardiography is both sensitive and specific for the diagnosis of cardiac amyloidosis. Heart. 2012;98(19):1442–8. https://doi.org/10.1136/heartjnl-2012-302353.
38. Fontana M, Corovic A, Scully P, Moon JC. Myocardial amyloidosis: the exemplar interstitial disease. JACC Cardiovasc Imaging. 2019;12(11 Pt 2):2345–56. https://doi.org/10.1016/j.jcmg.2019.06.023.
39. Karamitsos TD, Piechnik SK, Banypersad SM, et al. Noncontrast T1 mapping for the diagnosis of cardiac amyloidosis. JACC Cardiovasc Imaging. 2013;6(4):488–97. https://doi.org/10.1016/j.jcmg.2012.11.013.
40. Wechalekar AD, Schonland SO, Kastritis E, et al. A European collaborative study of treatment outcomes in 346 patients with cardiac stage III AL amyloidosis. Blood. 2013;121(17):3420–7. https://doi.org/10.1182/blood-2012-12-473066.
41. Dispenzieri A, Gertz MA, Kyle RA, et al. Serum cardiac troponins and N-terminal pro-brain natriuretic peptide: a staging system for primary systemic amyloidosis. J Clin Oncol. 2004;22(18):3751–7. https://doi.org/10.1200/JCO.2004.03.029.
42. Kumar S, Dispenzieri A, Lacy MQ, et al. Revised prognostic staging system for light chain amyloidosis incorporating cardiac biomarkers and serum free light chain measurements. J Clin Oncol. 2012;30(9):989–95. https://doi.org/10.1200/JCO.2011.38.5724.
43. Palladini G, Hegenbart U, Milani P, et al. A staging system for renal outcome and early markers of renal response to chemotherapy in AL amyloidosis. Blood. 2014;124(15):2325–32. https://doi.org/10.1182/blood-2014-04-570010.
44. Staron A, Zheng L, Doros G, et al. Marked progress in AL amyloidosis survival: a 40-year longitudinal natural history study. Blood Cancer J. 2021;11(8):139. https://doi.org/10.1038/s41408-021-00529-w.

Hereditary Transthyretin Amyloidosis

Laura Obici, Giorgia Panichella, and Roberta Mussinelli

6.1 Epidemiology

Transthyretin amyloidosis (ATTR) is a highly disabling and fatal systemic disease characterized by the extracellular deposition of amyloid fibrils composed of transthyretin (TTR). TTR, or prealbumin, is a tetrameric transport protein composed of four identical monomers of 127 amino acids. TTR is mainly secreted by the liver, by the choroid plexus of the brain and by the retinal pigment epithelium of the eye. This protein is highly conserved through vertebrate evolution. Its best characterized physiological functions are the co-transport of retinol (vitamin A) through retinol-binding protein in plasma and the transport of thyroxine, particularly in the cerebrospinal fluid (CSF) [1].

Based on the underlying genotype, ATTR amyloidosis is classified as either wild-type (ATTRwt) or hereditary (mutated or variant, ATTRv) [2]. In ATTRwt, which will be addressed in a dedicated chapter, TTR aggregates as amyloid in its wild-type form in the presence of conditions that are likely to promote the fibrillogenesis process, such as aging, tissue biomechanical forces, or oxidative stress. On the contrary, ATTRv amyloidosis is a severe, adult-onset autosomal dominant inherited systemic disease caused by mutations in the *TTR* gene. The main ATTRv presentations include polyneuropathy (ATTRv-PN), cardiomyopathy (ATTRv-CM), leptomeningeal, renal, and ocular involvement [2, 3].

L. Obici (✉) · R. Mussinelli
Rare Diseases Unit and Amyloidosis Research and Treatment Centre, IRCCS Fondazione Policlinico San Matteo, Pavia, Italy
e-mail: l.obici@smatteo.pv.it; r.mussinelli@smatteo.pv.it

G. Panichella
Department of Experimental and Clinical Medicine, University of Florence, Florence, Italy
e-mail: giorgia.panichella@unifi.it

M. Emdin et al. (eds.), *Cardiac Amyloidosis*,
https://doi.org/10.1007/978-3-031-51757-0_6

ATTRv amyloidosis has long been considered as a rare disorder that was initially reported in Northern Portugal, Northern Sweden and in two regions of Japan [4], with an estimated prevalence in these regions of 1–10 in 10,000 [5, 6]. Since the 1990s, new geographical areas with a relatively high prevalence due to a founder effect have been identified. Besides, an increasing number of private mutations associated with a late-onset and often apparently sporadic presentation have been described [4]. ATTRv amyloidosis has now been reported in about 30 countries, including many in Europe, in North and South America, and in Asia, particularly Japan, China, and India [4]. However, the distribution of ATTRv amyloidosis is extremely heterogeneous across different geographical regions making it difficult to estimate a general incidence or prevalence. In Italy, a national registry for ATTRv launched in 2017 has allowed to estimate a global prevalence of 4.33/million at 1 January 2019, with higher rates in some regions such as Sicily, Lazio, and Tuscany where it reaches 9.3/million due to a local genetic founder effect [7]. A 2013 study conducted in England showed that the annual incidence of systemic amyloidosis is about eight new cases per million inhabitants per year, of which 7% and 10% would be attributable to ATTRv and ATTRwt, respectively [8]. A Swedish study estimated an incidence of ATTRv amyloidosis equal to two new cases per million inhabitants per year [9].

A 2018 study by Schimdt et al. estimated the global prevalence of ATTRv-PN to be 10,186, with a range of 5526–38,468 [10]. A Portuguese nationwide study reported a mean incidence of ATTRv equal to 0.87/100,000 over the 2010–2016 period, corresponding to 71 new patients per year [11]. The Val30Met (c.148G>A, p.Val50Met) mutation in the *TTR* gene is the most common pathogenic mutation worldwide, typically leading to a predominantly neurological phenotype. In Portugal, the Val30Met mutation has an estimated prevalence of 1/538 individuals [12]. Other mutations associated with ATTRv-PN include Thr60Ala in Northern Ireland, Glu89Gln in Bulgaria, Ser50Arg in Mexico, Phe64Leu in Sicily, Ser77Tyr and Ser77Phe in France, and Ala97Ser in Taiwan [4].

The epidemiology of hereditary ATTR-CM is still largely unknown. Leu111Met, Ile68Leu, Val122Ile, and late-onset Val30Met mutations are among the most common found in ATTRv-CM patients [13]. A retrospective study on the epidemiology of ATTRv-CM in Northern countries showed that the Swedish ATTRv-CM population primarily consists of late-onset Val30Met patients, whereas Leu111Met is the most common variant found in Denmark [14]. Data from the Transthyretin Amyloid Outcome Survey (THAOS) registry showed that Val122Ile is the most represented TTR mutation in the United States. Val122Ile subjects are typically younger, more often female, and African Americans than patients with wild-type disease [15]. Finally, Ile68Leu mutation is a cause of ATTRv-CM endemic in Central-Northern regions of Italy [16].

With increasing awareness of this condition among clinicians, thanks to the increasing availability of effective therapeutic options and to the wider use of genetic testing, the incidence of ATTRv amyloidosis is likely to increase.

6.2   Genetic Basis of ATTRv

The gene encoding TTR is located on chromosome 18 (18q12.1) and spans 6956 bases, for a total of four exons and five introns. To date, more than 150 pathogenic mutations in the *TTR* gene have been reported [16, 17]. Single-base substitutions resulting in missense mutations represent the large majority of the amyloidogenic variants, while only a few small deletions and insertions are reported. The pattern of inheritance is Mendelian, autosomal dominant with variable expressivity and incomplete penetrance [18]. Penetrance varies according to specific mutations and populations suggesting that additional genetic factors and/or potential epigenetic mechanisms might play a role. In Northern Sweden, for example, carrier frequency is 1.95% and the estimated penetrance is 29% at the age of >60 years [19]. In Portugal, endemic areas carrier frequency is 0.18% [5] and the estimated prevalence is 91% at 70 years old [20].

There are also reported cases of mutation carrier who remained asymptomatic for life [21].

6.3   The Amyloidogenic Cascade

In physiological conditions, TTR is a globular homo-tetramer composed of four identical 127 amino acid subunits (named A, B, C, D) and organized as a dimer of dimers (AB and CD) [1]. In the native TTR tetramer, two symmetrical hydrophobic channels are generated at the dimer–dimer interface accommodating one thyroxine molecule each [1]. TTR is mainly secreted by the liver, by the choroid plexus of the brain, and by the retinal pigment epithelium of the eye. Except for a few highly unstable variants, such as Asp18Gly, amyloidogenic TTR mutations overcome the intracellular quality control mechanisms and are found at normal concentrations in plasma and CSF, where the protein plays its physiological functions [23].

TTR amyloidogenesis requires the dissociation of the native homotetrameric quaternary structure into misfolded monomers which aggregate into soluble oligomeric species, protofibrils, and finally insoluble amyloid fibrils [22]. Tetramer dissociation is the rate-limiting step in TTR amyloidogenesis [22]. A number of factors may trigger TTR misfolding and aggregation in vitro, such as exposure to low pH, biomechanical forces, proteolytic remodeling, and posttranslational modifications [24]. Mutations lead to a kinetically unstable tetrameric protein with an increased propensity to dissociate into monomers leading to misfolding. For example, the Val122Ile variant destabilizes the TTR tetramer by lowering the kinetic barrier for tetramer dissociation. On the contrary, some TTR mutations (i.e., Thr119Met [25], Arg104His [26], Ala108Val [27]) have been shown to increase TTR stability. Such mutations induce new hydrophobic contacts between the dimer–dimer interface, which increase the kinetic stability of TTR tetramers and the binding affinity for thyroxine, which further stabilize the tetramer [1]. Interestingly, individuals carrying both the Thr119Met and the ATTRv-PN associated Val30Met mutation present a more benign evolution of the disease than heterozygotes carrying the Val30Met mutation alone, indicating that Thr119Met may act as an inter-allelic trans-suppressor [28].

According to several observations, TTR amyloid fibrils obtained from patients are predominantly formed by both full-length and fragmented TTR species, mostly consisting of C-terminal fragments spanning residues 49–127 [29, 30]. This has suggested that TTR cleavage could be a key event in TTR amyloidogenesis in vivo and has prompted several investigations. The results of these studies support a mechano-enzymatic mechanism of TTR fibrillogenesis under physiological conditions [31]. According to this mechanism, TTR dissociation is primed by the sequential action of biomechanical forces that destabilize the TTR tetramer and expose protease sensitive loops, followed by cleavage by specific proteases. Importantly, these forces are in the range of magnitude of forces found in the extracellular space of tissues such as the heart or the joints.

Studies aimed at the identification of the putative enzyme responsible for this process in vivo have shown that plasmin cleaves TTR with efficiency, generating fibrils indistinguishable from those obtained ex vivo [32]. The recently published transgenic mouse model of cardiac ATTR amyloidosis expressing the highly Ser52Pro amyloidogenic variant recapitulates crucial molecular events predicted by in vitro studies [33]. This model confirms that TTR amyloidogenesis depends on proteolytic cleavage and, importantly, that plasmin activity promotes amyloid deposition.

Less is known about the mechanisms of organ dysfunction induced by amyloid deposition. Ongoing studies suggest a multifactorial process, resulting from a combination of mechanical disruption of tissue structure, as well as proteotoxicity induced by fibrils or putative prefibrillar aggregates leading to inflammation, reactive oxygen species generation, apoptosis, and autophagy [24, 34]. Another unsolved question in TTR amyloid pathology is related to the molecular basis of the tissue specificity of the different TTR variants. Based on clinical observations, it is possible to trace a continuous spectrum of mutations whose extremes consist of an exclusively neurological or cardiac phenotype, respectively (Fig. 6.1). However,

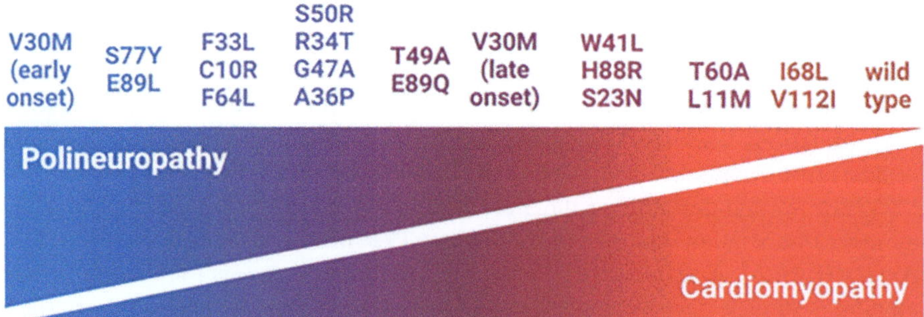

Fig. 6.1 Genotype–phenotype correlation in ATTRv amyloidosis. TTR mutations are associated with a wide spectrum of clinical manifestations ranging from predominantly neuropathic (e.g., early-onset V30M) to cardiac (e.g., V122I, I68L) phenotypes, and mixed forms in between. (Modified with permission from Castaño et al. [22])

there is no established relationship between the structural characteristics of the different TTR mutations and the pattern of amyloid deposits in cardiac, nervous, or other tissues. It has been speculated that several factors could be involved in driving tissue targeting including protein stability, interaction with extracellular components such as matrix constituents and chaperones, and/or the proteolytic remodeling by tissue-specific proteases [35]. Moreover, even if the overall degree of genotype-phenotype correlation is consistent, there is a high intra-mutational and intra-familial heterogeneity indicating that each single TTR mutation does not account exclusively for the specific phenotype.

6.4 Clinical Manifestations

ATTRv amyloidosis is a systemic and multifaceted disease. Key signs and symptoms mainly reflect involvement of the peripheral nervous system and the heart but virtually any tissue and organ can be involved, including the eyes, the kidneys, and the leptomeninges (Fig. 6.2). As a result, the clinical presentation of ATTRv is quite heterogeneous. Phenotype largely depends on the underlying mutation. It is well recognized that some variants are associated with a predominant cardiac phenotype, namely Val122Ile and Ile68Leu, and others invariably manifest with a sensorimotor and/or autonomic neuropathy. However, when patients are thoroughly investigated by a multidisciplinary team, the large majority can be classified as having a mixed phenotype. Therefore, the distinction between ATTRv-PN and ATTRv-CM does not allow to fully capture the systemic burden of this complex disease.

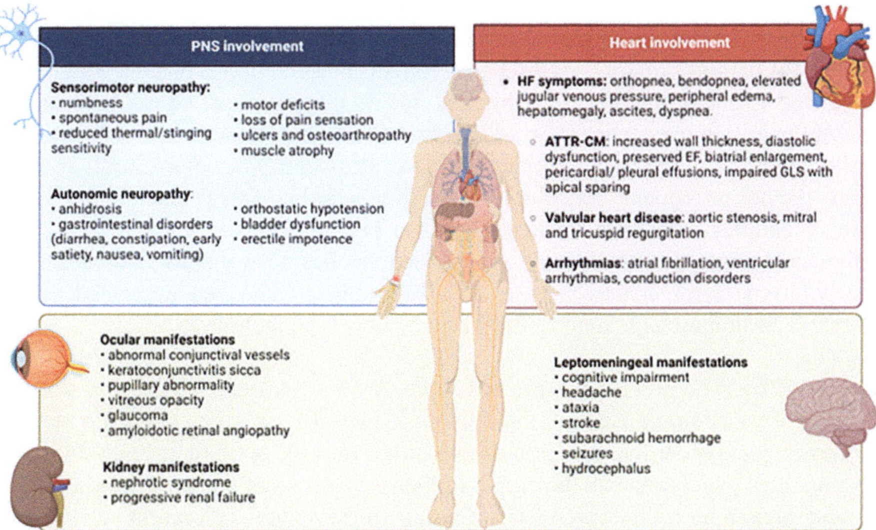

Fig. 6.2 Clinical manifestations of ATTRv amyloidosis. *ATTR-CM* transthyretin amyloidosis cardiomyopathy, *EF* ejection fraction, *GLS* global longitudinal strain, *HF* heart failure, *PNS* peripheral nervous system

Genotype is not the only factor affecting expression. The mechanisms driving tissue tropism, organ damage, and age of onset are not clarified yet. Gender, maternal or paternal inheritance, and putative environmental factors have been advocated as potential disease modifiers, together with still undiscovered genetic factors [22]. The most striking example of the contribution of additional modifying factor to phenotypic expression is the variable natural history of the Val30Met mutation, for which two completely distinct diseases have been described [36]. Early-onset Val30Met disease manifests with small-fiber peripheral neuropathy and autonomic dysfunction. Gastrointestinal manifestations and renal involvement are common and may represent the first clinical findings. The penetrance is high, and sex has limited impact on disease expression. Conduction abnormalities are observed in the early stages, with need for pacemaker implantation occurring since the fourth decade of life. On the contrary, in late-onset V30M, penetrance is higher in males, patients invariably present with bilateral carpal tunnel syndrome, a sensorimotor axonal polyneuropathy affecting both large and small nerve fibers, limited autonomic dysfunction and a typical infiltrative cardiac involvement [22].

6.4.1 Heart Involvement

Cardiac involvement is a common manifestation of ATTRv amyloidosis. ATTR can potentially infiltrate any cardiovascular structure, including the conduction system, atrial and ventricular myocardium, valvular tissue, coronary arteries, and great vessels [37]. Myocardial amyloid infiltration leads to a progressive increases in the thickness of the ventricular walls and the interventricular septum. Cardiac involvement typically manifests with signs and symptoms of restrictive cardiomyopathy and/or heart failure with preserved ejection fraction (HFpEF), which significantly impact the patient's quality of life. However, this presentation is usually observed in advanced stages of the disease, while cardiac involvement can be milder and even asymptomatic in the earlier stages [38]. Since the conduction system is frequently infiltrated by amyloid, bundle branch blocks, atrioventricular block, and sinoatrial block are not infrequent. The involvement of the cardiac valves leads to the formation of nodules or diffuse thickening of the leaflets, causing variable degrees of valvular regurgitation or stenosis. Aortic stenosis has been mainly associated with the wild-type form; however, cases in ATTRv amyloidosis are described as well [39]. Major mutations related to the cardiac phenotype include:

- **Val122Ile**. The mutation is present in up to 4% of African Americans, where it represents a common cause of misdiagnosed HFpEF [40]. The allele has no obvious impact on cardiac function or outcomes until the sixth or seventh decade of life, after which patients develop a higher prevalence of congestive heart failure and higher mortality rates [41]. Cardiac involvement is present in 100% of patients with this mutation, associated with none to minimal neuropathic involvement. Due to the high prevalence of hypertension and left ventricular hypertrophy in the African American elderly population, cardiac amyloidosis can often be misdiagnosed as hypertensive heart disease [42].

- **Ile68Leu**. The populations carrying this mutation are predominantly Caucasian, namely Italian and German. The cardiac phenotype is similar to ATTRwt amyloidosis, with concentric increase in left ventricular (LV) wall thickness and preserved LV ejection fraction. However, Ile68Leu ATTRv patients typically present younger and are more likely to have symptomatic neurological involvement than ATTRwt. Male preponderance is observed in affected patients but, as expected, not in unaffected mutation carriers [16].
- **Leu111Met**. This mutation is typically found in Caucasian patients, predominantly Danish. Cardiac involvement is present in 100% of cases with clinical onset in the fourth or fifth decade of life, often accompanied by gastrointestinal symptoms [43, 44].
- **Thr60Ala**. This is the most common variant in the United Kingdom [45]. Cardiac involvement is almost always present at diagnosis and is a major determinant of Thr60Ala ATTRv poor prognosis. It is frequently associated with neuropathic symptoms [45].

As discussed in other chapters, cardiac imaging plays a major role for the diagnosis and in disease monitoring. Echocardiography is typically the first approach to evaluate patients with cardiac symptoms and can be suggestive of amyloidosis in the presence of unexplained left ventricular (LV) thickening with normal to small LV cavity size, diastolic dysfunction and preserved ejection fraction, biatrial enlargement, thickened valves, right ventricular and interatrial septum, pericardial or pleural effusions [46]. The finding of impaired global longitudinal strain with characteristic sparing of the apex may help differentiate amyloidosis from other non-amyloid causes of LV thickening. Similar morphological and functional alterations can be seen with cardiac magnetic resonance (CMR). Moreover, this imaging technique allows a better tissue characterization showing elevated native T1, increased extracellular volume fraction, unique late gadolinium enhancement pattern with abnormal gadolinium kinetics [47]. Neither echocardiography nor CMR can be diagnostic for cardiac amyloidosis, whereas bone tracer scintigraphy allows the noninvasive diagnosis of ATTR-CM in the absence of a plasma cell clone. ATTRv infiltrated cardiac tissues display a grade 2 or 3 cardiac uptake of the tracer DPD (99m technetium 3,3-diphosphono-1,2 propanodicarboxylic acid), PYP (99m technetium pyrophosphate), or HMDP (99m technetium hydroxymethylene diphosphonate) [48]. Notably, in some TTR mutations, such as Phe64Leu, cardiac uptake can be low or absent even in the presence of clear clinical, biochemical, and echocardiographical signs of cardiac involvement [49].

Together with cardiac imaging, a persistent increase in the biomarkers N-terminal pro-brain natriuretic peptide and troponins is suggestive of cardiac amyloidosis [50].

6.4.2 PNS Involvement

Polyneuropathy in ATTRv reflects the involvement of both somatic and autonomic nerve fibers and typically manifests with a combination of signs and symptoms resulting from sensory, motor, and autonomic impairment [18]. TTR accumulates predominantly in the endoneurial vessels, causing progressive axonal degeneration with a length-dependent pattern. In early-onset Val30Met ATTRv, which can be regarded as the prototype of ATTRv polyneuropathy since its initial description by Corino de Andrade in 1952, both unmyelinated and small myelinated nerve fibers are initially affected, particularly in the lower limbs. Patients present with pain and thermal sensory loss [51]. The sensory damage subsequently proceeds proximally and progressively affects the upper limbs. Involvement of large nerve fibers causes progressive impairment of light touch and deep sensations associated with weakness and muscle waste. Loss of pain perception leads to painless trauma and the development of plantar ulcers and osteoarthropathy of the foot (i.e., Charcot osteoarthropathy) [52]. In the end stage of the disease, sensory loss, muscle atrophy, and weakness of the extremities result in complete inability to walk even assisted [18].

Autonomic neuropathy is frequently observed, particularly in early-onset phenotypes [51]. It characterized by an extremely wide range of manifestations, including anhidrosis, gastrointestinal motility disorders (most commonly diarrhea alternating with constipation, but also early satiety, nausea, and vomiting), orthostatic hypotension, bladder and erectile dysfunction [53].

Assessment of neurological involvement in ATTRv relies on multiple tests and composite scoring systems to fully capture the disease burden and to monitor disease progression and response to therapy. Validated measures include the composite mNIS+7 score that quantifies sensation loss, impaired muscle stretch reflexes, and weakness in upper and lower limbs in combination with autonomic dysfunction, the latter assessed either by heart rate deep breathing or postural hypotension [54].

Noninvasive investigation of small-fiber neuropathy includes quantitative sensory testing and assessment of sudomotor function either by sympathetic skin response (SSR) or electrochemical skin conductance. Although more invasive, measurement of intraepidermal nerve fiber density in skin biopsy performed both at the ankle and the thigh has demonstrated a proximal-distal gradient in small nerve fiber derangement which closely correlates with disease severity and duration [55].

Patients' reported outcome measures including quality of life and ability in performing activities of daily living represent an important tool in assessing disease burden and in tracking progression and response to therapy. The Norfolk-QoL-DN score, a 35-item measure sensitive to small fiber, large fiber, and autonomic nerve function initially developed for diabetic neuropathy, has been validated for ATTRv showing that either its total score and its five individual domains strongly correlate with disease progression.

The Rasch-built Overall Disability Scale is a 24-item scale developed to capture limitations on everyday activities and social participation, allowing measurement of physical function by providing information complementary to the assessment of gait speed (10-m walk test) and performance status.

Tools for assessing autonomic symptoms include the Composite Autonomic Symptom Scale-31 (COMPASS-31) and Compound Autonomic Dysfunction Test (CADT).

Finally, several novel tools for monitoring disease onset progression are under investigation. A promising biomarker is the plasma neurofilament light chain, that has been proved to quantitate neuro-axonal damage in several disorders and recently shown to correlate with disease severity [56] and with response to treatment [57] in ATTRv polyneuropathy.

More recently, imaging approaches such as nerve ultrasound and advanced nerve and muscle magnetic resonance have been suggested as innovative tools for assessment of disease onset and progression [58–60].

6.5 Other Clinical Manifestations

Most patients complain of systemic unspecific symptoms, such as fatigue, hoarseness, or unintentional weight loss, as the initial manifestations of the disease. Bilateral carpal tunnel syndrome frequently occurs in most patients with late-onset ATTRv amyloidosis as the first sign and may anticipate other clinical findings up to 10 years [61].

Ophthalmologic involvement due to transthyretin production by the retinal pigment epithelium is observed in association with several variants and typically manifests with abnormal conjunctival vessels, sicca keratoconjunctivitis, loss of corneal sensitivity and neurotrophic corneal ulcers, pupillary abnormality (e.g., scalloped iris), vitreous opacities, chronic open-angle glaucoma, and retinal angiopathy. The incidence of such manifestations increases as ATTRv-PN progresses and is high in long surviving V30M patients after liver transplantation [62].

Kidney involvement is more common than previously recognized and may affect most patients with ATTRv regardless of the underlying genetic variant [63]. However, it is significantly more frequent in patients with early-onset Val30Met, being reported in up to 30% of cases, than in late-onset, non V30M cases [51, 64]. It usually presents with proteinuria that may evolve to nephrotic syndrome and/or progressive renal failure.

Leptomeningeal amyloidosis represents a rare subtype of ATTRv amyloidosis, characterized by amyloid deposition in cranial and spinal leptomeninges, sometimes in combination with eye impairment (oculoleptomeningeal amyloidosis) [51]. To date 15 mutations have been found to be associated with leptomeningeal amyloidosis [65]. Symptoms include cognitive impairment, headache, ataxia, stroke, subarachnoid hemorrhage, seizures, and hydrocephalus [65].

6.6 Prognosis

The availability of effective therapeutic options is significantly changing the natural history and the prognosis of ATTRv amyloidosis. In the absence of treatment, however, progression may be extremely rapid and death may occur within 7–12 years from onset, depending on mutation and phenotype, with longer survival reported in patients with early-onset Val30Met [52]. Mortality is mostly influenced by the presence of cardiac involvement. In some patients, heart involvement may be quite aggressive reducing survival to 3.4 years, with death usually due to progressive heart failure or life-threatening arrhythmias [45]. It is also important to highlight how symptoms and progressive associated disabilities substantially decrease patient's quality of life [66]. As discussed in other chapters, clinical strategies, such as close follow-up of asymptomatic carriers, prompt diagnosis and early treatment would slow the progressive decline of the disease, thus reducing mortality and morbidity rates, and improving patients-reported quality of life. Finally, due to the rarity of the disease and its complex management, specialized centers and patients support groups play a crucial role in providing the best care and support for patients and their families.

6.7 Presymptomatic Genetic Testing and Monitoring of Carriers

Prompt detection of the earliest signs of the disease is of outmost importance to initiate effective therapy, preventing disability and irreversible organ damage. Best response is observed when treatment is started in the initial stages. Cascade genetic testing in at-risk relatives is therefore a valuable approach to systematically identify presymptomatic mutation carriers and to start a structured monitoring program. However, considering the potential psychological impact associated with the predictive test for a late-onset disease, it is recommended that presymptomatic testing (PST) for ATTRv is always offered in the context of a non-directive genetic counseling process. At-risk subjects should be provided with all information useful to fully appreciate the advantages and disadvantages of PST. For example, unmet needs related to untreatable, long-term complications such as ocular and leptomeningeal involvement, require thorough discussion. Potentially, subjects might also choose to undergo clinical monitoring without performing genetic test, until symptoms consistent with the disease arise. Expert recommendations for performing genetic counseling and PST in ATTRv have been proposed that particularly emphasize the importance of bridging the counseling protocol to an easily accessible clinical monitoring program, performed by a multidisciplinary team, when a positive result is disclosed. Close follow-up has been recommended to start within 10 years from the predicted age of onset (PADO) of the disease based on family and natural disease history according to the specific mutation/phenotype [67]. An annual follow-up is then established which includes a panel of evaluations tailored to detect the early signs of the expected phenotype. The frequency of controls can be increased when PADO approaches or a change in a single parameter occurs. Recommended investigations for neurological involvement include NIS, nerve conduction studies, neurophysiological tests to detect small nerve fiber neuropathy and autonomic dysfunction such as SSR, heart rate variability, sudomotor testing, postural hypotension, and questionnaires to investigate specific symptoms and quality of life (Norfolk QoL-DN, EuroQol-5 Dimension (EQ-5D), CADT and COMPASS-31). Cardiac assessments should include biomarkers, echocardiography, ECG, CMR, and bone tracer scintigraphy.

Skin biopsy is increasingly recognized as a sensitive test to detect early disease onset across different genotypes and phenotypes, providing early evidence of intraepidermal nerve fiber density reduction and dermal amyloid deposition. Several innovative approaches have also recently been proposed for early detection of measurable organ impairment associated with ATTRv, such as nerve ultrasound, magnetic resonance neurography, muscle magnetic resonance imaging, serum neurofilament light chain concentration, and corneal confocal in vivo microscopy.

6.8 Conclusions

The increasing availability of effective disease-modifying treatments for ATTRv is progressively spreading awareness of this systemic disease across many different specialties. Diagnostic delay is thus progressively reducing, paralleled by initial evidence of improved survival [68]. Early diagnosis and prompt treatment start are key for preventing significant organ damage and disability and for preserving quality of life. However, in spite of these major advancements, patients still experience several unmet needs. These not only include the lack of effective treatment options for severe complications such as progressive visual impairment and central nervous system involvement, already observed in long-term survivors after liver transplantation. A significant psychosocial burden is reported by patients and their caregivers, even in the early disease stages, that deserves a more comprehensive, multidimensional approach to long-term care. New frontiers in the management of this debilitating disease should therefore address also mental health, emotional well-being, and spiritual dimensions as well as provide occupational and social support.

References

1. Sanguinetti C, Minniti M, Susini V, Caponi L, Panichella G, Castiglione V, Aimo A, Emdin M, Vergaro G, Franzini M. The journey of human transthyretin: synthesis, structure stability, and catabolism. Biomedicines. 2022;10:1906.
2. Carroll A, Dyck PJ, de Carvalho M, Kennerson M, Reilly MM, Kiernan MC, Vucic S. Novel approaches to diagnosis and management of hereditary transthyretin amyloidosis. J Neurol Neurosurg Psychiatry. 2022;93:668–78.
3. Benson MD. Leptomeningeal amyloid and variant transthyretins. Am J Pathol. 1996;148:351–4.
4. Adams D, Koike H, Slama M, Coelho T. Hereditary transthyretin amyloidosis: a model of medical progress for a fatal disease. Nat Rev Neurol. 2019;15:387–404.

5. Sousa A, Coelho T, Barros J, Sequeiros J. Genetic epidemiology of familial amyloidotic polyneuropathy (FAP)-type I in Póvoa do Varzim and Vila do Conde (north of Portugal). Am J Med Genet. 1995;60:512–21.

6. Kato-Motozaki Y, Ono K, Shima K, Morinaga A, Machiya T, Nozaki I, Shibata-Hamaguchi A, Furukawa Y, Yanase D, Ishida C, Sakajiri K, Yamada M. Epidemiology of familial amyloid polyneuropathy in Japan: identification of a novel endemic focus. J Neurol Sci. 2008;270:133–40.

7. Russo M, Obici L, Bartolomei I, Cappelli F, Luigetti M, Fenu S, Cavallaro T, Chiappini MG, Gemelli C, Pradotto LG, Manganelli F, Leonardi L, My F, Sampaolo S, Briani C, Gentile L, Stancanelli C, Di Buduo E, Pacciolla P, Salvi F, Casagrande S, Bisogni G, Calabrese D, Vanoli F, Di Iorio G, Antonini G, Santoro L, Mauro A, Grandis M, Di Girolamo M, Fabrizi GM, Pareyson D, Sabatelli M, Perfetto F, Rapezzi C, Merlini G, Mazzeo A, Vita G. ATTRv amyloidosis Italian Registry: clinical and epidemiological data. Amyloid. 2020;27:259–65.

8. Pinney JH, Smith CJ, Taube JB, Lachmann HJ, Venner CP, Gibbs SD, Dungu J, Banypersad SM, Wechalekar AD, Whelan CJ, Hawkins PN, Gillmore JD. Systemic amyloidosis in England: an epidemiological study. Br J Haematol. 2013;161:525–32.

9. Hemminki K, Li X, Försti A, Sundquist J, Sundquist K. Incidence of hereditary amyloidosis and autoinflammatory diseases in Sweden: endemic and imported diseases. BMC Med Genet. 2013;14:88.

10. Schmidt HH, Waddington-Cruz M, Botteman MF, Carter JA, Chopra AS, Hopps M, Stewart M, Fallet S, Amass L. Estimating the global prevalence of transthyretin familial amyloid polyneuropathy. Muscle Nerve. 2018;57:829–37.

11. Inês M, Coelho T, Conceição I, Duarte-Ramos F, de Carvalho M, Costa J. Epidemiology of transthyretin familial amyloid polyneuropathy in Portugal: a Nationwide study. Neuroepidemiology. 2018;51:177–82.

12. Conceição I, De Carvalho M. Clinical variability in type I familial amyloid polyneuropathy (Val30Met): comparison between late- and early-onset cases in Portugal. Muscle Nerve. 2007;35:116–8.

13. Waddington-Cruz M, Wixner J, Amass L, Kiszko J, Chapman D, Ando Y. Characteristics of patients with late- vs. early-onset Val30Met transthyretin amyloidosis from the Transthyretin Amyloidosis Outcomes Survey (THAOS). Neurol Ther. 2021;10:753–66.

14. Lauppe R, Liseth Hansen J, Fornwall A, Johansson K, Rozenbaum MH, Strand AM, Väkeväinen M, Kuusisto J, Gude E, Smith JG, Gustafsson F. Prevalence, characteristics, and mortality of patients with transthyretin amyloid cardiomyopathy in the Nordic countries. ESC Heart Fail. 2022;9:2528–37.

15. Maurer MS, Hanna M, Grogan M, Dispenzieri A, Witteles R, Drachman B, Judge DP, Lenihan DJ, Gottlieb SS, Shah SJ, Steidley DE, Ventura H, Murali S, Silver MA, Jacoby D, Fedson S, Hummel SL, Kristen AV, Damy T, Planté-Bordeneuve V, Coelho T, Mundayat R, Suhr OB, Waddington Cruz M, Rapezzi C. Genotype and phenotype of transthyretin cardiac amyloidosis: THAOS (Transthyretin Amyloid Outcome Survey). J Am Coll Cardiol. 2016;68:161–72.

16. Gagliardi C, Perfetto F, Lorenzini M, Ferlini A, Salvi F, Milandri A, Quarta CC, Taborchi G, Bartolini S, Frusconi S, Martone R, Cinelli MM, Foffi S, Reggiani MLB, Fabbri G, Cataldo P, Cappelli F, Rapezzi C. Phenotypic profile of Ile68Leu transthyretin amyloidosis: an underdiagnosed cause of heart failure. Eur J Heart Fail. 2018;20:1417–25.

17. Rowczenio DM, Noor I, Gillmore JD, Lachmann HJ, Whelan C, Hawkins PN, Obici L, Westermark P, Grateau G, Wechalekar AD. Online registry for mutations in hereditary amyloidosis including nomenclature recommendations. Hum Mutat. 2014;35:E2403–12.

18. Sekijima Y. Hereditary transthyretin amyloidosis. GeneReviews; 2001.

19. Olsson M, Jonasson J, Cederquist K, Suhr OB. Frequency of the transthyretin Val30Met mutation in the northern Swedish population. Amyloid. 2014;21:18–20.

20. Planté-Bordeneuve V, Carayol J, Ferreira A, Adams D, Clerget-Darpoux F, Misrahi M, Said G, Bonaïti-Pellié C. Genetic study of transthyretin amyloid neuropathies: carrier risks among French and Portuguese families. J Med Genet. 2003;40:e120.

21. Schmidt HH, Barroso F, González-Duarte A, Conceição I, Obici L, Keohane D, Amass L. Management of asymptomatic gene carriers of transthyretin familial amyloid polyneuropathy. Muscle Nerve. 2016;54:353–60.
22. Castaño A, Drachman BM, Judge D, Maurer MS. Natural history and therapy of TTR-cardiac amyloidosis: emerging disease-modifying therapies from organ transplantation to stabilizer and silencer drugs. Heart Fail Rev. 2015;20:163–78.
23. Ton VK, Mukherjee M, Judge DP. Transthyretin cardiac amyloidosis: pathogenesis, treatments, and emerging role in heart failure with preserved ejection fraction. Clin Med Insights Cardiol. 2014;8:39–44.
24. Griffin JM, Rosenblum H, Maurer MS. Pathophysiology and therapeutic approaches to cardiac amyloidosis. Circ Res. 2021;128:1554–75.
25. Sebastião MP, Lamzin V, Saraiva MJ, Damas AM. Transthyretin stability as a key factor in amyloidogenesis: X-ray analysis at atomic resolution. J Mol Biol. 2001;306:733–44.
26. Sekijima Y, Dendle MT, Wiseman RL, White JT, D'Haeze W, Kelly JW. R104H may suppress transthyretin amyloidogenesis by thermodynamic stabilization, but not by the kinetic mechanism characterizing T119 interallelic trans-suppression. Amyloid. 2006;13:57–66.
27. Sant'Anna R, Almeida MR, Varejão N, Gallego P, Esperante S, Ferreira P, Pereira-Henriques A, Palhano FL, de Carvalho M, Foguel D, Reverter D, Saraiva MJ, Ventura S. Cavity filling mutations at the thyroxine-binding site dramatically increase transthyretin stability and prevent its aggregation. Sci Rep. 2017;7:44709.
28. Coelho T, Carvalho MG, Saraiva M, Alves C, Almeida MR, Costa PP. A strikingly benign evolution of FAP in an individual found to be a compound heterozygote for two TTR mutations: TTR MET 30 and TTR MET 119. J Rheumatol. 1993;20:179.
29. Bergström J, Gustavsson A, Hellman U, Sletten K, Murphy CL, Weiss DT, Solomon A, Olofsson BO, Westermark P. Amyloid deposits in transthyretin-derived amyloidosis: cleaved transthyretin is associated with distinct amyloid morphology. J Pathol. 2005;206:224–32.
30. Ihse E, Ybo A, Suhr O, Lindqvist P, Backman C, Westermark P. Amyloid fibril composition is related to the phenotype of hereditary transthyretin V30M amyloidosis. J Pathol. 2008;216:253–61.
31. Marcoux J, Mangione PP, Porcari R, Degiacomi MT, Verona G, Taylor GW, Giorgetti S, Raimondi S, Sanglier-Cianférani S, Benesch JL, Cecconi C, Naqvi MM, Gillmore JD, Hawkins PN, Stoppini M, Robinson CV, Pepys MB, Bellotti V. A novel mechano-enzymatic cleavage mechanism underlies transthyretin amyloidogenesis. EMBO Mol Med. 2015;7:1337–49.
32. Mangione PP, Verona G, Corazza A, Marcoux J, Canetti D, Giorgetti S, Raimondi S, Stoppini M, Esposito M, Relini A, Canale C, Valli M, Marchese L, Faravelli G, Obici L, Hawkins PN, Taylor GW, Gillmore JD, Pepys MB, Bellotti V. Plasminogen activation triggers transthyretin amyloidogenesis in vitro. J Biol Chem. 2018;293:14192–9.
33. Slamova I, Adib R, Ellmerich S, Golos MR, Gilbertson JA, Botcher N, Canetti D, Taylor GW, Rendell N, Tennent GA, Verona G, Porcari R, Mangione PP, Gillmore JD, Pepys MB, Bellotti V, Hawkins PN, Al-Shawi R, Simons JP. Plasmin activity promotes amyloid deposition in a transgenic model of human transthyretin amyloidosis. Nat Commun. 2021;12:7112.
34. Sousa MM, Yan SD, Stern D, Saraiva MJ. Interaction of the receptor for advanced glycation end products (RAGE) with transthyretin triggers nuclear transcription factor kB (NF-kB) activation. Lab Invest. 2000;80:1101–10.
35. Sekijima Y, Wiseman RL, Matteson J, Hammarström P, Miller SR, Sawkar AR, Balch WE, Kelly JW. The biological and chemical basis for tissue-selective amyloid disease. Cell. 2005;121:73–85.
36. Suhr OB, Lundgren E, Westermark P. One mutation, two distinct disease variants: unravelling the impact of transthyretin amyloid fibril composition. J Intern Med. 2017;281:337–47.
37. Shah KB, Inoue Y, Mehra MR. Amyloidosis and the heart: a comprehensive review. Arch Intern Med. 2006;166:1805–13.

38. González-López E, Gagliardi C, Dominguez F, Quarta CC, de Haro-Del Moral FJ, Milandri A, Salas C, Cinelli M, Cobo-Marcos M, Lorenzini M, Lara-Pezzi E, Foffi S, Alonso-Pulpon L, Rapezzi C, Garcia-Pavia P. Clinical characteristics of wild-type transthyretin cardiac amyloidosis: disproving myths. Eur Heart J. 2017;38:1895–904.

39. Ripoll-Vera T, Álvarez Rubio J, Iglesias M, Losada López I, Ferrer-Nadal A, González Moreno J. Association between aortic stenosis and hereditary transthyretin amyloidosis. Revista Esp Cardiol (English ed). 2021;74:185–7.

40. Quarta CC, Buxbaum JN, Shah AM, Falk RH, Claggett B, Kitzman DW, Mosley TH, Butler KR, Boerwinkle E, Solomon SD. The amyloidogenic V122I transthyretin variant in elderly black Americans. N Engl J Med. 2015;372:21–9.

41. Jenne DE, Denzel K, Blätzinger P, Winter P, Obermaier B, Linke RP, Altland K. A new isoleucine substitution of Val-20 in transthyretin tetramers selectively impairs dimer-dimer contacts and causes systemic amyloidosis. Proc Natl Acad Sci U S A. 1996;93:6302–7.

42. Falk RH, Dubrey SW. Amyloid heart disease. Prog Cardiovasc Dis. 2010;52:347–61.

43. Nelson LM, Penninga L, Sander K, Hansen PB, Villadsen GE, Rasmussen A, Gustafsson F. Long-term outcome in patients treated with combined heart and liver transplantation for familial amyloidotic cardiomyopathy. Clin Transpl. 2013;27:203–9.

44. Ranløv I, Alves IL, Ranløv PJ, Husby G, Costa PP, Saraiva MJ. A Danish kindred with familial amyloid cardiomyopathy revisited: identification of a mutant transthyretin-methionine111 variant in serum from patients and carriers. Am J Med. 1992;93:3–8.

45. Sattianayagam PT, Hahn AF, Whelan CJ, Gibbs SD, Pinney JH, Stangou AJ, Rowczenio D, Pflugfelder PW, Fox Z, Lachmann HJ, Wechalekar AD, Hawkins PN, Gillmore JD. Cardiac phenotype and clinical outcome of familial amyloid polyneuropathy associated with transthyretin alanine 60 variant. Eur Heart J. 2012;33:1120–7.

46. Mitchell C, Rahko PS, Blauwet LA, Canaday B, Finstuen JA, Foster MC, Horton K, Ogunyankin KO, Palma RA, Velazquez EJ. Guidelines for performing a comprehensive transthoracic echocardiographic examination in adults: recommendations from the American Society of Echocardiography. J Am Soc Echocardiogr. 2019;32:1–64.

47. Martinez-Naharro A, Treibel TA, Abdel-Gadir A, Bulluck H, Zumbo G, Knight DS, Kotecha T, Francis R, Hutt DF, Rezk T, Rosmini S, Quarta CC, Whelan CJ, Kellman P, Gillmore JD, Moon JC, Hawkins PN, Fontana M. Magnetic resonance in transthyretin cardiac amyloidosis. J Am Coll Cardiol. 2017;70:466–77.

48. Gillmore JD, Maurer MS, Falk RH, Merlini G, Damy T, Dispenzieri A, Wechalekar AD, Berk JL, Quarta CC, Grogan M, Lachmann HJ, Bokhari S, Castano A, Dorbala S, Johnson GB, Glaudemans AW, Rezk T, Fontana M, Palladini G, Milani P, Guidalotti PL, Flatman K, Lane T, Vonberg FW, Whelan CJ, Moon JC, Ruberg FL, Miller EJ, Hutt DF, Hazenberg BP, Rapezzi C, Hawkins PN. Nonbiopsy diagnosis of cardiac transthyretin amyloidosis. Circulation. 2016;133:2404–12.

49. Musumeci MB, Cappelli F, Russo D, Tini G, Canepa M, Milandri A, Bonfiglioli R, Di Bella G, My F, Luigetti M, Grandis M, Autore C, Perlini S, Perfetto F, Rapezzi C. Low sensitivity of bone scintigraphy in detecting Phe64Leu mutation-related transthyretin cardiac amyloidosis. J Am Coll Cardiol Img. 2020;13:1314–21.

50. Garcia-Pavia P, Rapezzi C, Adler Y, Arad M, Basso C, Brucato A, Burazor I, Caforio ALP, Damy T, Eriksson U, Fontana M, Gillmore JD, Gonzalez-Lopez E, Grogan M, Heymans S, Imazio M, Kindermann I, Kristen AV, Maurer MS, Merlini G, Pantazis A, Pankuweit S, Rigopoulos AG, Linhart A. Diagnosis and treatment of cardiac amyloidosis. A position statement of the European Society of Cardiology Working Group on Myocardial and Pericardial Diseases. Eur J Heart Fail. 2021;23:512–26.

51. Luigetti M, Romano A, Di Paolantonio A, Bisogni G, Sabatelli M. Diagnosis and treatment of hereditary transthyretin amyloidosis (hATTR) polyneuropathy: current perspectives on improving patient care. Ther Clin Risk Manag. 2020;16:109–23.

52. Koike H, Ando Y, Ueda M, Kawagashira Y, Iijima M, Fujitake J, Hayashi M, Yamamoto M, Mukai E, Nakamura T, Katsuno M, Hattori N, Sobue G. Distinct characteristics of amyloid

deposits in early- and late-onset transthyretin Val30Met familial amyloid polyneuropathy. J Neurol Sci. 2009;287:178–84.

53. Ando Y, Coelho T, Berk JL, Cruz MW, Ericzon BG, Ikeda S, Lewis WD, Obici L, Planté-Bordeneuve V, Rapezzi C, Said G, Salvi F. Guideline of transthyretin-related hereditary amyloidosis for clinicians. Orphanet J Rare Dis. 2013;8:31.

54. Dyck PJB, González-Duarte A, Obici L, Polydefkis M, Wiesman JF, Antonino I, Litchy WJ, Dyck PJ. Development of measures of polyneuropathy impairment in hATTR amyloidosis: from NIS to mNIS + 7. J Neurol Sci. 2019;405:116424.

55. Leonardi L, Adam C, Beaudonnet G, Beauvais D, Cauquil C, Not A, Morassi O, Benmalek A, Trassard O, Echaniz-Laguna A, Adams D, Labeyrie C. Skin amyloid deposits and nerve fiber loss as markers of neuropathy onset and progression in hereditary transthyretin amyloidosis. Eur J Neurol. 2022;29:1477–87.

56. Maia LF, Maceski A, Conceição I, Obici L, Magalhães R, Cortese A, Leppert D, Merlini G, Kuhle J, Saraiva MJ. Plasma neurofilament light chain: an early biomarker for hereditary ATTR amyloid polyneuropathy. Amyloid. 2020;27:97–102.

57. Ticau S, Sridharan GV, Tsour S, Cantley WL, Chan A, Gilbert JA, Erbe D, Aldinc E, Reilly MM, Adams D, Polydefkis M, Fitzgerald K, Vaishnaw A, Nioi P. Neurofilament light chain as a biomarker of hereditary transthyretin-mediated amyloidosis. Neurology. 2021;96:e412–22.

58. Salvalaggio A, Coraci D, Obici L, Cacciavillani M, Luigetti M, Mazzeo A, Pastorelli F, Grandis M, Cavallaro T, Bisogni G, Lozza A, Gemelli C, Gentile L, Russo M, Ermani M, Fabrizi GM, Plasmati R, De Napoli F, Campagnolo M, Castellani F, Salvi F, Fenu S, Devigili G, Pareyson D, Gasparotti R, Rapezzi C, Martinoli C, Padua L, Briani C. Progressive brachial plexus enlargement in hereditary transthyretin amyloidosis. J Neurol. 2022;269:1905–12.

59. Gasparotti R, Salvalaggio A, Corbo D, Agazzi G, Cacciavillani M, Lozza A, Fenu S, De Vigili G, Tagliapietra M, Fabrizi GM, Pareyson D, Obici L, Briani C. Magnetic resonance neurography and diffusion tensor imaging of the sciatic nerve in hereditary transthyretin amyloidosis polyneuropathy. J Neurol. 2023;270:4827.

60. Vegezzi E, Cortese A, Bergsland N, Mussinelli R, Paoletti M, Solazzo F, Currò R, Ascagni L, Callegari I, Quartesan I, Lozza A, Deligianni X, Santini F, Marchioni E, Cosentino G, Alfonsi E, Tassorelli C, Bastianello S, Merlini G, Palladini G, Obici L, Pichiecchio A. Muscle quantitative MRI as a novel biomarker in hereditary transthyretin amyloidosis with polyneuropathy: a cross-sectional study. J Neurol. 2023;270:328–39.

61. Karam C, Dimitrova D, Christ M, Heitner SB. Carpal tunnel syndrome and associated symptoms as first manifestation of hATTR amyloidosis. Neurol Clin Pract. 2019;9:309–13.

62. Ando E, Ando Y, Okamura R, Uchino M, Ando M, Negi A. Ocular manifestations of familial amyloidotic polyneuropathy type I: long-term follow up. Br J Ophthalmol. 1997;81:295–8.

63. Ferraro PM, D'Ambrosio V, Di Paolantonio A, Guglielmino V, Calabresi P, Sabatelli M, Luigetti M. Renal involvement in hereditary transthyretin amyloidosis: an Italian single-Centre experience. Brain Sci. 2021;11:980.

64. Lobato L, Rocha A. Transthyretin amyloidosis and the kidney. Clin J Am Soc Nephrol. 2012;7:1337–46.

65. Qin Q, Wei C, Piao Y, Lian F, Wu H, Zhou A, Wang F, Zuo X, Han Y, Lyu J, Guo D, Jia J. Current review of leptomeningeal amyloidosis associated with transthyretin mutations. Neurologist. 2021;26:189–95.

66. Inês M, Coelho T, Conceição I, Ferreira L, de Carvalho M, Costa J. Health-related quality of life in hereditary transthyretin amyloidosis polyneuropathy: a prospective, observational study. Orphanet J Rare Dis. 2020;15:67.

67. Conceição I, Coelho T, Rapezzi C, Parman Y, Obici L, Galán L, Rousseau A. Assessment of patients with hereditary transthyretin amyloidosis—understanding the impact of management and disease progression. Amyloid. 2019;26:103–11.

68. Mejia Baranda J, Ljungberg J, Wixner J, Anan I, Oskarsson V. Epidemiology of hereditary transthyretin amyloidosis in the northernmost region of Sweden: a retrospective cohort study. Amyloid. 2022;29:120–7.

Federico Perfetto, Francesco Cappelli, Giorgia Panichella,
Alessia Argirò, and Mathew S. Maurer

Abbreviations

AF	Atrial fibrillation
AL	Amyloid light chain amyloidosis
AS	Aortic stenosis
ATTR	Amyloid transthyretin amyloidosis
ATTR-ACT	Tafamidis in Transthyretin Cardiomyopathy Clinical *Trial*
BBTR	Brachial biceps tendon rupture
CA	Cardiac amyloidosis
CTS	Carpal tunnel syndrome
HF	Heart failure
LSS	Lumbar spinal stenosis
PM	Pacemaker
TR	Trigger release

F. Perfetto (✉) · G. Panichella
Tuscan Regional Amyloidosis Centre, Careggi University Hospital, Florence, Italy

Department of Experimental and Clinical Medicine, Careggi University Hospital,
Florence, Italy
e-mail: federico.perfetto@unifi.it; giorgia.panichella@unifi.it

F. Cappelli · A. Argirò
Tuscan Regional Amyloidosis Centre, Careggi University Hospital, Florence, Italy
e-mail: f.cappelli@unifi.it; alessia.argiro@unifi.it

M. S. Maurer
Columbia University Irving Medical Center, New York, NY, USA
e-mail: msm10@cumc.columbia.edu

© The Author(s), under exclusive license to Springer Nature
Switzerland AG 2024
M. Emdin et al. (eds.), *Cardiac Amyloidosis*,
https://doi.org/10.1007/978-3-031-51757-0_7

7.1   Definition and Epidemiology

Transthyretin amyloidosis (ATTR amyloidosis) is a systemic disease characterized by the extracellular deposition of amyloid fibrils composed of misfolded transthyretin (TTR) [1]. There are two distinct types of ATTR amyloidosis: hereditary (mutated or variant, ATTRv) and wild type (ATTRwt, previously referred to as senile cardiac amyloidosis [SCA]). In ATTRv, an amyloidogenic variant in the *TTR* gene facilitates the dissociation of its tetramer into monomers and promotes subsequent misfolding, whereas in ATTRwt amyloidosis, the non-variant, wild-type TTR can cause amyloid formation in the presence of favorable conditions, such as aging and oxidative stress [2]. Accumulation of wild-type TTR amyloid fibrils leads to a progressive systemic disease with principal clinical manifestations involving the heart and producing arrhythmia, syncope, heart failure (HF), and ultimately death if not treated. The exact prevalence and incidence of ATTRwt amyloidosis are currently unknown. Historically, amyloidosis has been considered a rare disease, but recent evidence suggests that ATTRwt is probably more common than previously thought, especially in elderly patients with HF. This is related to the recent growing awareness of amyloidosis and especially thanks to the introduction of a bone scintigraphy-based algorithm for non-invasive diagnosis of ATTR amyloidosis and to the approval of effective disease-modifying therapies for the disease [3–6]. Data obtained from the United Kingdom National Amyloidosis Centre database on 11,000 patients who received a diagnosis of amyloidosis during the last 30 years showed that light chain (AL) amyloidosis remained the most common type, accounting for 55% of all cases, while ATTRwt amyloidosis accounted for 13% of all cases [7]. However, the incidence of ATTRwt amyloidosis is growing rapidly, from less than 3% of all cases in the period 1987–2009 to 14% in the period 2010–2015 and to 25% in the past 4 years [7]. The prevalence of ATTRwt amyloidosis increases with age and most patients are over the age of 70, although diagnoses younger than 60 are not uncommon [8]. In ATTRwt amyloidosis, the male to female ratio is about 8:1, and males also display an earlier age of onset of the disease [8, 9].

A recent systematic review has addressed the need to evaluate CA prevalence in specific settings [10]. For example, 1–3% of women and men over 75 years of age have demonstrable uptake on DPD bone scintigraphy, indicating ATTR-CA [11]. Moreover, ATTR amyloidosis is detected in approximately 12% of patients with HF with preserved ejection fraction (HFpEF) and 8% of sever aortic stenosis referred to surgery [10, 12].

TTR amyloid deposition in flexor tenosynovium and transverse ligament during carpal tunnel syndrome (CTS) represents an established red flag for ATTR amyloidosis. A study retrospectively evaluating the prevalence of CA among 233 patients who underwent CTS surgery found out that ATTRwt amyloidosis was present in 0.8% (2/233) cases, which rose to 9.1% (2/22) among patients with bilateral CTS and left ventricular hypertrophy (LVH) on echocardiogram, when known occupational risks were excluded [13]. Finally, in a *post-mortem* study on 56 unselected patients aged more than 75 years, CA was found in 43% (50% AL amyloidosis, 50% ATTR amyloidosis) of the autopsied hearts [14].

7.2   Pathophysiology

7.2.1   Transthyretin

TTR, also known as prealbumin due to its electrophoretic properties, is a 55 kDa homotetrameric protein composed of four monomeric subunits of 127 amino acids each [15]. It is encoded by a 7 kb gene located at chromosome 18q11.2–q12.1, composed of four exon and three introns [16]. The protein is mainly produced by the liver and to a less extent in choroid plexus and by the retinal epithelium, then secreted into the bloodstream, cerebrospinal fluid, and the ocular chamber. Some production of TTR by pancreatic islet α-cells and Schwann cells has also been reported [17]. TTR serves as a transporter of thyroid hormone T4 and retinol-binding protein 4 (RBP4) bound to retinol (vitamin A), hence its name (TRANSporter of THYroxine and RETINol) [18]. TTR is the second major T4 transporter in the blood, following thyroxine-binding globulin (TBG). However, less than 1% of plasma circulating TTR is normally involved in T4 transport [17].

The X-ray crystal structure of human TTR was determined by Colin Blake in 1971. TTR displays an unusually β-strand rich secondary structure, which makes it highly amyloidogenic. Each TTR monomer consists of eight β-strands, identified by the letters A to H, and one short α-helix of nine residues included between strands E and F (Fig. 7.1) [17]. Interstrand hydrogen bonds allow the organization of a tertiary structure of β-strands constituted by an inner (strands DAGH) and an outer (strands CBEF) β-sheet, which are orthogonal to one another [17, 19]. The monomers of TTR they interact with each other to form a dimer thanks to the hydrogen bonds that are formed between two F (F, F′) and two H (H, H′) strands from adjacent monomers. The quaternary structure of TTR is characterized by the presence of four identical monomeric subunits (A, B, C, and D) which associate with each other to generate two hydrophobic pockets which serve as binding sites for thyroxine (T4) [20]. The tetramer of TTR has two dimeric interfaces: one interface is located between the subunits A–C and B–D, supported by an extensive network of hydrogen bonds involving the β F and H strands, while the other interface is located between the subunits A–B and C–D, stabilized by multiple hydrophobic interactions [21].

The binding of a T4 molecule stabilizes the native TTR tetramer. One of the current therapeutic strategies for ATTR amyloidosis involves enhancing the kinetic stability of the native TTR tetramers by small molecules able to bind the T4 pocket (i.e., tafamidis), thus preventing the early stage of TTR dissociation [22].

7.2.2   The TTR Amyloid Cascade

ATTRwt amyloidosis is caused by the deposition of misfolded TTR in the cardiac extracellular space. The conversion of native TTR tetramer into insoluble amyloid fibrils is a dynamic, largely unknown, multi-step process [23]. Initially, the TTR tetramer becomes unstable and dissociates into dimers and monomers, acquiring a

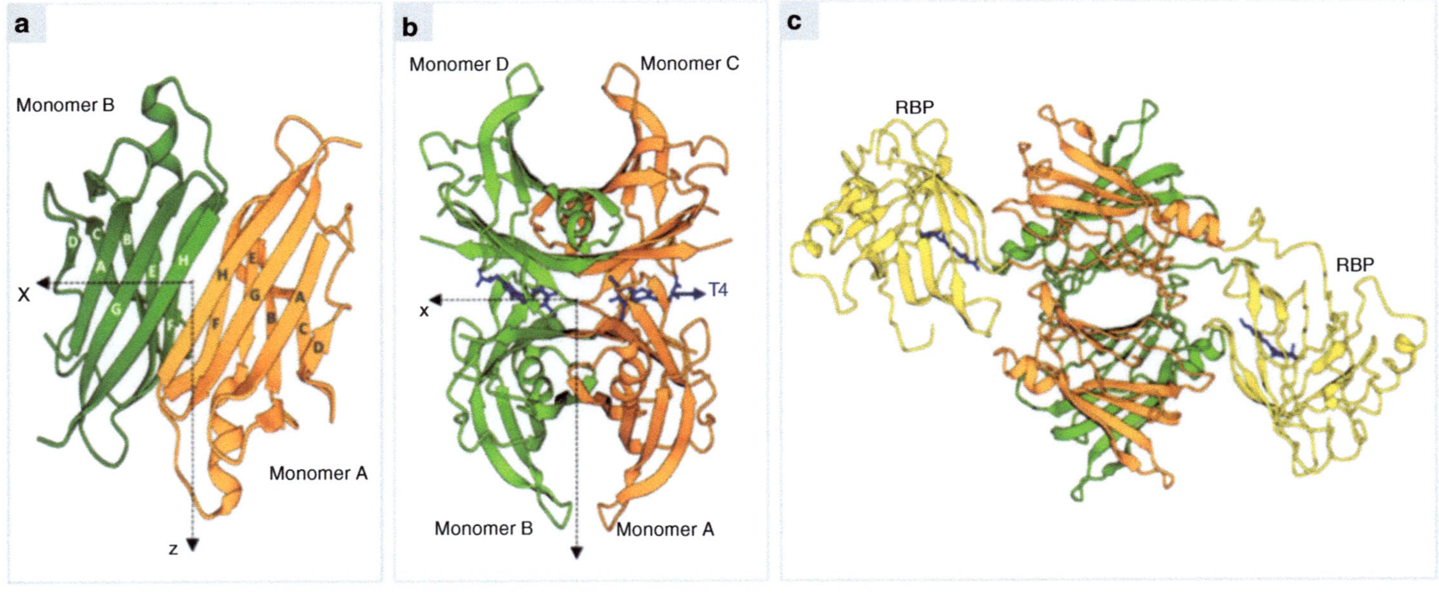

Fig. 7.1 Transthyretin (TTR) structure. (**a**) TTR dimer is composed of two monomers (A and B). Each monomer is composed of eight β-strands, identified by the letters A to H. (**b**) TTR tetramer. The *X*-axis passes through the thyroid hormone T4 (T4) binding channels, which are formed at the interface of monomers D–B and C–A. T4 is represented in blue. (**c**) Structure of TTR–retinol binding protein (RBP) complex. Retinol is represented in blue. (Figure modified with permission from Sanguinetti et al. [17])

partially misfolded conformation and self-assembling into soluble oligomeric aggregates and, subsequently, into protofibrils and insoluble fibrils which accumulate in the form of amyloid deposits in the extracellular matrix (ECM) of different tissue, including the heart and peripheral nervous system (PNS) [23].

The dissociation of the TTR tetramer into monomers represents the initial, as well as the rate-limiting step of the entire process [24]. The mechanisms underlying the misfolding in ATTRwt amyloidosis are not fully understood, although deficits in proteostasis, environmental factors, aging, and proteolysis-induced fragmentation of TTR seem to play a key role [24]. The residue 49–127 C-terminal fragment is a major component of ex vivo TTR amyloid fibrils [25], regardless of the presence of any amyloidogenic mutation [26]. Several studies suggest that a proteolytic cleavage of TTR could be enhanced by increased mechanical forces such as shear stress, that occur in vivo into the heart and/or at the weight-bearing joints, or into tenosynovial tissues subjected to heavy gravitational loading combined with continuous repetitive vigorous movement, such as carpal tunnel o lumbar spine [27–29].

Amyloidogenesis is generally considered to be a nucleation-dependent process, in which the growth of fibrils requires the formation of a high-energy quaternary structure before the addition of an additional monomer becomes energetically favorable; however, once the limiting step has been passed, the addition of subsequent monomers proceeds energetically favorably (Fig. 7.2) [30].

Several steps forward have been made in defining the structural characteristics of amyloid fibrils. Amyloid fibrils originating from TTR show two different morphologies, named as type A and type B [31]. Type A amyloid substance contains fragmented ATTR monomers as well as full-length monomers, which form short, closely related and spatially disoriented fibers; this type of fibrils is usually present in ATTRwt patients; on the contrary, type B amyloid substance is composed of non-fragmented TTR, which makes relatively long fibrils arranged in parallel bundles [31]. The type of ATTR fibril deposited also seems segregate with the degree of cardiac uptake on bone scintigraphy and Congo red affinity. Type A fibrils display low affinity for Congo red staining and high ^{99m}Tc-DPD uptake at scintigraphy, whereas type B fibrils show high Congo red affinity and low or absent radiotracer heart retention at bone scan [32].

At present, the association between the different types of amyloid and the different types of ATTR amyloidosis variants is unknown. Nonetheless, all organs of a patient with ATTR amyloidosis exhibit type A or B deposits, and the amyloid type remains unchanged over time [31].

Historically, it was assumed that the mere accumulation of amyloid fibrils in tissues was at the basis of TTR amyloid toxicity. Such fibrils in fact induce direct tissue damage linked to the compressive effect and vascular damage [30]. However, recent studies indicate that monomers, low-molecular weight oligomers, and protofibrils are equally toxic species [33, 34]. Furthermore, aging-induced oxidation of TTR would appear to increase its cytotoxicity [35]. This might, in part, explain the increased incidence of ATTR amyloidosis with age, especially for the wild form type.

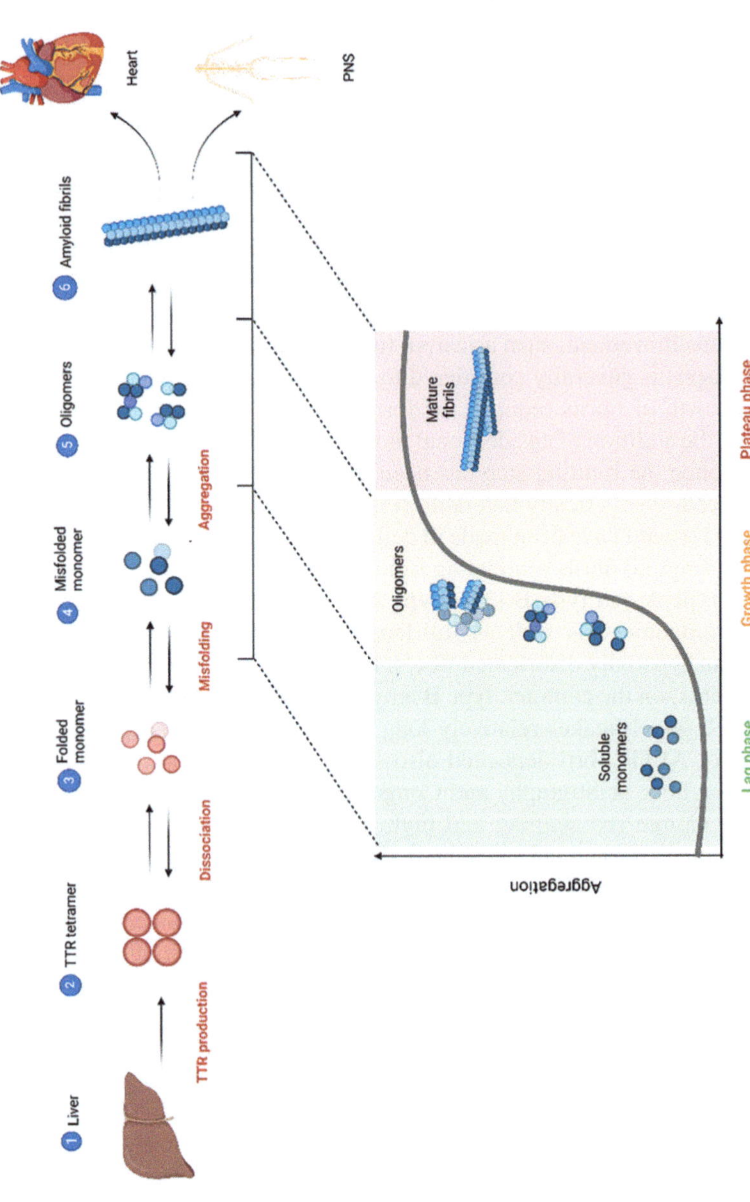

Fig. 7.2 Pathophysiology of transthyretin (TTR) amyloidosis. Initially, the TTR tetramer produced by the liver may become unstable and dissociate into monomers, further acquiring a partially misfolded conformation and self-assembling into soluble oligomeric aggregates and, subsequently, into insoluble fibrils which accumulate in the form of amyloid deposits in different organs. The amyloid formation follows a sigmoid kinetic. During the lag phase, monomers undergo conformational changes and bond with each other to form an oligomeric nucleus. The transition to the growth phase is determined by the accumulation of oligomeric nuclei, which serve as seeds for the formation of protofibrils and mature fibrils. *PNS* peripheral nervous system, *TTR* transthyretin

7.3   Clinical Manifestations

7.3.1   Cardiac Manifestations

Amyloid fibrils can infiltrate every cardiac structure, including atrial and ventricular myocardium, the conduction system, valves and vessels (Fig. 7.3). In this paragraph we will discuss the most common cardiac complications in ATTRwt amyloidosis.

7.3.1.1 Heart Failure

Ventricular infiltration leads to chambers' progressive thickening and development of a pseudo-hypertrophic phenotype. Thus, ventricular stiffening and diastolic dysfunction are one of the first manifestations of the disease and the severity of diastolic dysfunction increases with left ventricular mass [36, 37]. Diastolic dysfunction and limited chamber's capacity may cause a reduction in stroke volume and consequent exercise intolerance, determining the development of heart failure with preserved ejection fraction. Progressively, amyloid deposition may cause right ventricular dysfunction that may present with orthopnea, bendopnea, elevated jugular venous pressure, peripheral edema, hepatomegaly, and ascites. Eventually, left ventricular ejection fraction may progressively decline, with resulting heart failure

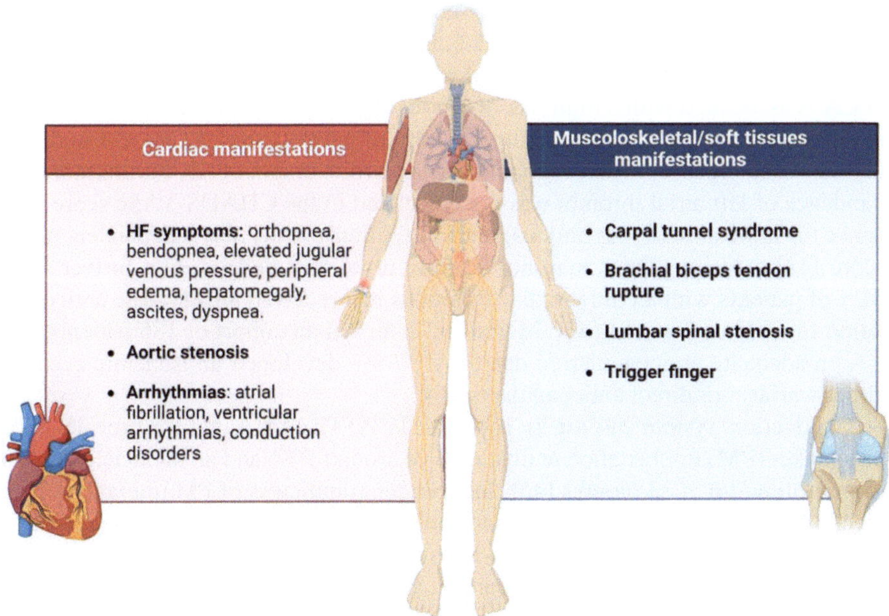

Fig. 7.3 Clinical manifestations of wild-type transthyretin (ATTRwt) amyloidosis. ATTRwt amyloidosis typically affects elderly men. Patients present more frequently with symptoms related to the involvement of the cardiovascular system and/or musculoskeletal or soft tissues. *HF* heart failure

with reduced ejection fraction and systemic hypoperfusion in late stages of the disease [37]. The treatment of heart failure in CA needs to be individualized and will be discussed in Chap. 20.

7.3.1.2 Aortic Stenosis

ATTR-CA has a prevalence that ranges from 13% to 16% among candidates for transcatheter aortic valve replacement (AVR) with significant aortic stenosis (AS) [38]. The pathophysiology of AS in ATTR-CA is complex and still not completely understood. Probably, the age-related aortic calcifications create an environment of elevated shear stress favoring amyloid deposition following the mechano-enzymatic hypothesis [29]. Amyloid deposition in turn may increase valve stiffening and worsen the valvulopathy severity. The co-existence of AS and ATTR-CA compared to lone AS is characterized by a more frequent low-flow, low-gradient pattern, greater concentric hypertrophy, worse left ventricular systolic function, more severe diastolic dysfunction, and more blunted right ventricular function [38]. Transcatheter aortic valve replacement is capable of improving outcome compared to medical management in ATTR-CA with AS and is preferable to surgical AVR in ATTR-CA patients, and after a median follow-up of 2 years, mortality is similar between patients with and without ATTR-CA who underwent transcatheter AVR [39].

7.3.1.3 Arrhythmias

Atrial fibrillation (AF) is the most common sustained arrhythmia in ATTR-CA and has been reported in 40%, 9%, and 11%, respectively in ATTRwt, AL, and ATTRv CA. AF in ATTR-CA is not associated with a reduced survival [40]. However, AF in CA is associated with a high risk of intracardiac thrombi and stroke. A thrombus in left atrial appendage was identified in 30% of patients with ATTR-CA undergoing transesophageal echocardiography before cardioversion of AF. Furthermore, the incidence of left atrial thrombi was not correlated to the CHADS-VASc score [41], hence the indication to start anticoagulants in patients with AF is independent of this score [42]. Anticoagulants may not be fully protective, indeed, in a further study 31% of patients with an intracardiac thrombus had received an adequate anticoagulation for at least 3 weeks [43]. Moreover, in an Italian cohort of 186 patients with CA on adequate anticoagulation due to AF, 7.6% developed an ischemic event on either warfarin or direct anticoagulants [44].

Conduction system disease is common in ATTRwt-CA with a prevalence of pacemaker (PM) implantation at diagnosis of around 30% and an incidence of 8.9% over a follow-up of 33 months [45]. Independent predictors of PM implantation are signs of a more advanced disease and include a history of AF, first degree atrioventricular block, and a wide QRS (>120 ms) [14].

Non-sustained ventricular tachycardias are common in ATTR-CA being identified in about 65% of patients during hospital monitoring [46] and are associated with advanced stages of the disease [47].

7.3.2 Extracardiac Manifestations

ATTRwt-CA is also characterized by amyloid deposition in musculoskeletal soft tissues [48]. The musculoskeletal involvement may precede cardiac symptoms and serve as a diagnostic red flag [42]. Musculoskeletal involvement include:

- **Carpal tunnel syndrome (CTS)**: CTS may be found in about half of patients with ATTR-CA and may precede the disease onset from 5 to 15 years [49]. CTS is caused by amyloid deposition in the tenosynovial tissues of the carpal tunnel, leading to median nerve compression and typical symptoms like pain, numbness, and tingling in the first three hand fingers and the radial side of the ring finger [48]. CTS is particularly suspect for CA when found in an elderly male without professional risk factors for this condition, being unilateral CTS associated with a 12-fold increased risk of ATTRwt-CA, that rises to 31-fold when bilateral [50]. Among 98 men aged $\geq$50 and women $\geq$60 years who underwent carpal tunnel release surgery, 10% had a positive biopsy for amyloid and four had a definitive amyloidosis diagnosis (two ATTRv, one AL, one ATTRwt) [51]. Among 67 patients referred for CTS surgery aged $\geq$60 years with at least one red flag for CA (elevated cardiac biomarkers, left ventricular hypertrophy, apical sparing) that underwent bone scintigraphy, 10 (8.3%) have been eventually diagnosed with early ATTRwt-CA [52].
- **Brachial biceps tendon rupture (BBTR)**: BBTR is very uncommon in the general population, while it is often encountered in ATTRwt-CA representing a further pivotal extra cardiac red flag [42]. Out of 111 patients with ATTRwt-CA, 33% had BBTR, in 95% of cases involved the dominant limb and was bilateral in 24% [53]. BBTR usually occurs spontaneously or after light exertion, patients are often unaware of the injury, that can be easily identified on physical examination [54]. In fact, biceps contraction against a resistance may trigger the bulging of the muscle belly after the rupture of the tendon defining the "Popeye sign" (Fig. 7.4) [53].
- **Lumbar spinal stenosis (LSS)**: LSS is due to amyloid deposition in the ligamentum flavum [55] leading to lower extremity aching, weakness, and paresthesia. Among 324 patients referred for surgery for symptomatic LSS, 13% ($n = 43$) had ATTRwt deposits. Thirty-seven of them underwent bone scintigraphy and 4 had intense myocardial uptake (Perugini 2 or 3), while 33 had no or slight positivity and underwent clinical follow-up to identify early signs of CA.
- **Hip, shoulder, and knee osteoarthritis**: Hip and knee arthroplasty are common among patients with ATTRwt. In particular, total hip and knee arthroplasties have been performed in 23% of patients with ATTR and 9% of patients with AL, furthermore lower extremity arthroplasty was about four times more common in ATTR-CA compared to the general population. On average, arthroplasty occurred 7 years before ATTR-CA diagnosis [56, 57].

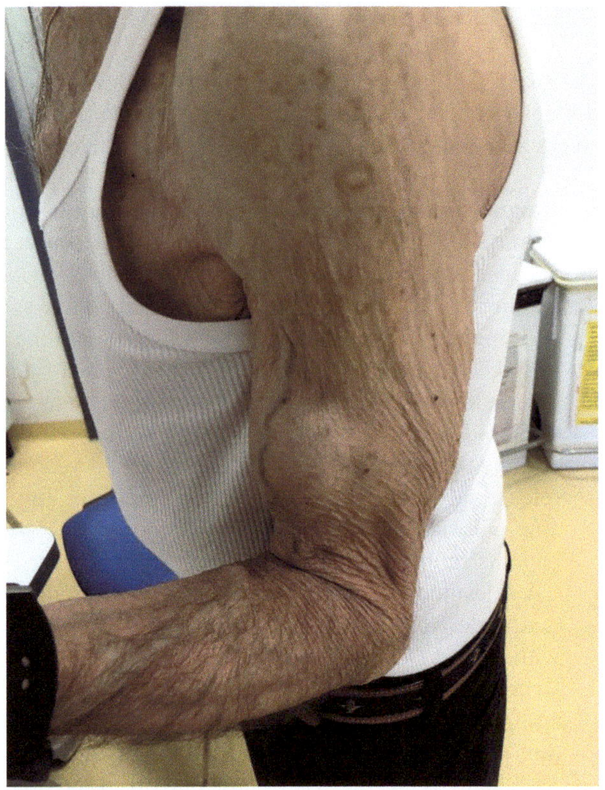

Fig. 7.4 Brachial biceps tendon rupture evident as the "Popeye sign" during bicep's contraction. (The picture is reproduced from Perfetto et al. [48] published under creative commons CC-BY license)

- **Trigger finger**: In this condition, one or more fingers are locked in a bent or straightened position due to thickening of the flexor tendons. In a recent study, patients who underwent digit-trigger release (TR) and/or CTS release showed a higher risk of amyloidosis with an adjusted hazard ratio of 4.8 (95% CI: 7.74–13.6) for lone TR and 15 (95% CI: 9.87–22) for TR and CTS release [58]. Independent risk predictor for amyloidosis included: age, black race, prior CTS release, heart failure, and the number of digits released [58].
- **Rotator cuff disease**: Beside the shoulder pad sign, a progressive shoulder enlargement pathognomonic for AL amyloidosis, thickening of the tendons of the rotator cuff is common also in ATTR amyloidosis. Sonographic findings of amyloid deposition include: thickening of the supraspinatus tendon, thickening of the synovial sheath around the long head of the biceps tendon, and the thickening of the subdeltoid bursa [59]. Data on the prevalence of ATTR amyloidosis in patients with rotator cuff disease are still lacking, the only study addressing this issue showed that among 21 samples of rotator cuff tears, 5 (24%) was ATTR-positive [60].

References

1. Ando Y, Coelho T, Berk JL, Cruz MW, Ericzon B-G, Ikeda S-i, et al. Guideline of transthyretin-related hereditary amyloidosis for clinicians. Orphanet J Rare Dis. 2013;8:31.
2. Obi CA, Mostertz WC, Griffin JM, Judge DP. ATTR epidemiology, genetics, and prognostic factors. Methodist Debakey Cardiovasc J. 2022;18:17–26.
3. Gillmore JD, Maurer MS, Falk RH, Merlini G, Damy T, Dispenzieri A, et al. Nonbiopsy diagnosis of cardiac transthyretin amyloidosis. Circulation. 2016;133:2404–12.
4. Maurer MS, Schwartz JH, Gundapaneni B, Elliott PM, Merlini G, Waddington-Cruz M, et al. Tafamidis treatment for patients with transthyretin amyloid cardiomyopathy. N Engl J Med. 2018;379:1007–16.
5. Adams D, Gonzalez-Duarte A, O'Riordan WD, Yang C-C, Ueda M, Kristen AV, et al. Patisiran, an RNAi therapeutic, for hereditary transthyretin amyloidosis. N Engl J Med. 2018;379:11–21.
6. Benson MD, Waddington-Cruz M, Berk JL, Polydefkis M, Dyck PJ, Wang AK, et al. Inotersen treatment for patients with hereditary transthyretin amyloidosis. N Engl J Med. 2018;379:22–31.
7. Ravichandran S, Lachmann HJ, Wechalekar AD. Epidemiologic and survival trends in amyloidosis, 1987–2019. N Engl J Med. 2020;382:1567–8.
8. Maurer MS, Hanna M, Grogan M, Dispenzieri A, Witteles R, Drachman B, et al. Genotype and phenotype of transthyretin cardiac amyloidosis: THAOS (Transthyretin Amyloid Outcome Survey). J Am Coll Cardiol. 2016;68:161–72.
9. González-López E, Gagliardi C, Dominguez F, Quarta CC, de Haro-Del Moral FJ, et al. Clinical characteristics of wild-type transthyretin cardiac amyloidosis: disproving myths. Eur Heart J. 2017;38:1895–904.
10. Aimo A, Merlo M, Porcari A, Georgiopoulos G, Pagura L, Vergaro G, et al. Redefining the epidemiology of cardiac amyloidosis. A systematic review and meta-analysis of screening studies. Eur J Heart Fail. 2022;24:2342–51.
11. Longhi S, Guidalotti PL, Quarta CC, Gagliardi C, Milandri A, Lorenzini M, et al. Identification of TTR-related subclinical amyloidosis with 99mTc-DPD scintigraphy. JACC Cardiovasc Imaging. 2014;7:531–2.
12. AbouEzzeddine OF, Davies DR, Scott CG, Fayyaz AU, Askew JW, McKie PM, et al. Prevalence of transthyretin amyloid cardiomyopathy in heart failure with preserved ejection fraction. JAMA Cardiol. 2021;6:1267–74.
13. Zegri-Reiriz I, de Haro-del Moral FJ, Dominguez F, Salas C, de la Cuadra P, et al. Prevalence of cardiac amyloidosis in patients with carpal tunnel syndrome. J Cardiovasc Transl Res. 2019;12:507–13.
14. Porcari A, Bussani R, Merlo M, Varrà GG, Pagura L, Rozze D, et al. Incidence and characterization of concealed cardiac amyloidosis among unselected elderly patients undergoing postmortem examination. Front Cardiovasc Med. 2021;8:749523.
15. Kanda Y, Goodman DS, Canfield RE, Morgan FJ. The amino acid sequence of human plasma prealbumin. J Biol Chem. 1974;249:6796–805.
16. Tsuzuki T, Mita S, Maeda S, Araki S, Shimada K. Structure of the human prealbumin gene. J Biol Chem. 1985;260:12224–7.
17. Sanguinetti C, Minniti M, Susini V, Caponi L, Panichella G, Castiglione V, et al. The journey of human transthyretin: synthesis, structure stability, and catabolism. Biomedicine. 2022;10:1906.
18. Ingbar SH. Observations concerning the binding of thyroid hormones by human serum prealbumin. J Clin Invest. 1963;42:143–60.
19. He S, He X, Liu L, Zhang W, Yu L, Deng Z, et al. The structural understanding of transthyretin misfolding and the inspired drug approaches for the treatment of heart failure associated with transthyretin amyloidosis. Front Pharmacol. 2021;12:628184.

20. Kelly JW, Colon W, Lai Z, Lashuel HA, McCulloch J, McCutchen SL, et al. Transthyretin quaternary and tertiary structural changes facilitate misassembly into amyloid. Adv Prot Chem. 1997;50:161–81.
21. Wojtczak A, Cody V, Luft JR, Pangborn W. Structures of human transthyretin complexed with thyroxine at 2.0 A resolution and 3′,5′-dinitro-N-acetyl-L-thyronine at 2.2 A resolution. Acta Crystallogr. 1996;52:758–65.
22. Johnson SM, Connelly S, Fearns C, Powers ET, Kelly JW. The transthyretin amyloidoses: from delineating the molecular mechanism of aggregation linked to pathology to a regulatory-agency-approved drug. J Mol Biol. 2012;421:185–203.
23. Bezerra F, Saraiva MJ, Almeida MR. Modulation of the mechanisms driving transthyretin amyloidosis. Front Mol Neurosci. 2020;13:592644.
24. Ruberg FL, Grogan M, Hanna M, Kelly JW, Maurer MS. Transthyretin amyloid cardiomyopathy: JACC state-of-the-art review. J Am Coll Cardiol. 2019;73:2872–91.
25. Ihse E, Rapezzi C, Merlini G, Benson MD, Ando Y, Suhr OB, et al. Amyloid fibrils containing fragmented ATTR may be the standard fibril composition in ATTR amyloidosis. Amyloid. 2013;20:142–50.
26. Bergström J, Gustavsson A, Hellman U, Sletten K, Murphy CL, Weiss DT, et al. Amyloid deposits in transthyretin-derived amyloidosis: cleaved transthyretin is associated with distinct amyloid morphology. J Pathol. 2005;206:224–32.
27. Mangione PP, Porcari R, Gillmore JD, Pucci P, Monti M, Porcari M, et al. Proteolytic cleavage of Ser52Pro variant transthyretin triggers its amyloid fibrillogenesis. Proc Natl Acad Sci U S A. 2014;111:1539–44.
28. Marcoux J, Mangione PP, Porcari R, Degiacomi MT, Verona G, Taylor GW, et al. A novel mechano-enzymatic cleavage mechanism underlies transthyretin amyloidogenesis. EMBO Mol Med. 2015;7:1337–49.
29. Mangione PP, Verona G, Corazza A, Marcoux J, Canetti D, Giorgetti S, et al. Plasminogen activation triggers transthyretin amyloidogenesis in vitro. J Biol Chem. 2018;293:14192–9.
30. Sekijima Y. Transthyretin (ATTR) amyloidosis: clinical spectrum, molecular pathogenesis and disease-modifying treatments. J Neurol Neurosurg Psychiatry. 2015;86:1036–43.
31. Suhr OB, Lundgren E, Westermark P. One mutation, two distinct disease variants: unravelling the impact of transthyretin amyloid fibril composition. J Intern Med. 2017;281:337–47.
32. Suhr OB, Wixner J, Anan I, Lundgren HE, Wijayatunga P, Westermark P, Ihse E. Amyloid fibril composition within hereditary Val30Met (p. Val50Met) transthyretin amyloidosis families. PLoS One. 2019;14:e0211983.
33. Monteiro FA, Sousa MM, Cardoso I, do Amaral JB, Guimarães A, Saraiva MJ. Activation of ERK1/2 MAP kinases in familial amyloidotic polyneuropathy. J Neurochem. 2006;97:151–61.
34. Dasari AKR, Hughes RM, Wi S, Hung I, Gan Z, Kelly JW, et al. Transthyretin aggregation pathway toward the formation of distinct cytotoxic oligomers. Sci Rep. 2019;9:33.
35. Zhao L, Buxbaum JN, Reixach N. Age-related oxidative modifications of transthyretin modulate its amyloidogenicity. Biochemistry. 2013;52:1913–26.
36. Oghina S, Bougouin W, Kharoubi M, Bonnefous L, Galat A, Guendouz S, et al. Echocardiographic patterns of left ventricular diastolic function in cardiac amyloidosis: an updated evaluation. J Clin Med. 2021;10:4888.
37. Knight DS, Zumbo G, Barcella W, Steeden JA, Muthurangu V, Martinez-Naharro A, et al. Cardiac structural and functional consequences of amyloid deposition by cardiac magnetic resonance and echocardiography and their prognostic roles. JACC Cardiovasc Imaging. 2019;12:823–33.
38. Nitsche C, Scully PR, Patel KP, Kammerlander AA, Koschutnik M, Dona C, et al. Prevalence and outcomes of concomitant aortic stenosis and cardiac amyloidosis. J Am Coll Cardiol. 2021;77:128–39.

39. Rosenblum H, Masri A, Narotsky DL, Goldsmith J, Hamid N, Hahn RT, et al. Unveiling outcomes in coexisting severe aortic stenosis and transthyretin cardiac amyloidosis. Eur J Heart Fail. 2021;23:250–8.
40. Longhi S, Quarta CC, Milandri A, Lorenzini M, Gagliardi C, Manuzzi L, et al. Atrial fibrillation in amyloidotic cardiomyopathy: prevalence, incidence, risk factors and prognostic role. Amyloid. 2015;22:147–55.
41. Donnellan E, Elshazly MB, Vakamudi S, Wazni OM, Cohen JA, Kanj M, et al. No association between CHADS-VASc score and left atrial appendage thrombus in patients with transthyretin amyloidosis. JACC Clin Electrophysiol. 2019;5:1473–4.
42. Garcia-Pavia P, Rapezzi C, Adler Y, Arad M, Basso C, Brucato A, et al. Diagnosis and treatment of cardiac amyloidosis: a position statement of the ESC Working Group on Myocardial and Pericardial Diseases. Eur Heart J. 2021;42:1554–68.
43. El-Am EA, Dispenzieri A, Melduni RM, Ammash NM, White RD, Hodge DO, et al. Direct current cardioversion of atrial arrhythmias in adults with cardiac amyloidosis. J Am Coll Cardiol. 2019;73:589–97.
44. Cappelli F, Tini G, Russo D, et al. Arterial thrombo-embolic events in cardiac amyloidosis: a look beyond atrial fibrillation. Amyloid. 2021;28:12–8.
45. Cappelli F, Vignini E, Martone R, Perlini S, Mussinelli R, Sabena A, et al. Baseline ECG features and arrhythmic profile in transthyretin versus light chain cardiac amyloidosis. Circ Heart Fail. 2020;13:e006619.
46. Thakkar S, Patel HP, Chowdhury M, Patel K, Kumar A, Arora S, et al. Impact of arrhythmias on hospitalizations in patients with cardiac amyloidosis. Am J Cardiol. 2021;143:125–30.
47. Cappelli F, Cipriani A, Russo D, Tini G, Zampieri M, Zocchi C, et al. Prevalence and prognostic role of nonsustained ventricular tachycardia in cardiac amyloidosis. Amyloid. 2022;29:211–2.
48. Perfetto F, Zampieri M, Bandini G, Fedi R, Tarquini R, Santi R, et al. Transthyretin cardiac amyloidosis: a cardio-orthopedic disease. Biomedicine. 2022;10:3226.
49. Sekijima Y, Uchiyama S, Tojo K, Sano K, Shimizu Y, Imaeda T, et al. High prevalence of wild-type transthyretin deposition in patients with idiopathic carpal tunnel syndrome: a common cause of carpal tunnel syndrome in the elderly. Hum Pathol. 2011;42:1785–91.
50. Fosbøl EL, Rørth R, Leicht BP, Schou M, Maurer MS, Kristensen SL, et al. Association of carpal tunnel syndrome with amyloidosis, heart failure, and adverse cardiovascular outcomes. J Am Coll Cardiol. 2019;74:15–23.
51. Sperry BW, Reyes BA, Ikram A, Donnelly JP, Phelan D, Jaber WA, et al. Tenosynovial and cardiac amyloidosis in patients undergoing carpal tunnel release. J Am Coll Cardiol. 2018;72:2040–50.
52. Ladefoged B, Clemmensen T, Dybro A, Hartig-Andreasen C, Kirkeby L, Gormsen LC, et al. Identification of wild-type transthyretin cardiac amyloidosis in patients with carpal tunnel syndrome surgery (CACTuS). ESC Heart Fail. 2023;10:234–44.
53. Geller HI, Singh A, Alexander KM, Mirto TM, Falk RH. Association between ruptured distal biceps tendon and wild-type transthyretin cardiac amyloidosis. JAMA. 2017;318:962–3.
54. Cappelli F, Zampieri M, Fumagalli C, Nardi G, Del Monaco G, Matucci Cerinic M, et al. Tenosynovial complications identify TTR cardiac amyloidosis among patients with hypertrophic cardiomyopathy phenotype. J Intern Med. 2021;289:831–9.
55. Godara A, Riesenburger RI, Zhang DX, Varga C, Fogaren T, Siddiqui NS, et al. Association between spinal stenosis and wild-type ATTR amyloidosis. Amyloid. 2021;28:226–33.
56. Rubin J, Alvarez J, Teruya S, Castano A, Lehman RA, Weidenbaum M, et al. Hip and knee arthroplasty are common among patients with transthyretin cardiac amyloidosis, occurring years before cardiac amyloid diagnosis: can we identify affected patients earlier? Amyloid. 2017;24:226–30.

57. Basdavanos A, Maurer MS, Ives L, Derwin K, Ricchetti ET, Seitz W, et al. Prevalence of orthopedic manifestations in patients with cardiac amyloidosis with a focus on shoulder pathologies. Am J Cardiol. 2023;190:67–74.
58. Sood RF, Lipira AB. Risk of amyloidosis and heart failure among patients undergoing surgery for trigger digit or carpal tunnel syndrome: a nationwide cohort study with implications for screening. J Hand Surg. 2022;47:517–525.e4.
59. Sommer R, Valen GJ, Ori Y, Weinstein T, Katz M, Hendel D, et al. Sonographic features of dialysis-related amyloidosis of the shoulder. J Ultrasound Med. 2000;19:765–70.
60. Sueyoshi T, Ueda M, Jono H, Irie H, Sei A, Ide J, et al. Wild-type transthyretin-derived amyloidosis in various ligaments and tendons. Hum Pathol. 2011;42:1259–64.

Electrocardiographic Patterns

Stefano Perlini, Lucio Teresi, Andrea Rossi,
and Gianluca Mirizzi

Abbreviations

AL	Amyloid light chain amyloidosis
ATTR	Amyloid transthyretin amyloidosis (ATTRv, variant form; ATTRwt, wild-type form)
CA	Cardiac amyloidosis
ECG	Electrocardiogram
fQRS	QRS complex fragmentation
LBBB	Left bundle branch block
LV	Left ventricle
NSVT	Non-sustained ventricular tachycardia
NT-proBNP	N-terminal fragment of pro-B-type natriuretic peptide
NYHA	New York Heart Association
RBBB	Right bundle branch block
SAECG	Signal averaged electrocardiogram
SCD	Sudden cardiac death
VT	Ventricular tachycardia

S. Perlini
Emergency Medicine Unit and Emergency Medicine Postgraduate Training Program,
Department of Internal Medicine, IRCCS Policlinico San Matteo Foundation, University of
Pavia, Pavia, Italy
e-mail: stefano.perlini@unipv.it

L. Teresi
Azienda Ospedaliera Universitaria "Gaetano Martino", Messina, Italy
e-mail: lucio.teresi@studenti.unime.it

A. Rossi · G. Mirizzi (✉)
Fondazione Toscana Gabriele Monasterio, Pisa, Italy
e-mail: rossi79@ftgm.it; gmirizzi@ftgm.it

The electrocardiogram (ECG) plays a crucial role in raising the suspicion of cardiac amyloidosis (CA), as part of a comprehensive clinical evaluation that takes into account personal and family history, comorbidities, and findings from physical examination and other diagnostic imaging techniques such as echocardiography.

The first description of ECG patterns specifically associated with CA dates back to the 1950s, when Berneiter described the findings on 6 patients with heart failure and biopsy- (or autopsy-) proven CA. Unfortunately, the amyloidosis type was not reported [1]. The author described the presence of low QRS voltages in the peripheral leads, an abnormal deviation of the QRS axis, atrial fibrillation, and disturbances of atrioventricular conduction. The frequent finding of poor R wave progression in precordial leads, simulating an anteroseptal infarction, was also noted. Interestingly enough, these patterns, although described in such a small population, became almost pathognomonic for the diagnosis of CA (Fig. 8.1). ECG patterns are commonly attributed to direct infiltration of the conduction tissue by amyloid fibrils, although such hypothesis was not confirmed by histological examination. Ridolfi and coworkers studied the conduction system in a necropsy series of 23 CA patients with a 91% prevalence of rhythm and conduction disturbances, namely atrial arrhythmias (39%), atrioventricular block (43%), and bundle branch block (30%). "Senile" CA was diagnosed in 18 patients, whereas CA was related to a plasma cell dyscrasia in 3 subjects and to an unspecified "systemic" form in 1 patient. In the latter subject, amyloidosis was primarily affecting the peripheral

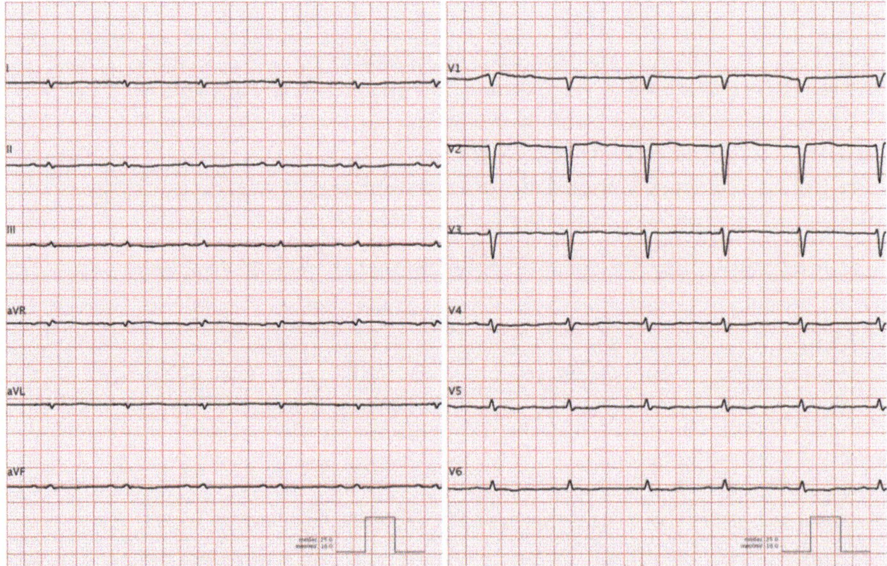

Fig. 8.1 Typical ECG findings in a patient with cardiac amyloidosis. ECG tracing of a 69-year-old man with light chain cardiac amyloidosis. Note the low QRS voltages, particularly in the peripheral leads, and the poor R wave progression in the precordial leads with deep Q waves in V1–V2

nervous system. The prevalence of peripheral lead low voltages was 35%, and of poor R-wave progression was 30%, respectively [2]. Despite the presence of these ECG changes and the stratification of patients based on the severity of myocardial amyloid infiltration (limited in 7, moderate in 5, and severe in 11 patients, respectively), involvement of specialized conduction tissue (sinoatrial and atrioventricular nodes, main branches) was surprisingly low. Notably, only 3 patients out of 23 (13%) had extensive amyloidosis of the conduction system, associated with first-degree atrioventricular block and left anterior hemiblock. A more common morphologic abnormality of the conduction system was severe sinoatrial node fibrosis ($n = 7$; 30%) and idiopathic atrophy and fibrosis of the bundle branches ($n = 6$; 26%). At variance with fibrosis of the sinus node, that was more frequent in patients with severe or moderate amyloid myocardial infiltration, bundle branch fibrosis was not related to the amount of amyloid elsewhere in the heart. Moreover, varying degrees of atrioventricular and bundle branch block were also present in 6 patients without any morphologic abnormality of the conduction system. The authors conclude that although conduction and rhythm disturbances are common in CA, direct amyloid infiltration of the specialized conduction tissue of the heart does not account for the majority of these alterations [2]. A possible (albeit speculative) explanation might be a reactive and/or toxic damage at the interface between the conduction and working myocardial tissue. However these hypotheses are yet to be proven.

8.1 Relevance of ECG Patterns for Diagnosis and Risk Stratification

The pseudonecrosis pattern consists in the presence of Q waves measuring at least 1 mV in at least 2 contiguous leads, in the absence of history of ischemic heart disease and/or akinetic or dyskinetic segments in the left ventricle (LV) (Fig. 8.2). Among patients with amyloid light chain (AL) amyloidosis, those with pseudonecrosis waves have higher N-terminal fraction of pro-B-type natriuretic peptide (NT-proBNP) levels and were more symptomatic for dyspnea. Only Q waves and New York Heart Association (NYHA) class emerged as independent predictors of survival [3].

Patients with CA might also have low QRS voltages, that is widely recognized as an important "red flag" of the disease [4]. This finding is much more common in AL amyloidosis than in other types of CA [5], although some authors believe that the different frequencies of the low-voltage pattern are not related to the different forms of CA, but rather reflect a different prevalence of cardiac involvement in these patients [6]. When comparing the prevalence of low voltages in CA, attention should be taken in clearly defining this pattern. As expected, the prevalence of low voltage can indeed vary in the same patient population when using different criteria, i.e., Sokolow-Lyon index $\leq$15 mV, peripheral low voltages (QRS $\leq$5 mV in every leads), or low voltages in all leads (QRS $\leq$5 mV in the peripheral and $\leq$10 mV in the precordial leads, respectively) [7]. A decrease in QRS voltage amplitude across repeated ECG tracings should also be emphasized (Fig. 8.3).

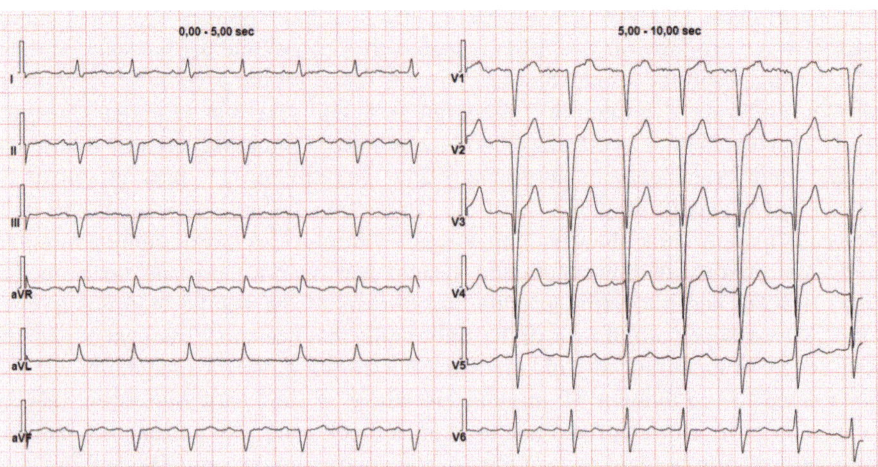

Fig. 8.2 Q waves. CG of a 54-year-old man with variant transthyretin amyloidosis (mutation Glu89Gln) showing left bundle branch block and anterior pseudonecrosis with Q waves in V1–V4 measuring at least 1 mV, without a history of ischemic heart disease and/or kinetic alterations at echocardiography

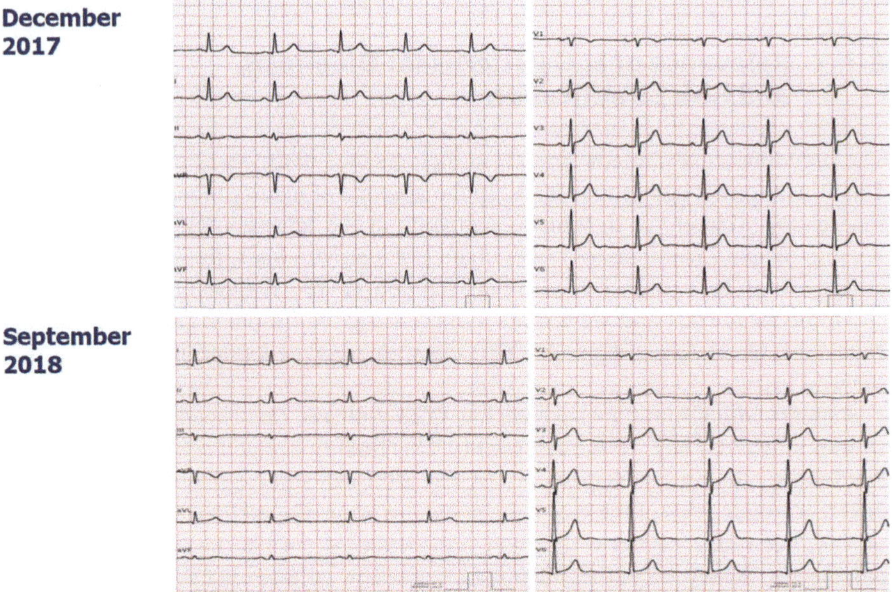

Fig. 8.3 Decrease in QRS voltages over less than 1 year as an early manifestation of cardiac amyloidosis. ECG tracings of a 77-year-old man with cardiac transthyretin amyloidosis. Note the slight decrease in QRS voltages, particularly evident in some leads (e.g., aVF)

Nonetheless, despite these caveats in a common definition of these patterns, it is agreed that the combined presence of low voltages and pseudonecrosis is a powerful red flag for CA. Indeed, the concomitant presence of both ECG patterns is more common when comparing patients with systemic amyloidosis with or without cardiac involvement (28.0% vs. 2.3%), with 28% sensitivity, 98% specificity, 96% positive predictive value, and 39% negative predictive value [8]. The diagnostic performance further improves when considering the amplitude of specific QRS waves: a sum of S-wave amplitude in V1 plus R-wave amplitude in V6 lower than 1.2 mV allows diagnosing CA with a 91% sensitivity and an 89% specificity. As expected, the combination of ECG and echocardiographic findings yielded the best results, since a ratio <0.4 between R-wave amplitude in lead I and posterior wall thickness has 91% sensitivity and 89% specificity [9].

As to prognosis, the relevance of ECG findings in stratifying the risk of events in patients with CA is less clear. Although in some studies, low-voltage [7] or pseudonecrosis pattern [3] was associated with mortality, in other studies NYHA class [10] or the presence of heart failure and history of recent syncope [11] emerged as independent predictors of cardiac death. It has been therefore proposed to combine ECG findings with other clinical and instrumental variables. Seven continuous variables associated with CA (systolic arterial pressure <130 mmHg; PR duration >200 ms; Sokolow index <12 mV; diastolic LV posterior thickness >13 mm; E/E' ratio >10; global longitudinal strain > −12% and sum of basal longitudinal strain > −47%) were selected and dichotomized according to the best cutoff value, providing a diagnostic score for CA with a 90% sensitivity and 81% specificity. A score >3 was also associated with a higher risk of mortality, specificity becoming 100% with a score >5 [12].

Notably, the commonly recognized factors related to QRS voltages in the general population (such as LV mass index, age, gender, hypertension, body surface area, and smoking habit) are no longer predictive of voltage amplitude in patients with CA. This can be explained by considering that wall thickening is caused by myocardial infiltration of non-conductive material, thereby abolishing the relationship between QRS voltages and LV mass. The diagnosis of CA should be therefore suspected whenever a discrepancy between LV mass and QRS voltages is noted [13].

8.2 ECG Patterns in AL Vs. ATTR Amyloidosis

The two most common forms of CA, i.e., AL and transthyretin (ATTR) amyloidosis, are associated with different ECG manifestations (Tables 8.1 and 8.2).

In AL amyloidosis, low peripheral voltages, pseudoinfarction pattern, and conduction anomalies (with different degrees of fascicular block or atrioventricular blocks) are more commonly observed [14]. Another finding, commonly described in patients with previous myocardial infarction, is QRS complex fragmentation (fQRS), defined as a notch of QRS and a RsR' pattern in the absence of QRS prolongation. A higher prevalence of fQRS has been found in patients with AL and CA than those without cardiac involvement (28.5 vs. 11.7%). Furthermore, the presence

Table 8.1 Pseudonecrosis patterns in patients with cardiac amyloidosis

		Pseudoinfarction location												
		Any location				Anterior			Inferior			Lateral		
	N	AL	ATTRv	ATTRwt	AL + ATTR	AL	ATTRv	ATTRwt	AL	ATTRv	ATTRwt	AL	ATTRv	ATTRwt
Zhao et al. [3]	110	/	/	/		/	/	/	/	/	/	/	/	/
Rapezzi et al. [5]	186	/	55	33		/	/	/	/	/	/	/	/	/
Cyrille et al. [6]	200	25	18	18		16	10	9	7	13	12	3	0	3
Mussinelli et al. [7]	233	/	/	/		/	/	/	/	/	/	/	/	/
Cheng et al. [8]	276	/	/	/		/	/	/	/	/	/	/	/	/
Austin et al. [10]	45	/	/	/		/	/	/	/	/	/	/	/	/
Finocchiaro et al. [11]	48	/	/	/		/	/	/	/	/	/	/	/	/
Cariou et al. [12]	114	/	/	/	68	/	/	/	/	/	/	/	/	/
Perlini et al. [15]	375	/	/	/		/	/	/	/	/	/	/	/	/
Dungu et al. [16]	64	/	52	/		/	/	/	/	/	/	/	/	/
Di Bella et al. [17]	35	/	28	/		/	/	/	/	/	/	/	/	/
Gonzalez-Lopez et al. [18]	149	/	/	63		/	/	/	/	/	/	/	/	/
Rapezzi et al. [19]	233	69	69	66		/	/	/	/	/	/	/	/	/
Murtagh et al. [25]	127	/	/	/	47	/	/	/	/	/	/	/	/	/

Data are reported as percentages. *AL* amyloid light chain amyloidosis, *ATTR* amyloid transthyretin amyloidosis (ATTRv, variant form; ATTRwt, wild-type form)

Table 8.2 Low-voltage patterns in patients with cardiac amyloidosis

| | | Low voltages | | | | | | | | Sokolow index < 1.5 mV | | | Abnormal voltage/mass ratio | | |
| | | Peripheral | | | | Precordial | | | | | | | | | |
	N	AL	ATTRv	ATTRwt	AL + ATTR	AL	ATTRv	ATTRwt	AL + ATTR	AL	ATTRv	ATTRwt	AL	ATTRv	ATTRwt
Zhao et al. [3]	110	54	/	/		54	/	/		/	/	/	/	/	/
Rapezzi et al. [5]	186	/	/	/		/	/	/		/	/	/	/	/	/
Cyrille et al. [6]	200	37	38	18		16	10	6		64	53	58	78	73	80
Mussinelli et al. [7]	233	66	/	/		38	/	/		84	/	/	/	/	/
Cheng et al. [8]	276	/	/	/	54	/	/	/		/	/	/	/	/	/
Austin et al. [10]	45	/	/	/		/	/	/	42	/	/	/	/	/	/
Finocchiaro et al. [11]	48	/	/	/	53	/	/	/		/	/	/	/	/	/
Cariou et al. [12]	114	/	/	/	40	/	/	/	10	/	/	/	/	/	/
Perlini et al. [15]	375	64	/	/		/	/	/		/	/	/	/	/	/
Dungu et al. (2012)	64	/	25	/		/	49	/		/	11	/	/	/	/
Di Bella et al. [16]	35	/	53	/		/	/	/		/	/	/	/	/	/
Gonzalez-Lopez et al. [18]	149	/	/	22		/	/	22		/	/	48	/	/	/
Rapezzi et al. [19]	233	60	25	40		/	/	/		/	/	/	/	/	/
Murtagh et al. [25]	127	/	/	/	45	/	/	/	4	/	/	/	/	/	/

Data are reported as percentages. *AL* amyloid light chain amyloidosis, *ATTR* amyloid transthyretin amyloidosis (ATTRv, variant form; ATTRwt, wild-type form)

of fQRS was associated with higher mortality, independently of other prognostic predictors such as PQ and QTc intervals, or wall thickness [15].

Since the clinical manifestations of variant ATTR (ATTRv) depend on the specific transthyretin mutation, any comparison with cardiac AL should be based on the presence of cardiac involvement, that is much more prevalent in a portfolio of mutations [5]. In V142I patients, Dungu and coworkers reported a 56.7% prevalence of low QRS voltages. However, 25% of patients met the ECG criteria for LV hypertrophy. Moreover, the prevalence first-degree atrioventricular block was 56%, much higher than the 20% frequency observed in AL amyloidosis, as reported in other studies [16]. As for cardiac AL, the association between ECG measures and other non-invasive measures can effectively identify the presence of CA in patients affected by ATTRv. Among echocardiographic parameters, a >14 mm interventricular wall thickness had a 78% sensitivity and an 89% specificity for the identification of patients with cardiac involvement. By combining septal thickness with an abnormal ECG tracing (poor R-wave progression, pseudonecrosis pattern, left bundle branch block (LBBB), QRS <15 mV), an 89% sensitivity was reached [17]. In the much more common wild-type ATTR (ATTRwt), a study showed that 22% of patients (but 48% according to a low Sokolow-Lyon index) had low-voltage QRS, and only 11% had LV hypertrophy, based on ECG criteria. In the same study, 63% of patients had a pseudoinfarction pattern and 56% had atrial fibrillation [18].

ECG findings might also differentiate between AL and ATTR CA, although such a diagnosis should be based on amyloid typing. Some comparison studies reported a 25% prevalence of low voltages in ATTRwt versus 60% in AL patients, despite a higher LV wall thickness at echocardiography. Therefore, the voltage-to-mass ratio is expected to be higher in the former as compared to the latter CA patients. Indeed, the greater cardiomyocyte damage induced by amyloidogenic light chains plays a relevant role in explaining these differences. Another difference between the two forms is related to the prevalence of left bundle branch block, that was much higher in ATTRwt- than in AL CA [19].

8.3 Bradyarrhythmias and Tachyarrhythmias

8.3.1 Ventricular Arrhythmias

Patients with CA may experience ventricular arrhythmias, from isolated ventricular ectopic beats to life-threatening arrhythmias, particularly in the most advanced forms. Among patients with biopsy-proven AL amyloidosis undergoing autologous stem cell transplantation, a high incidence of ventricular arrhythmias was recorded (326 events in 24 patients over 24 days), mostly represented by non-sustained ventricular tachycardia (NSVT), with only one case of sustained VT [20]. Despite patient population was small, the cumulative number of ventricular arrhythmias (NSVT, sustained VT, ventricular fibrillation) per each patient, normalized for the length of hospital stay, was correlated with indexes of cardiac function such as stroke volume [20].

In a study on 51 patients with AL amyloidosis, the majority of whom having signs of cardiac involvement (55% with increased wall thickness, 23% with heart failure), a high frequency of ventricular arrhythmias was observed on Holter recording. The majority were complex ventricular arrhythmias (Lown class 3–4a–4b: 57%, class 4a–4b: 33%). Over a median 23-month follow-up, a high mortality was observed (70%), with 25% of patients experiencing sudden cardiac death. Complex arrhythmias were associated with a worse prognosis, as well as a greater impairment of echocardiographic parameters [21].

The cause of such a high incidence of sudden cardiac death (SCD) among patients with CA as well as the specific arrhythmias causing this event is still poorly understood. Diffuse amyloid infiltration of myocardial tissue may cause inhomogeneities in impulse propagation in the ventricles, during both depolarization and repolarization phases, making the ventricles more vulnerable to arrhythmogenic stimuli. Additionally, the formation of macroscopically evident protein formations in the ventricular myocardium could produce anatomical and/or functional barriers able to sustain reentrant arrhythmias. Moreover, electromechanical dissociation can also be triggered by amyloid infiltration. In 133 cardiac AL patients, signal averaged ECG (SAECG), a technique that can provide information on the heterogeneity in ventricular activation and the presence of delayed potentials [22] showed a prevalence of abnormalities ranging from 15% to 22%, according to the different criteria. During follow-up, 71 patients died (53%), 68% of whom for cardiac causes; SCD represented the 31% of all events. Abnormal SAECG signals were associated with cardiac mortality and SCD, suggesting a role for tachyarrhythmias. However, as pointed out by the authors, since 53% of patients experiencing SCD did not show alterations on SAECG, other mechanisms should be taken into account, namely bradyarrhythmias. It is important to note that since the study protocol did not include invasive electrophysiological studies, heterogeneous ventricular activation was not confirmed. On the other hand, studies based on the interrogation of implanted devices (defibrillators or loop recorders) showed a high prevalence of electromechanical dissociation or bradyarrhythmias as the precipitating cause of SCD [23, 24]. To the best of our knowledge, data on the incidence of ventricular arrhythmias in patients with other forms of CA are still lacking.

8.3.2 Atrial Arrhythmias

Atrial arrhythmias are quite common in patients with CA (Table 8.3). Based on historical cohorts of CA patients, atrial fibrillation (AF) is the most frequently diagnosed arrhythmia [1, 2], with a prevalence that is highly variable according to the etiology of CA. AF prevalence is lower in AL (between 15 and 20%) [8, 10, 23, 25], than in ATTR patients, being up to 67% in the latter [26, 27]. Such discrepancy might be partly explained by the more advanced age and greater burden of comorbidities, such as hypertension and diabetes, associated with a higher incidence and prevalence of AF. Specific arrhythmic substrates have been investigated in a single invasive study. Among 7 patients with CA (4 ATTRwt and 3 AL) and persistent AF

Table 8.3 Atrial arrhythmias in patients with cardiac amyloidosis

		Sinus rhythm				Atrial fibrillation			
	N	AL	ATTRv	ATTRwt	AL + ATTR	AL	ATTRv	ATTRwt	AL + ATTR
Zhao et al. [3]	110	81	/	/		12	/	/	
Rapezzi et al. [5]	186	/	/	/		/	29	37	
Cyrille et al. [6]	200	86	76	48		6	17	38	
Cheng et al. [8]	276	/	/	/		/	/	/	16
Austin et al. [10]	45	/	/	/		/	/	/	18
Finocchiaro et al. [11]	48	/	/	/	70	/	/	/	25
Cariou et al. [12]	114	/	/	/		/	/	/	28
Sperry et al. [13]	389	/	/	/		32	24	75	
Dungu et al. [16]	64	/	62	/		/	/	/	69
Gonzalez-Lopez et al. [18]	149	/	/	52		/	/	56	
Rapezzi et al. [5]	233	/	/	/		12	5	27	
Murtagh et al. [25]	127	/	/	/	86	/	/	/	10
Mints et al. [26]	146	/	/	/		/	/	70	

Data are reported as percentages. *AL* amyloid light chain amyloidosis, *ATTR* amyloid transthyretin amyloidosis (ATTRv, variant form; ATTRwt, wild-type form)

undergoing an electrophysiological study with electroanatomical mapping of the left atrium for arrhythmia ablation, mean voltages per atrial segments explored (measured while on AF) were significantly lower than the same measures performed in patients with persistent AF but without CA [28] (Fig. 8.4).

8.3.3 Bradyarrhythmias and Conduction Disturbances

Conduction abnormalities are some of the most commonly reported findings in patients with CA and involve particularly the atrioventricular node and the ventricular myocardium, despite a relative preservation of specialized conduction tissue (as explained above) (Table 8.4). In a cohort of 127 patients with AL amyloidosis and cardiac involvement demonstrated by endomyocardial biopsy, 76% had a normal atrioventricular conduction, while 24% had an atrioventricular block, most commonly a first-degree block (21%). A right bundle branch block (RBBB) was present in 9% (Fig. 8.5), and 5% displayed a LBBB. These findings were not influenced by the degree of myocardial infiltration, that was indirectly estimated (albeit with limited specificity) from the degree of wall thickness [25]. The prognostic significance of these abnormalities is still uncertain, because of diverging conclusions from published studies. In a study on 59 patients with CA (43 with AL and 16 with ATTRv), a shorter PQ interval and a longer QRS duration were associated with a worse prognosis. When comparing survivors ($n = 41$) and non-survivors ($n = 18$), PQ intervals were 166.0 ± 4.8 vs. 164.1 ± 5.6 ms, respectively ($p < 0.01$), and QRS intervals were

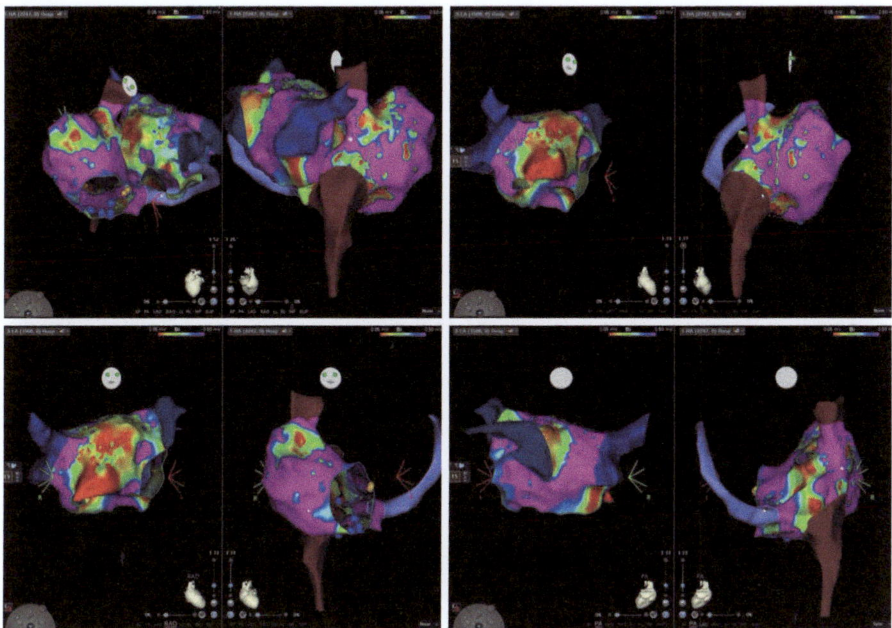

Fig. 8.4 Electroanatomic mapping in a patient with cardiac amyloidosis. Electroanatomic mapping of the left and right atrium of a 72-year-old patient with light chain cardiac amyloidosis and no history of atrial fibrillation or other atrial arrhythmias. Electrical abnormalities are similar to those observed in patients with longstanding atrial fibrillation

95.7 ± 3.4 vs. 115.1 ± 6.7 ms ($p < 0.05$). No significant differences were noted between patients with the 2 forms of amyloidosis. Significant proportions of patients had right ventricle conduction disturbances (32%) or a left anterior hemiblock (20%), while LBBB was rare (only 1 patient). In another study, ECG findings of patients with AL amyloidosis were examined to assess the prevalence and prognostic significance of conduction disturbances [14]. Patients with AL CA displayed a mean prolongation of PQ and QRS intervals compared to patients with AL amyloidosis but no cardiac disease (179 ± 37 vs. 169 ± 30 ms, $p = 0.023$, and 90 ± 21 vs. 85 ± 20 ms, $p = 0.022$, respectively), together with a longer QTc interval (456 ± 37 vs. 425 ± 30, $p < 0.001$). An atrioventricular conduction disturbance was present in 18% of patients with AL CA, compared to 13% of patients with isolated AL (almost exclusively first-degree block). A fascicular conduction disturbance was found in 28% of patients with AL CA, mostly RBBB, compared with 17% of patients with AL amyloidosis but no cardiac disease. Significantly, the study also showed that a fascicular conduction disturbance, but not an atrioventricular conduction disturbance, was associated with worse survival, regardless of other predictors such as NT-proBNP or troponin. As noted by the authors, these observations do not indicate a causal relationship, but provide a tool for risk stratification and a mean to interpret the observation that a significant proportion of terminal events in these patients is

Table 8.4 Conduction disturbances and prolongation of the QT interval in the different forms of amyloidosis

| | | RBBB | | | | LBBB | | | | LAH | | | LPH | | | QTc prolongation | | | AV block I degree | | | | II degree | | | |
	N	AL	ATTRv	ATTRwt	AL + ATTR	AL	ATTRv	ATTRwt	AL + ATTR	AL	ATTRv	ATTRwt	AL	ATTRv	ATTRwt	AL	ATTRv	ATTRwt	AL	ATTRv	ATTRwt	AL + ATTR	AL	ATTRv	ATTRwt	AL + ATTR
Cyrille et al. [6]	200	/	/	/		/	/	/		/	/	/	/	/	/	55	63	56	26	33	45		0	10	10	
Cheng et al. [8]	276	/	/	/	7	/	/	/	2	/	/	/	/	/	/	/	/	/	/	/	/	13	/	/	/	
Finocchiaro et al. [11]	48	/	/	/	14	/	/	/	9	/	/	/	/	/	/	/	/	/	/	/	/	21	/	/	/	
Cariou et al. [12]	114	/	/	/		/	14	/		/	/	/	/	/	/	/	/	/	/	/	/		/	/	/	
Boldrini et al. [14]	344	/	/	/		/	/	/		/	/	/	/	/	/	/	/	/	15	/	/		/	/	/	
Perlini et al. [15]	375	/	/	/		/	/	/		/	/	/	/	/	/	/	/	/	25	/	/		/	/	/	
Dungu et al. [16]	64	/	13	/		/	7	/		/	/	/	/	/	/	/	/	/	/	56	/		/	/	/	
Di Bella et al. [17]	35	/	/	/		/	11	/		/	/	/	/	/	/	/	/	/	/	/	/		/	/	/	
Gonzalez-Lopez et al. [18]	149	/	/	15		/	/	17		/	/	/	/	/	/	/	/	/	/	/	31		/	/	/	
Rapezzi et al. [19]	233	19	12	13		4	7	40		29	30	20	/	/	/	/	/	/	18	25	33		/	/	/	
Murtagh et al. [25]	127	/	/	/	9	/	/	/	5	/	/	/	/	/	/	/	/	/	/	/	/	21	/	/	/	1

Data are reported as percentages. *AL* amyloid light chain amyloidosis, *ATTR* amyloid transthyretin amyloidosis (ATTRv, variant form; ATTRwt, wild-type form), *AV* atrioventricular, *LAH* left anterior hemiblock, *LBBB* left bundle branch block, *LPH* left posterior hemiblock, *RBBB* right bundle branch block

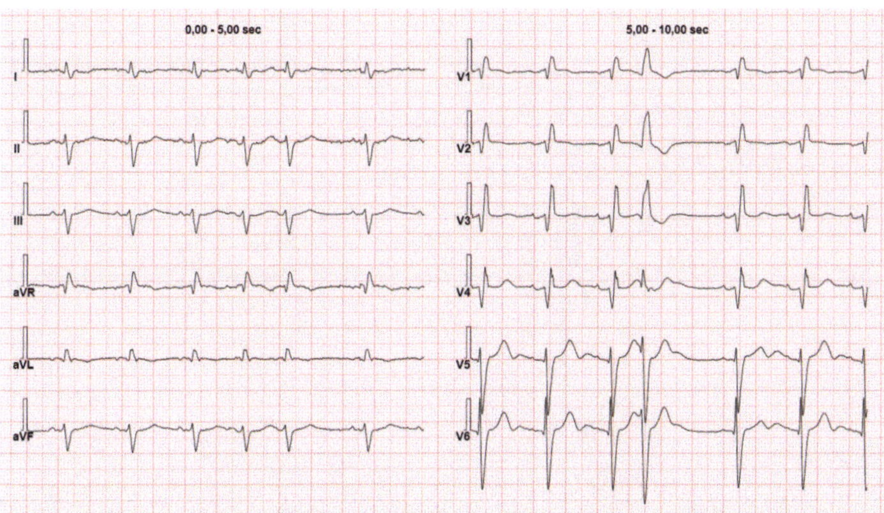

Fig. 8.5 Conduction alterations in light chain amyloidosis. ECG of a 65-year-old man with light chain amyloidosis with first-degree atrioventricular block and right ventricular block. A pair of atrial ectopic beats and a single ventricular ectopic beat can be observed

represented by pulseless electrical activity or electromechanical dissociation [23, 24, 29].

Very limited data derive from invasive measurements. Reisinger et al. examined 25 patients with AL CA diagnosed by low QRS voltages in the precordial leads and/ or LV hypertrophy in the setting of histologically proven AL amyloidosis (with an endomyocardial biopsy in 4 patients) [30]. A first-degree atrioventricular block was found in 52% of patients, QRS prolongation in 20%, with equal prevalence of LBBB and RBBB (8% each), while the anterior fascicular block was highly prevalent (24%). No information regarding the combinations of these disorders was provided. Both AH and HV intervals were prolonged (121 ± 33 and 79 ± 18 ms, respectively). QRS prolongation >120 ms was found in all patients with prolongation of the HV interval. Among 5 patients with marked prolongation of the HV interval (>80 ms), a prolongation of intra-Hisian conduction was found (>30 ms with fragmented potentials) (Fig. 8.6). Prolongation of the HV interval displayed an independent association with SCD during follow-up (odds ratio 2.26 per each 10 ms prolongation).

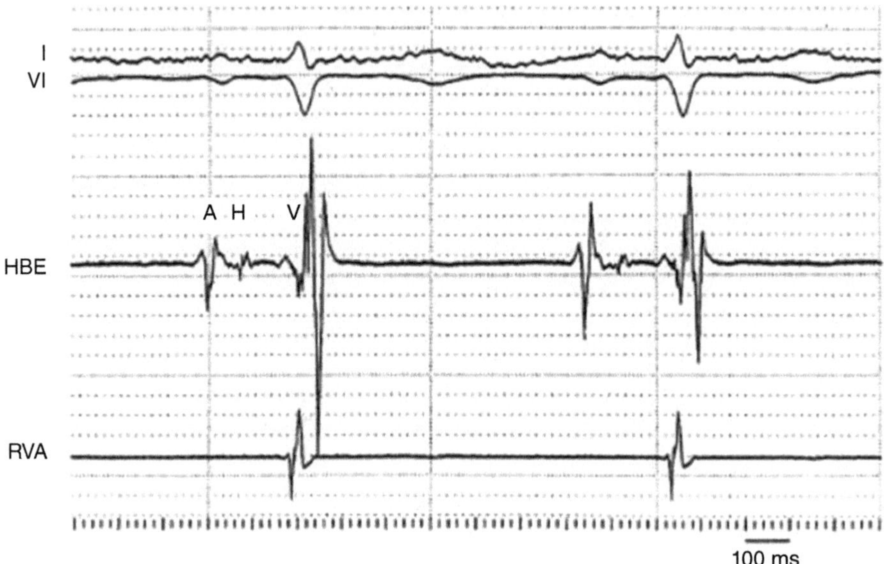

Fig. 8.6 Impaired atrioventricular conduction. Intra-cavitary electrophysiological recording of a patient with light chain amyloidosis showing split His potential and prolonged HV interval (90 ms). *A* atrium, *H* His, *HBE* His bundle electrogram, *RVA* right ventricular apex, *V* ventricle. Adapted with permission from: Reisinger et al. [30]

8.4 Conclusions

The ECG is one of the simplest, yet very informative diagnostic tools able to suggest the presence of CA. It can provide several diagnostic red flags, especially if interpreted together with imaging findings, and can allow to refine prognostic stratification. Associate with prolonged ECG monitoring, it prompts the decision of prophylactic device implantation. Therefore, ECG cannot but be an integral part of the initial diagnostic workup in every patient with suspected CA.

References

1. Bernreiter M. Cardiac amyloidosis; electrocardiographic findings. Am J Cardiol. 1958;1:644–7.
2. Ridolfi RL, Bulkley BH, Hutchins GM. The conduction system in cardiac amyloidosis. Clinical and pathologic features of 23 patients. Am J Med. 1977;62:677–86.
3. Zhao L, Li J, Tian Z, Fang Q. Clinical correlates and prognostic values of pseudoinfarction in cardiac light-chain amyloidosis. J Cardiol. 2016;68:426–30.
4. Rapezzi C, Aimo A, Serenelli M, Barison A, Vergaro G, Passino C, et al. Critical comparison of documents from scientific societies on cardiac amyloidosis: JACC state-of-the-art review. J Am Coll Cardiol. 2022;79:1288–303.

5. Rapezzi C, Quarta CC, Obici L, Perfetto F, Longhi S, Salvi F, et al. Disease profile and differential diagnosis of hereditary transthyretin-related amyloidosis with exclusively cardiac phenotype: an Italian perspective. Eur Heart J. 2013;34:520–8.
6. Cyrille NB, Goldsmith J, Alvarez J, Maurer MS. Prevalence and prognostic significance of low QRS voltage among the three main types of cardiac amyloidosis. Am J Cardiol. 2014;114:1089–93.
7. Mussinelli R, Salinaro F, Alogna A, Boldrini M, Raimondi A, Musca F, et al. Diagnostic and prognostic value of low QRS voltages in cardiac AL amyloidosis. Ann Noninv Electrocardiol. 2013;18:271–80.
8. Cheng Z, Zhu K, Tian Z, Zhao D, Cui Q, Fang Q. The findings of electrocardiography in patients with cardiac amyloidosis. Ann Noninv Electrocardiol. 2013;18:157–62.
9. Cheng Z, Kang L, Tian Z, Chen W, Guo W, Xu J, et al. Utility of combined indexes of electrocardiography and echocardiography in the diagnosis of biopsy proven primary cardiac amyloidosis. Ann Noninv Electrocardiol. 2011;16:25–9.
10. Austin BA, Duffy B, Tan C, Rodriguez ER, Starling RC, Desai MY. Comparison of functional status, electrocardiographic, and echocardiographic parameters to mortality in endomyocardial-biopsy proven cardiac amyloidosis. Am J Cardiol. 2009;103:1429–33.
11. Finocchiaro G, Pinamonti B, Merlo M, Giannini F, Barbati G, Pivetta A, et al. Focus on cardiac amyloidosis: a single-center experience with a long-term follow-up. J Cardiovasc Med. 2013;14(4):281–8.
12. Cariou E, Bennani Smires Y, Victor G, Robin G, Ribes D, Pascal P, et al. Diagnostic score for the detection of cardiac amyloidosis in patients with left ventricular hypertrophy and impact on prognosis. Amyloid. 2017;24:101–9.
13. Sperry BW, Vranian MN, Hachamovitch R, Joshi H, McCarthy M, Ikram A, et al. Are classic predictors of voltage valid in cardiac amyloidosis? A contemporary analysis of electrocardiographic findings. Int J Cardiol. 2016;214:477–81.
14. Boldrini M, Salinaro F, Mussinelli R, Raimondi A, Alogna A, Musca F, et al. Prevalence and prognostic value of conduction disturbances at the time of diagnosis of cardiac AL amyloidosis. Ann Noninv Electrocardiol. 2013;18:327–35.
15. Perlini S, Salinaro F, Cappelli F, Perfetto F, Bergesio F, Alogna A, et al. Prognostic value of fragmented QRS in cardiac AL amyloidosis. Int J Cardiol. 2013;167:2156–61.
16. Dungu J, Sattianayagam PT, Whelan CJ, Gibbs SD, Pinney JH, Banypersad SM, et al. The electrocardiographic features associated with cardiac amyloidosis of variant transthyretin isoleucine 122 type in Afro-Caribbean patients. Am Heart J. 2012;164:72–9.
17. Di Bella G, Minutoli F, Piaggi P, Casale M, Mazzeo A, Zito C, et al. Usefulness of combining electrocardiographic and echocardiographic findings and brain natriuretic peptide in early detection of cardiac amyloidosis in subjects with transthyretin gene mutation. Am J Cardiol. 2015;116:1122–7.
18. Gonzalez-Lopez E, Gagliardi C, Dominguez F, Quarta CC, de Haro-Del Moral FJ, Milandri A, et al. Clinical characteristics of wild-type transthyretin cardiac amyloidosis: disproving myths. Eur Heart J. 2017;38:1895–904.
19. Rapezzi C, Merlini G, Quarta CC, Riva L, Longhi S, Leone O, et al. Systemic cardiac amyloidoses: disease profiles and clinical courses of the 3 main types. Circulation. 2009;120:1203–12.
20. Goldsmith YB, Liu J, Chou J, Hoffman J, Comenzo RL, Steingart RM. Frequencies and types of arrhythmias in patients with systemic light-chain amyloidosis with cardiac involvement undergoing stem cell transplantation on telemetry monitoring. Am J Cardiol. 2009;104:990–4.
21. Palladini G, Malamani G, Co F, Pistorio A, Recusani F, Anesi E, et al. Holter monitoring in AL amyloidosis: prognostic implications. Pacing Clin Electrophysiol. 2001;24:1228–33.
22. Dubrey SW, Bilazarian S, LaValley M, Reisinger J, Skinner M, Falk RH. Signal-averaged electrocardiography in patients with AL (primary) amyloidosis. Am Heart J. 1997;134:994–1001.
23. Kristen AV, Dengler TJ, Hegenbart U, Schonland SO, Goldschmidt H, Sack FU, et al. Prophylactic implantation of cardioverter-defibrillator in patients with severe cardiac amyloidosis and high risk for sudden cardiac death. Heart Rhythm. 2008;5:235–40.

24. Sayed RH, Rogers D, Khan F, Wechalekar AD, Lachmann HJ, Fontana M, et al. A study of implanted cardiac rhythm recorders in advanced cardiac AL amyloidosis. Eur Heart J. 2015;36:1098–105.
25. Murtagh B, Hammill SC, Gertz MA, Kyle RA, Tajik AJ, Grogan M. Electrocardiographic findings in primary systemic amyloidosis and biopsy-proven cardiac involvement. Am J Cardiol. 2005;95:535–7.
26. Mints YY, Doros G, Berk JL, Connors LH, Ruberg FL. Features of atrial fibrillation in wild-type transthyretin cardiac amyloidosis: a systematic review and clinical experience. ESC Heart Fail. 2018;5:772–9.
27. Connors LH, Sam F, Skinner M, Salinaro F, Sun F, Ruberg FL, et al. Heart failure resulting from age-related cardiac amyloid disease associated with wild-type transthyretin: a prospective, observational cohort study. Circulation. 2016;133:282–90.
28. Barbhaiya CR, Kumar S, Baldinger SH, Michaud GF, Stevenson WG, Falk R, et al. Electrophysiologic assessment of conduction abnormalities and atrial arrhythmias associated with amyloid cardiomyopathy. Heart Rhythm. 2016;13:383–90.
29. Hess EP, White RD. Out-of-hospital cardiac arrest in patients with cardiac amyloidosis: presenting rhythms, management and outcomes in four patients. Resuscitation. 2004;60:105–11.
30. Reisinger J, Dubrey SW, Lavalley M, Skinner M, Falk RH. Electrophysiologic abnormalities in AL (primary) amyloidosis with cardiac involvement. J Am Coll Cardiol. 1997;30:1046–51.

Echocardiography: A Gatekeeper to Diagnosis

Iacopo Fabiani, Vladyslav Chubuchny, Federico Landra, and Matteo Cameli

Abbreviations

AL	Amyloid light chain amyloidosis
ATTR	Amyloidosis related to transthyretin
ATTRv	Variant transthyretin amyloidosis
ATTRwt	Wild-type transthyretin amyloidosis
CA	Cardiac amyloidosis
EF	Ejection fraction
GLS	Global longitudinal strain
HCM	Hypertrophic cardiomyopathy
IWT	Increased wall thickness
LA	Left atrium
LS	Longitudinal strain
LV	Left ventricle
PACS	Left atrial contractile strain
PALS	Left atrial reservoir strain
RA	Right atrium
RRSR	Relative regional strain ratio
RV	Right ventricle
SAB	Septal apical-to-basal ratio

I. Fabiani (✉) · V. Chubuchny
UO Cardiologia e Medicina Cardiovascolare, Fondazione Toscana Gabriele Monasterio, Pisa, Italy
e-mail: ifabiani@ftgm.it; vlad@ftgm.it

F. Landra · M. Cameli
Cardiology Division, University Hospital of Siena, Siena, Italy
e-mail: f.landra@studenti.unisi.it; matteo.cameli@unisi.it

M. Emdin et al. (eds.), *Cardiac Amyloidosis*,
https://doi.org/10.1007/978-3-031-51757-0_9

STE	Speckle tracking echocardiography
TAPSE	Tricuspid annular plane systolic excursion
TDI	Tissue Doppler imaging

Echocardiography is a first-line examination in the diagnostic algorithm of cardiac amyloidosis (CA). CA is most commonly characterized by increased wall thickness with restrictive physiology and diastolic stiffening, causing a rapid increase in intraventricular pressures [1, 2]. Increased wall thickness leading to restrictive cardiomyopathy may suggest hypertrophic cardiomyopathy (HCM), but since the pathophysiology and treatment of the two conditions differ, making a correct diagnosis is crucially important. Amyloid also accumulates in the atria, promoting the development of supraventricular arrhythmias, thrombus formation, and valves, leading to different degrees of regurgitation. Furthermore, amyloidogenic light chains may be toxic to cardiomyocytes, as discussed in Chap. 3. As part of a comprehensive evaluation that includes clinical history and electrocardiography, echocardiography can raise the suspicion of CA [1]. Echocardiography can highlight morphological and functional abnormalities even in the earliest disease phases and provide elements for risk stratification [2]. Typical echocardiographic findings suggestive of CA are concentric left ventricular (LV) wall thickness, biatrial enlargement, preserved ejection fraction (EF), and diastolic dysfunction up to a restrictive filling pattern [3]. Apparent preservation or even exaggeration of systolic function in some patients may be explained by reduced wall stress due to small chamber volume, thickened walls, and low systolic pressure leading to arterial hypotension. However, the LV EF can progressively decline in the late stages of CA. Dynamic obstruction of LV outflow is also possible but rare [4].

9.1   M-mode Echocardiography

The M-mode technique can be used for acquiring linear measures of the LV, such as end-diastolic diameter, interventricular septum, and posterior wall from the parasternal long-axis view. The echocardiographic beam must be aligned perpendicularly to the LV long axis and placed just above the end of the mitral valve leaflets [5]. The typical features of CA at M-mode analysis include increased LV wall thickness, normal or reduced LV dimensions, left atrial (LA) dilation, and occasionally pericardial effusion. A reduced LV fractional shortening can be observed in the most advanced disease stages, but LV dilation is rare even in this phase [5, 6].

9.2   2D Echocardiography

The introduction of bidimensional echocardiography has allowed identifying numerous features suggestive of CA (Figs. 9.1 and 9.2). Wall thickness, particularly in the LV, is markedly increased because of amyloid infiltration in the cardiac wall (so-called pseudohypertrophy). LV thickening in the absence of hypertension suggests an infiltrative cardiac disease, but this is not specific to amyloidosis and can also be found in other conditions, including sarcoidosis, glycogen storage diseases, and hemochromatosis. This condition must be differentiated from other conditions where increased afterload leads to true LV hypertrophy, e.g., aortic stenosis, hypertensive heart disease, or renal disease [7]. Also, CA may frequently coexist in up to 15% of patients presenting with aortic stenosis, which could potentially mask the underlying infiltrative process [8]. To distinguish hypertrophy from pseudohypertrophy, echocardiographic evaluation can be coupled to electrocardiographic

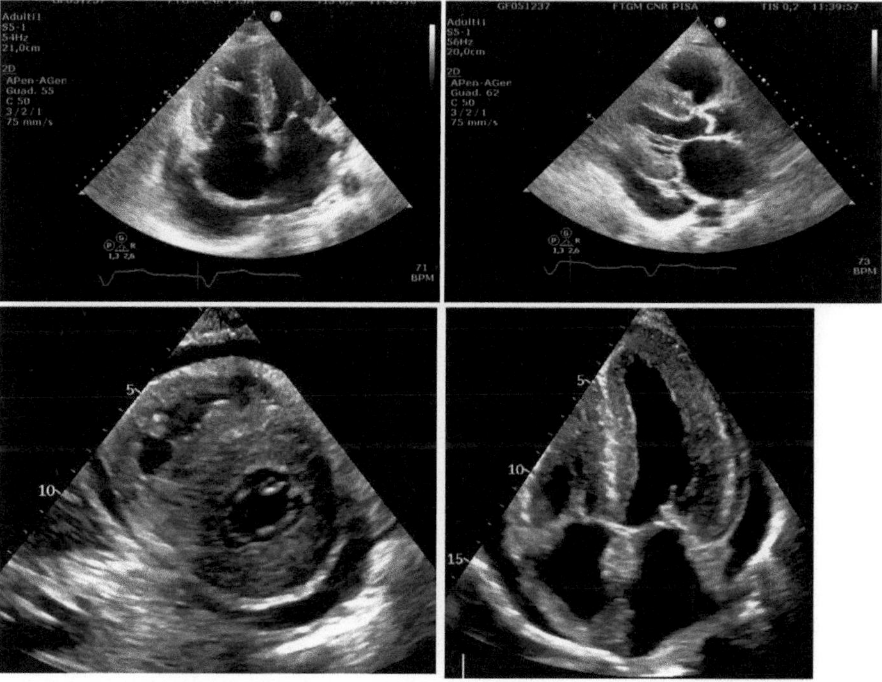

Fig. 9.1 Cardiac amyloidosis. Left upper panel showing an apical four chamber view with relevant hypertrophy, biatrial enlargement, pleuro-pericardial effusion. Right upper panel of a parasternal view showing severe pseudohypertrophy, left atrial enlargement, and pericardial effusion. In the left lower panel, typical left and right ventricular hypertrophy, with pericardial effusion, in the right lower panel, from the same patient, severe hypertrophy with interatrial septum thickening, valve thickening, and pleural effusion

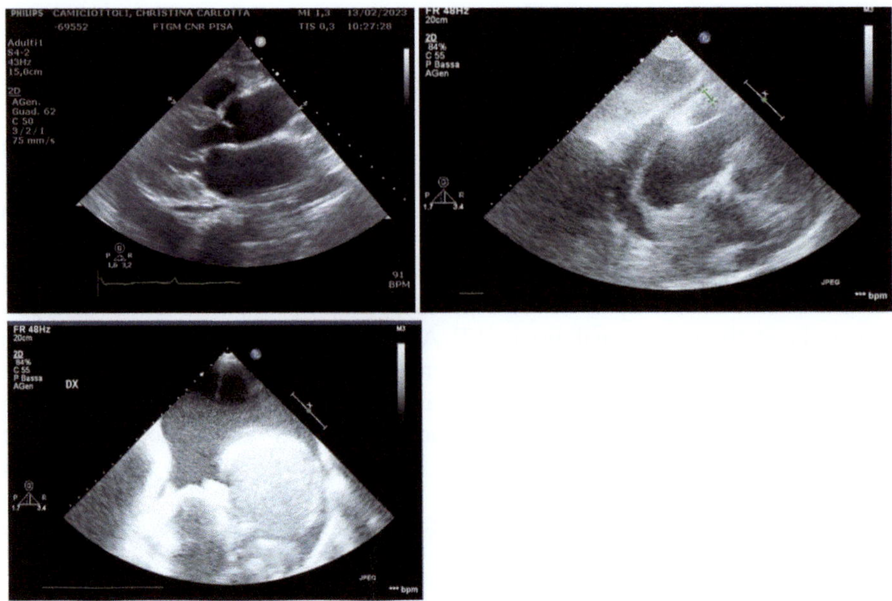

Fig. 9.2 Congestion in cardiac amyloidosis. Evidence of congestion in amyloidotic patients (left panel): upper, pleural effusion from parastenal view; lower, pleural effusion with atelectasia from a chest scan. In the right panel, a relevant sign of amyloidotic heart disease, right ventricular free-wall hypertrophy

assessment: low or normal QRS voltages and increased LV mass induce suspect CA [10–14]. The combination of a low-voltage electrocardiographic pattern and septal thickness ≥2 cm amyloid light chain amyloidosis (AL)-dependent CA with a 72% sensitivity and 91% specificity [9, 10].

In an analysis on patients from the transthyretin amyloidosis outcomes survey registry, including patients with amyloid transthyretin (ATTR) CA, women had more often a septal wall thickness ≥13 mm, while men usually had a thickness ≥14 mm. In addition, patients with wild-type disease, those without the Val30Met mutation and those with the Val30Met mutation but late disease onset displayed higher wall thickness values [6, 11, 12]. The pseudohypertrophy pattern is often symmetrical, but asymmetrical patterns have been described in up to one-fifth of patients with ATTR-CA [12]. A normal wall thickness does not exclude the diagnosis of CA, particularly in the early disease stages. LV volumes are usually normal or reduced, and LV EF is often preserved, although it can be moderately or severely reduced in the most advanced cases. The interventricular and interatrial septa are often thickened as well. Hypertrophy of the right ventricular (RV) free wall (usually >7 mm) and impaired RV function at the Doppler examination with RV enlargement are often found [13]. RV dilation in CA patients is associated with a more severe prognosis [14]. Furthermore, in CA, atria are often enlarged, with the LA area usually >20 cm^2 and LA volume index >28 mL/m^2. This is due to diastolic dysfunction, increased filling pressures, and ventricular infiltration by amyloid causing a mechanical standstill. Similarly, amyloid-dependent ineffective atrial contraction may lead to the formation of atrial thrombi even in patients in sinus rhythm [15].

The thickened wall may have a speckled or granular appearance. These highly refractile echoes are believed to be caused by hyperechogenic collagen and amyloid nodules in the heart. These findings are non-specific and have been observed in many other conditions, such as advanced kidney disease failure, left heart hypoplastic syndrome, and HCM [16]. Furthermore, this pattern is less specific for CA when using the harmonic imaging mode since this technique increases the presence of speckles in the myocardium [7]. This pattern also has poor sensitivity and is found only in about a quarter of patients [17], but the combination of this echocardiographic finding, low-voltage electrocardiographic pattern, and atrial septum thickening is strongly suggestive of CA.

Other possible echocardiographic findings are thickened the cardiac valves (Figs. 9.3 and 9.4). Cardiac valves are often involved, but the resulting dysfunction is usually mild and does not lead to significant regurgitation, and heart failure derives primarily from diastolic dysfunction [6]. However, the thickening of left heart valves in AL patients has been associated with LV systolic and diastolic dysfunction, worse functional class, more advanced disease stage, and all-cause mortality [18].

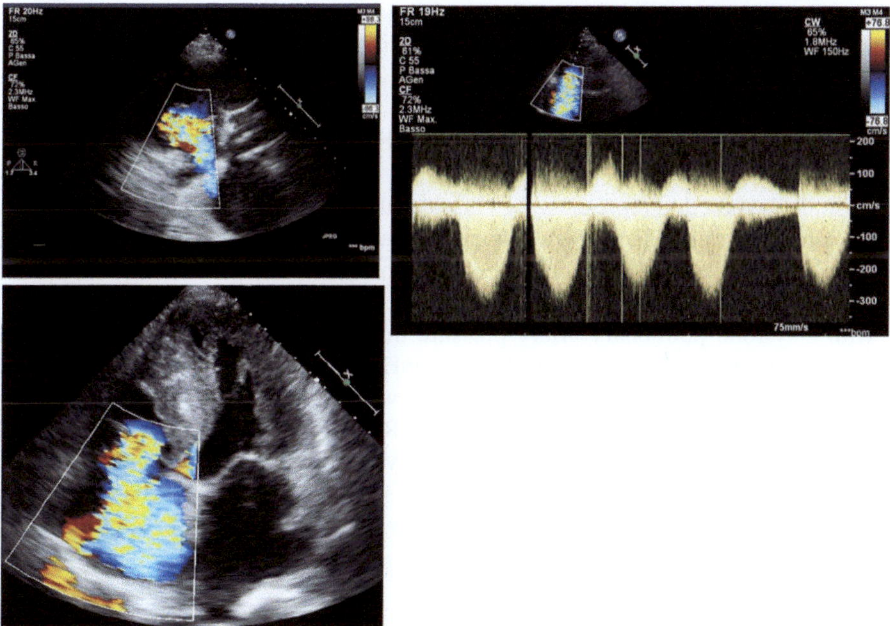

Fig. 9.3 Tricuspid regurgitation. Severe tricuspid regurgitation in an amyloidotic patient, with prominent right ventricular dilation (left upper and lower panel; inflow view from modified parasternal view) and holosystolic Doppler jet form continuous wave Doppler (right)

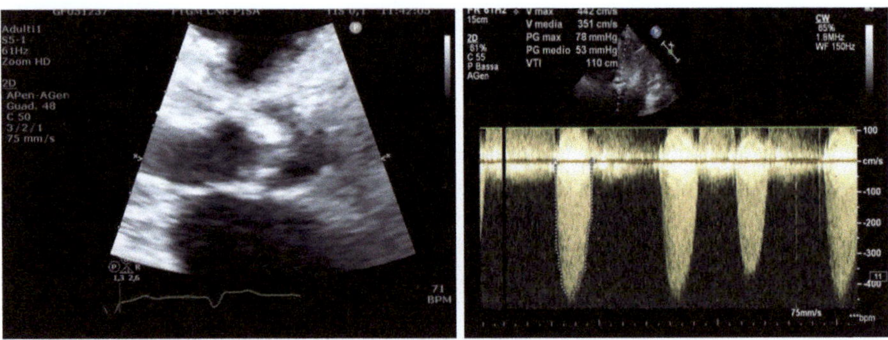

Fig. 9.4 Severe valvular stenosis in amyloidosis. Particular (left) of a severely calcified aortic valve, with reduced cusps excursion. On the right panel, continuous wave Doppler tracing showing increased transvalvular velocity

A slight pericardial effusion is present in 50% of cases and is associated with a worse prognosis. Disease onset with pericardial tamponade has been described but is very rare [19].

All the characteristics above are non-specific for diagnosing CA but can be highly suggestive when combined with other echocardiographic parameters and clinical and laboratory findings. Furthermore, it is not possible to distinguish the different forms of CA from the simple analysis of morphological echocardiographic abnormalities, although some differences have been reported, such as a greater LV and RV wall thickness in ATTR- than AL-CA [20].

9.3 Diastolic Function and Right Heart Involvement

Diastolic dysfunction represents the classical abnormality of CA and is possibly the earliest alteration evidenced by echocardiography (Fig. 9.5). A grade 2 or higher diastolic dysfunction can be documented in many cases, while an impaired relaxation pattern can be evidenced in earlier cases. Pulmonary pressures can be elevated (with a systolic pulmonary artery pressure that is usually >35 mmHg), and right atrial (RA) pressure can be elevated (>10 mmHg), particularly in the most advanced disease stages. RA involvement is associated with a worse prognosis. Some authors have recommended measuring end-diastolic RA wall thickness from the subcostal window [21, 22]. While LV dilation is rare, RV dilation can be observed, and is correlated to pulmonary hypertension and RV systolic dysfunction due to amyloid accumulation. RV dysfunction is associated with a worse prognosis [23].

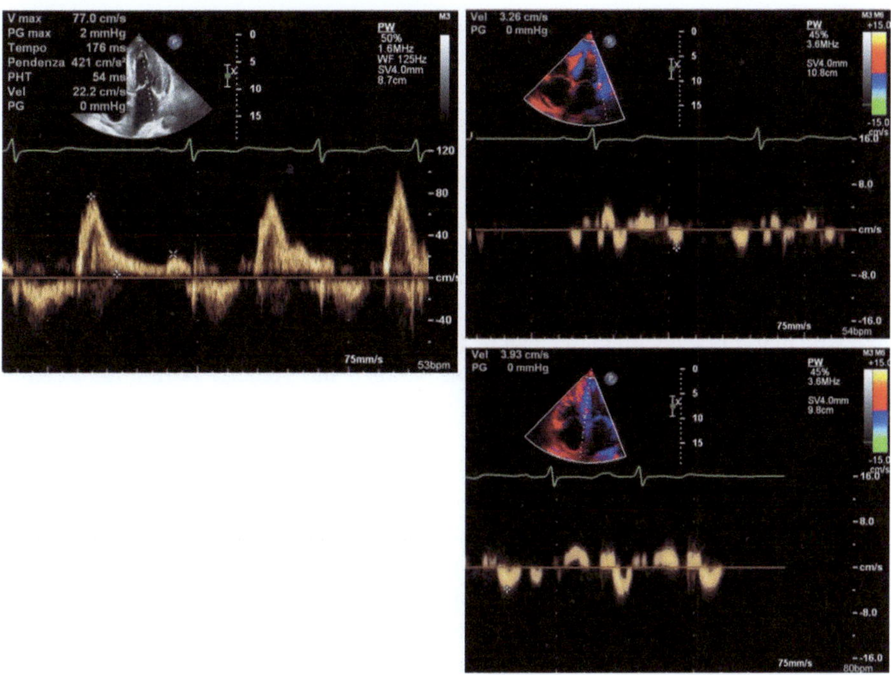

Fig. 9.5 Diastolic dysfunction in cardiac amyloidosis. In the left panel, transmitral flow evaluated with pulsed wave Doppler, showing an E/A ratio > 2 (restrictive filling pattern). In the right upper and lower panel, tissue Doppler velocities at mitral annulus, showing e' wave reduction

9.4 Tissue Doppler Imaging

Tissue Doppler Imaging (TDI) relies on the measurement of myocardial tissue motion, providing parameters that are not preload-dependent, contrary to traditional measures of diastolic dysfunction. TDI allows, for example, to derive curves of systolic and diastolic velocities measured at the mitral annulus level. These velocities are significantly reduced in CA (usually less than 6 cm/s) (Fig. 9.5) with a mismatch between the severity of TDI abnormalities and the degree of wall thickening and systolic dysfunction, as opposite to hypertrophic or hypertensive cardiomyopathies [7].

Patients with CA often show a reduction of systolic (s'), early diastolic (e'), and atrial contraction (a') velocities. When all these velocities are lower than 5 cm/s (5-5-5 sign), the suspicion of CA is high. This sign is highly specific, but poorly sensitive, being found only in the most advanced disease stages [19]. Recent literature suggests that diastolic dysfunction parameters such as a short E-wave deceleration time [24] or the average ratio between early transmitral inflow and mitral annular TDI velocities [25, 26] might become abnormal early stages of CA or help distinguish CA from other forms of cardiac hypertrophy [4]. TDI can also show prolonged isovolumetric relaxation and contraction and shortened LV ejection times in CA patients [27].

9.5 Speckle Tracking Echocardiography

Bidimensional speckle tracking echocardiography (STE) is a technique that provides a quantitative assessment of the global and regional ventricular and atrial myocardium function. The interaction of ultrasounds with the myocardium causes acoustic markers (speckles) that can be tracked during cardiac cycles by a dedicated software. The displacement, deformation (strain), and velocity (strain rate) can be calculated as objective and quantitative measures of myocardial thickening, shortening, and rotation. The results do not depend on the ultrasound angle and, to a certain extent, on translational movements of the heart.

STE is useful for diagnosis, identification of the etiology, and functional assessment of CA. It is a sensitive and specific tool for early detection of CA. Indeed, longitudinal LV function can be altered in early disease stages when radial thickening and circumferential shortening are preserved [10, 28, 29]. Longitudinal strain (LS) is myocardial shortening along its longitudinal axis. It has negative values during systole and positive values during diastole. The average of segmental strain values can be calculated, providing the global LS (GLS), an important metric of LV function. A GLS > −15.0% denotes subclinical cardiac disease.

For similar degrees of LV hypertrophy, patients with HCM have better-preserved GLS values than those with CA. GLS is commonly reduced in CA. While in a healthy heart myocardial contractility gradually increases from the basis to the apex, patients with CA show basal hypokinesis and a relative increase in apical contractility (apical sparing; Fig. 9.6). This is likely due to preferential amyloid

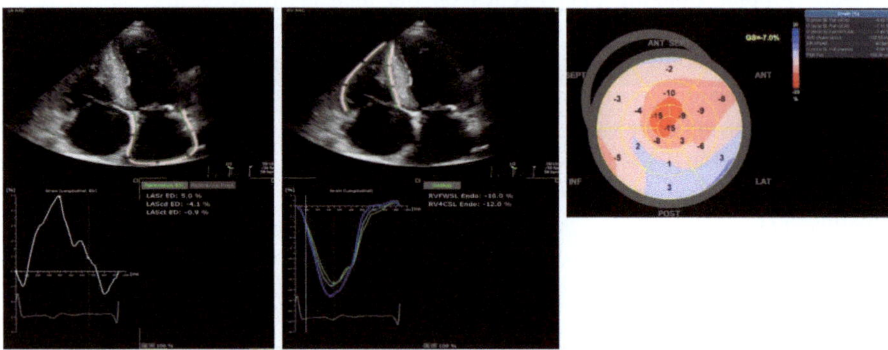

Fig. 9.6 Speckle tracking evaluation in cardiac amyloidosis. From the left panel, left atrial strain showing relevant reduction of reservoir (PALS), conduction and contractile phases (PACS) values (%). In the middle panel, right ventricular strain (global, %) impairment. In the right panel, the typical cherry on top sign: severe middle and basal segments left ventricular longitudinal strain reduction with apical segments relative preservation

accumulation in the basal portions of the LV. However, a recent paper based on histopathological evaluation of 27 hearts, partly refuted this hypothesis, since this pattern at echocardiography is not always explained by a base-to-apex gradient of amyloid burden at histopathology, suggesting that apical sparing might be an epiphenomenon of complex interactions among amyloid infiltration, myocardial structure, and adaptation [30]. Disorders that cause LV hypertrophy (aortic stenosis, HCM) are typically characterized by a maximal impairment of LS in the most severely hypertrophied regions, while this association is not found in CA [31]. In particular, a deformation parameter that has been found to differentiate CA from other hypertrophic cardiac diseases is the LVEF to GLS ratio. This index is significantly higher in CA patients than in those with mild hypertrophy or normal EF [32].

The ratio of apical strain to mid and basal strain, or relative regional strain ratio (RRSR, cutoff >1), the septal apical-to-basal (SAB) ratio (cutoff >2.1), which uses the septal apical and basal segmental longitudinal strain values and the EF-to-strain ratio (cutoff >4.1), although not validated in large populations, represent useful parameters for discriminating CA from other conditions with increased wall thickness [32]. The apical sparing pattern can also be present in the RV. A free-wall RV longitudinal strain worse than 21.2% is typical [33].

As for other cardiac chambers, LA strain curves are diffusely reduced and show a pattern of altered shortening during atrial systole and impairment of LA relaxation during diastole. Compared to relative LV apical sparing, LA strain reduction has higher diagnostic accuracy in discrimination for CA, particularly reservoir strain. However, even in patients with sinus rhythm, atrial contraction can be absent in many patients, and this atrial electromechanical dissociation confers a poorer prognosis [34]. Aimo et al. showed that LA reservoir strain <6.65% and/or LA contractile strain <3.62% are associated with the diagnosis of CA when this condition is suspected [35]. Even abnormal RA conduit and reservoir strain are associated with worse survival [36]. Furthermore, RV free-wall strain can highlight RV systolic dysfunction, although few data from the literature are available. A longitudinal RV strain $< -16\%$ indicates patients with severe RV dysfunction and at high risk of death [33]. In particular, RV strain had a higher prognostic role than GLS in ATTR-CA [37]. Interestingly, the systolic excursion of the tricuspid annulus, if below 14 mm, has a prognostic impact [38]. The global information from transthoracic echocardiography was recently combined in two specific multiparametric scores that include relative LV wall thickness, LV GLS, tricuspid annular plane systolic excursion (TAPSE), mitral Doppler E/e', and longitudinal strain (Systemic AL score). Adding apical-to-basal ratio identifies the second score, the increased wall thickness (IWT) [2]. A systemic AL score ≥ 5 points is highly suggestive of AL, instead an IWT score ≥ 8 points is highly suggestive of CA, with a good diagnostic performance of both. This scoring system can be used in patients with systemic AL amyloidosis to check for cardiac involvement or in those with increased LV wall thickness. In particular, the addition of septal apical-to-base ratio to the previous parameters yielded the best diagnostic accuracy in the increased heart wall thickness group. Second-level imaging modalities are encouraged in patients with an intermediate probability of CA. Another suggested score is the product of LV relative wall thickness and mitral E/e', and a value <2.22 in the overall population excluded the diagnosis in a group of patients that underwent a diagnostic screening for CA, a value <2.36 excludes AL-CA in a hematology subset of patients and a value <2.22 excludes ATTR-CA in an unexplained hypertrophy subset [39].

Over the last few years, greater attention has been paid to the use of 3D STE to diagnose CA. This technique relies on wall movement tracking, automatically calculates cavity volumes, and derives time-volume curves based on myocardial deformation. Contrary to 2D-STE, 3D-STE does not which require acquiring 2-, 3-, and 4-chamber views and does not have long elaboration times [40–42]. A 3D acquisition can measure LV end-systolic and end-diastolic volumes, LV mass and EF, and global longitudinal, circumferential and radial strains. Moreover, the 3D technique allows to detect even earlier abnormalities of systolic function than those identified by 2D techniques and to identify diastolic dysfunction and abnormalities in longitudinal strain in an earlier stage [43]. However, 3D technology has some limitations. Its temporal resolution is lower than 2D STE, which limits the possibility to assess anatomical details, and different software is needed to assess the two ventricles. Thus, 3D echocardiography is not commonly used in clinical practice.

9.6 Echocardiography for Differential Diagnosis Between Amyloidosis Subtypes

There are specific features that are useful to differentiate AL- from ATTR-CA, but their specificity is variable. In AL-CA, there is a proportional increase in LV wall thickness, with a substantial decline in deceleration time and early filling velocity by spectral transmitral Doppler flow [6, 10]. Pericardial effusion is also more common in this subtype. In ATTR-CA, the increase in LV wall thickness is usually asymmetrical, sometimes with a sigmoid septal morphology, with a much higher LV indexed mass. RV involvement and TAPSE reduction are also more frequent in ATTR-CA. STE can also be useful. In AL-CA, LV strain values are usually significantly worse, but apical LV strain in ATTR-CA is generally worse than in AL. RV GLS is reduced considerably in variant ATTR- compared to AL-CA. However, RV free-wall longitudinal strain (particularly in its basal and mid-segments) is significantly more impaired in AL-CA, followed by ATTRwt- and ATTRv-CA. On the other hand, LA reservoir and pump function on strain imaging are lower in ATTRwt-CA compared to AL- and ATTRv-CA [10, 37, 44].

9.7 Echocardiography to Assess the Response to Treatment

Disease-modifying therapies for ATTR-CA reduce myocardial deposition of amyloid by various mechanisms. Diflunisal improved LV function (rotation/torsion, GLS), without longitudinal and radial strain deterioration at 1 year [28, 45]. Patients on tafamidis showed less deterioration of stroke volume over 30 months [46], while patisiran and inotersen decreased mean LV wall thickness, maintained GLS, and higher cardiac output following 18-month therapy [47]. Patients with AL-CA showing a complete hematological response after first-line bortezomib therapy displayed an improvement of diastolic function (decrease in E/e' ratio and left atrial stiffness) and GLS, ultimately leading to an improved outcome and paralleled by a net reduction of natriuretic peptides and troponin [48]. The same results have been observed in patients undergoing stem cell transplantation [49].

9.8 Conclusions

Several abnormalities related to CA can be detected with echocardiography (Table 9.1), which is an essential tool for CA diagnosis and risk stratification. A classification of the degree of suspicion of CA based on different echocardiographic parameters has been proposed [11, 50]:

- Non-suggestive echocardiogram: normal LV wall thickness, LV mass, atrial dimensions, septal or lateral e' > 10 cm/s.

Table 9.1 Main echocardiographic findings in cardiac amyloidosis

Anatomic landmark	Echocardiographic variables
Left ventricle	
• Structure • Function	EDD, ESD, IVS, PW, RWT, EDV, ESV, LV mass, LVEF, SVi, GLS, RRSR, SAB, EFSR, E/e', e', a', s', IVCT, IVRT, ET, DecT
Right ventricle	
• Structure • Function	Free-wall thickness TAPSE, s', fwRVLS
Left atrium	
• Structure • Function	LAd, LA volume PALS, PACS
Right atrium	RA volume, RA wall thickness, estimated RA pressure
Valves	Diffuse valve thickening, aortic stenosis
Pericardium	Effusion
Others	sPAP, atrial septal thickness, pulmonary vein velocities, sparkling myocardium

EDD end-diastolic diameter, *ESD* end-systolic diameter, *IVS* interventricular septum, *PW* posterior wall, *RWT* relative wall thickness, *EDV* end-diastolic volume, *ESV* end-systolic volume, *LV* left ventricle, *LVEF* left ventricular ejection fraction, *SVi* stroke volume index, *GLS* global longitudinal strain, *RRSR* relative regional strain ratio, *SAB* septal apical-to-basal ratio, *EFSR* ejection fraction to strain ratio, *IVCT* isovolumic contraction time, *IVRT* isovolumic relaxation time, *ET* ejection time, *DecT* deceleration time, *TAPSE* tricuspid annular plane systolic excursion, *fwGLS* free-wall global longitudinal strain, *fwRVLS* free-wall right ventricular longitudinal strain, *LAd* left atrium diameter, *LA* left atrium, *PACS* left atrial contractile strain, *PALS* left atrial reservoir strain, *RA* right atrium, *sPAP* estimated systolic pulmonary artery pressure

- Suggestive echocardiogram: increased LV wall thickness and mass, typical longitudinal strain, e' < 5 cm/s, increased biatrial volume, small a wave (when patients are in sinus rhythm), pericardial effusion.
- Non-conclusive echocardiogram: other combinations of echocardiographic features.

Many other promising parameters are emerging thanks to new techniques, such as shear wave imaging. Cardiac shear wave imaging has been proposed as a noninvasive tool to assess myocardial stiffness. Shear waves occur after mechanical excitation of the myocardium, and their propagation velocity is theoretically related to stiffness. It has recently been shown that CA patients had significantly higher shear wave velocities, possibly because of myocardial stiffening [51]. Myocardial work, a relatively new STE method to non-invasively estimate pressure-volume loops, is another emerging technique currently under evaluation in the field of CA. Early studies have shown conflicting results in terms of diagnostic utility [52, 53], but potential role regarding evaluation of response to treatment and prognosis has already emerged [54, 55]. Overall, echocardiography is a crucial tool for assessing patients with CA. Echocardiographic findings must be integrated with all the available information: detailed clinical history, laboratory profile, other imaging techniques (cardiac magnetic resonance, diphosphonate scintigraphy), and, when needed, tissue biopsy.

References

1. Kyriakou P, Mouselimis D, Tsarouchas A, Rigopoulos A, Bakogiannis C, Noutsias M, et al. Diagnosis of cardiac amyloidosis: a systematic review on the role of imaging and biomarkers. BMC Cardiovasc Disord. 2018;18(1):221.
2. Boldrini M, Cappelli F, Chacko L, Restrepo-Cordoba MA, Lopez-Sainz A, Giannoni A, et al. Multiparametric echocardiography scores for the diagnosis of cardiac amyloidosis. J Am Coll Cardiol Img. 2020;13(4):909–20.
3. Weber N, Mollee P, Augustson B, Brown R, Catley L, Gibson J, et al. Management of systemic AL amyloidosis: recommendations of the Myeloma Foundation of Australia Medical and Scientific Advisory Group. Intern Med J. 2015;45(4):371–82.
4. Jurcuţ R, Onciul S, Adam R, Stan C, Coriu D, Rapezzi C, et al. Multimodality imaging in cardiac amyloidosis: a primer for cardiologists. Eur Heart J Cardiovasc Imaging. 2020;21(8):833–44.
5. Wechalekar AD, Gillmore JD, Hawkins PN. Systemic amyloidosis. Lancet (London, England). 2016;387(10038):2641–54.
6. Falk RH, Quarta CC. Echocardiography in cardiac amyloidosis. Heart Fail Rev. 2015;20(2):125–31.
7. Agha AM, Parwani P, Guha A, Durand JB, Iliescu CA, Hassan S, et al. Role of cardiovascular imaging for the diagnosis and prognosis of cardiac amyloidosis. Open Heart. 2018;5(2):e000881.
8. Ternacle J, Krapf L, Mohty D, Magne J, Nguyen A, Galat A, et al. Aortic stenosis and cardiac amyloidosis: JACC review topic of the week. J Am Coll Cardiol. 2019;74(21):2638–51.
9. Rahman JE, Helou EF, Gelzer-Bell R, Thompson RE, Kuo C, Rodriguez ER, et al. Noninvasive diagnosis of biopsy-proven cardiac amyloidosis. J Am Coll Cardiol. 2004;43(3):410–5.

10. Quarta CC, Solomon SD, Uraizee I, Kruger J, Longhi S, Ferlito M, et al. Left ventricular structure and function in transthyretin-related versus light-chain cardiac amyloidosis. Circulation. 2014;129(18):1840–9.
11. Dorbala S, Ando Y, Bokhari S, Dispenzieri A, Falk RH, Ferrari VA, et al. ASNC/AHA/ASE/EANM/HFSA/ISA/SCMR/SNMMI expert consensus recommendations for multimodality imaging in cardiac amyloidosis: part 2 of 2-diagnostic criteria and appropriate utilization. J Nucl Cardiol. 2020;27(2):659–73.
12. Damy T, Maurer MS, Rapezzi C, Planté-Bordeneuve V, Karayal ON, Mundayat R, et al. Clinical, ECG and echocardiographic clues to the diagnosis of TTR-related cardiomyopathy. Open Heart. 2016;3(1):e000289.
13. Klein AL, Hatle LK, Burstow DJ, Taliercio CP, Seward JB, Kyle RA, et al. Comprehensive Doppler assessment of right ventricular diastolic function in cardiac amyloidosis. J Am Coll Cardiol. 1990;15(1):99–108.
14. Patel AR, Dubrey SW, Mendes LA, Skinner M, Cupples A, Falk RH, et al. Right ventricular dilation in primary amyloidosis: an independent predictor of survival. Am J Cardiol. 1997;80(4):486–92.
15. Dubrey S, Pollak A, Skinner M, Falk RH. Atrial thrombi occurring during sinus rhythm in cardiac amyloidosis: evidence for atrial electromechanical dissociation. Br Heart J. 1995;74(5):541–4.
16. Bhandari AK, Nanda NC. Myocardial texture characterization by two-dimensional echocardiography. Am J Cardiol. 1983;51(5):817–25.
17. Porcari A, Falco L, Lio V, Merlo M, Fabris E, Bussani R, et al. Cardiac amyloidosis: do not forget to look for it. Eur Heart J Suppl. 2020;22(Suppl E):E142–e7.
18. Mohty D, Pradel S, Magne J, Fadel B, Boulogne C, Petitalot V, et al. Prevalence and prognostic impact of left-sided valve thickening in systemic light-chain amyloidosis. Clin Res Cardiol. 2017;106(5):331–40.
19. Bellavia D, Pellikka PA, Al-Zahrani GB, Abraham TP, Dispenzieri A, Miyazaki C, et al. Independent predictors of survival in primary systemic (Al) amyloidosis, including cardiac biomarkers and left ventricular strain imaging: an observational cohort study. J Am Soc Echocardiogr. 2010;23(6):643–52.
20. Tuzovic M, Yang EH, Baas AS, Depasquale EC, Deng MC, Cruz D, et al. Cardiac amyloidosis: diagnosis and treatment strategies. Curr Oncol Rep. 2017;19(7):46.
21. Lang RM, Badano LP, Mor-Avi V, Afilalo J, Armstrong A, Ernande L, et al. Recommendations for cardiac chamber quantification by echocardiography in adults: an update from the American Society of Echocardiography and the European Association of Cardiovascular Imaging. J Am Soc Echocardiogr. 2015;28(1):1–39.e14.
22. Lang RM, Bierig M, Devereux RB, Flachskampf FA, Foster E, Pellikka PA, et al. Recommendations for chamber quantification. Eur J Echocardiogr. 2006;7(2):79–108.
23. Cappelli F, Porciani MC, Bergesio F, Perlini S, Attanà P, Moggi Pignone A, et al. Right ventricular function in AL amyloidosis: characteristics and prognostic implication. Eur Heart J Cardiovasc Imaging. 2012;13(5):416–22.
24. Liu D, Hu K, Niemann M, Herrmann S, Cikes M, Störk S, et al. Effect of combined systolic and diastolic functional parameter assessment for differentiation of cardiac amyloidosis from other causes of concentric left ventricular hypertrophy. Circ Cardiovasc Imaging. 2013;6(6):1066–72.
25. Schiano-Lomoriello V, Galderisi M, Mele D, Esposito R, Cerciello G, Buonauro A, et al. Longitudinal strain of left ventricular basal segments and E/e' ratio differentiate primary cardiac amyloidosis at presentation from hypertensive hypertrophy: an automated function imaging study. Echocardiography (Mount Kisco, NY). 2016;33(9):1335–43.
26. Knight DS, Zumbo G, Barcella W, Steeden JA, Muthurangu V, Martinez-Naharro A, et al. Cardiac structural and functional consequences of amyloid deposition by cardiac magnetic resonance and echocardiography and their prognostic roles. J Am Coll Cardiol Img. 2019;12(5):823–33.

27. Tei C, Dujardin KS, Hodge DO, Kyle RA, Tajik AJ, Seward JB. Doppler index combining systolic and diastolic myocardial performance: clinical value in cardiac amyloidosis. J Am Coll Cardiol. 1996;28(3):658–64.
28. Koyama J, Minamisawa M, Sekijima Y, Ikeda SI, Kozuka A, Ebisawa S, et al. Left ventricular deformation and torsion assessed by speckle-tracking echocardiography in patients with mutated transthyretin-associated cardiac amyloidosis and the effect of diflunisal on myocardial function. Int J Cardiol Heart Vasc. 2015;9:1–10.
29. Voigt JU, Pedrizzetti G, Lysyansky P, Marwick TH, Houle H, Baumann R, et al. Definitions for a common standard for 2D speckle tracking echocardiography: consensus document of the EACVI/ASE/industry task force to standardize deformation imaging. Eur Heart J Cardiovasc Imaging. 2015;16(1):1–11.
30. De Gaspari M, Sinigiani G, De Michieli L, Della Barbera M, Rizzo S, Thiene G, et al. Relative apical sparing in cardiac amyloidosis is not always explained by an amyloid gradient. Eur Heart J Cardiovasc Imaging. 2023;24:1258–68.
31. Phelan D, Collier P, Thavendiranathan P, Popović ZB, Hanna M, Plana JC, et al. Relative apical sparing of longitudinal strain using two-dimensional speckle-tracking echocardiography is both sensitive and specific for the diagnosis of cardiac amyloidosis. Heart. 2012;98(19):1442–8.
32. Pagourelias ED, Mirea O, Duchenne J, Van Cleemput J, Delforge M, Bogaert J, et al. Echo parameters for differential diagnosis in cardiac amyloidosis: a head-to-head comparison of deformation and nondeformation parameters. Circ Cardiovasc Imaging. 2017;10(3):e005588.
33. Tjahjadi C, Fortuni F, Stassen J, Debonnaire P, Lustosa RP, Marsan NA, et al. Prognostic implications of right ventricular systolic dysfunction in cardiac amyloidosis. Am J Cardiol. 2022;173:120–7.
34. Aquaro GD, Morini S, Grigoratos C, Taborchi G, Di Bella G, Martone R, et al. Electromechanical dissociation of left atrium in patients with cardiac amyloidosis by magnetic resonance: prognostic and clinical correlates. Int J Cardiol Heart Vasc. 2020;31:100633.
35. Aimo A, Fabiani I, Giannoni A, Mandoli GE, Pastore MC, Vergaro G, et al. Multi-chamber speckle tracking imaging and diagnostic value of left atrial strain in cardiac amyloidosis. Eur Heart J Cardiovasc Imaging. 2022;24(1):130–41.
36. Singulane CC, Slivnick JA, Addetia K, Asch FM, Sarswat N, Soulat-Dufour L, et al. Prevalence of right atrial impairment and association with outcomes in cardiac amyloidosis. J Am Soc Echocardiogr. 2022;35(8):829–35.e1.
37. Binder C, Duca F, Stelzer PD, Nitsche C, Rettl R, Aschauer S, et al. Mechanisms of heart failure in transthyretin vs. light chain amyloidosis. Eur Heart J Cardiovasc Imaging. 2019;20(5):512–24.
38. Bodez D, Ternacle J, Guellich A, Galat A, Lim P, Radu C, et al. Prognostic value of right ventricular systolic function in cardiac amyloidosis. Amyloid. 2016;23(3):158–67.
39. Aimo A, Chubuchny V, Vergaro G, Barison A, Nicol M, Cohen-Solal A, et al. A simple echocardiographic score to rule out cardiac amyloidosis. Eur J Clin Investig. 2021;51(5):e13449.
40. Vitarelli A, Lai S, Petrucci MT, Gaudio C, Capotosto L, Mangieri E, et al. Biventricular assessment of light-chain amyloidosis using 3D speckle tracking echocardiography: differentiation from other forms of myocardial hypertrophy. Int J Cardiol. 2018;271:371–7.
41. Altman M, Bergerot C, Aussoleil A, Davidsen ES, Sibellas F, Ovize M, et al. Assessment of left ventricular systolic function by deformation imaging derived from speckle tracking: a comparison between 2D and 3D echo modalities. Eur Heart J Cardiovasc Imaging. 2014;15(3):316–23.
42. Mor-Avi V, Lang RM, Badano LP, Belohlavek M, Cardim NM, Derumeaux G, et al. Current and evolving echocardiographic techniques for the quantitative evaluation of cardiac mechanics: ASE/EAE consensus statement on methodology and indications endorsed by the Japanese Society of Echocardiography. Eur J Echocardiogr. 2011;12(3):167–205.
43. Pradel S, Magne J, Jaccard A, Fadel BM, Boulogne C, Salemi VMC, et al. Left ventricular assessment in patients with systemic light chain amyloidosis: a 3-dimensional speckle tracking transthoracic echocardiographic study. Int J Cardiovasc Imaging. 2019;35(5):845–54.

44. Geenty P, Sivapathan S, Stefani LD, Boyd A, Richards D, Kwok F, et al. Left ventricular mass-to-strain ratio predicts cardiac amyloid subtype. J Am Coll Cardiol Img. 2021;14(3):690–2.
45. Lohrmann G, Pipilas A, Mussinelli R, Gopal DM, Berk JL, Connors LH, et al. Stabilization of cardiac function with diflunisal in transthyretin (ATTR) cardiac amyloidosis. J Card Fail. 2020;26(9):753–9.
46. Maurer MS, Schwartz JH, Gundapaneni B, Elliott PM, Merlini G, Waddington-Cruz M, et al. Tafamidis treatment for patients with transthyretin amyloid cardiomyopathy. N Engl J Med. 2018;379(11):1007–16.
47. Solomon SD, Adams D, Kristen A, Grogan M, González-Duarte A, Maurer MS, et al. Effects of Patisiran, an RNA interference therapeutic, on cardiac parameters in patients with hereditary transthyretin-mediated amyloidosis. Circulation. 2019;139(4):431–43.
48. Cohen OC, Ismael A, Pawarova B, Manwani R, Ravichandran S, Law S, et al. Longitudinal strain is an independent predictor of survival and response to therapy in patients with systemic AL amyloidosis. Eur Heart J. 2022;43(4):333–41.
49. Hwang IC, Koh Y, Park JB, Yoon YE, Kim HL, Kim HK, et al. Time trajectory of cardiac function and its relation with survival in patients with light-chain cardiac amyloidosis. Eur Heart J Cardiovasc Imaging. 2021;22(4):459–69.
50. Dorbala S, Ando Y, Bokhari S, Dispenzieri A, Falk RH, Ferrari VA, et al. ASNC/AHA/ASE/EANM/HFSA/ISA/SCMR/SNMMI expert consensus recommendations for multimodality imaging in cardiac amyloidosis: part 1 of 2-evidence base and standardized methods of imaging. J Card Fail. 2019;25(11):e1–e39.
51. Petrescu A, Santos P, Orlowska M, Pedrosa J, Bézy S, Chakraborty B, et al. Velocities of naturally occurring myocardial shear waves increase with age and in cardiac amyloidosis. J Am Coll Cardiol Img. 2019;12(12):2389–98.
52. Henein MY, Lindqvist P. Myocardial work does not have additional diagnostic value in the assessment of ATTR cardiac amyloidosis. J Clin Med. 2021;10(19):4555.
53. Stassen J, Tjahjadi C, Adam R, Debonnaire P, Claeys M, Popescu BA, et al. Left ventricular myocardial work to differentiate cardiac amyloidosis from hypertrophic cardiomyopathy. J Am Soc Echocardiogr. 2023;36(2):252–4.
54. Giblin GT, Cuddy SAM, González-López E, Sewell A, Murphy A, Dorbala S, et al. Effect of tafamidis on global longitudinal strain and myocardial work in transthyretin cardiac amyloidosis. Eur Heart J Cardiovasc Imaging. 2022;23(8):1029–39.
55. Clemmensen TS, Eiskjær H, Ladefoged B, Mikkelsen F, Sørensen J, Granstam SO, et al. Prognostic implications of left ventricular myocardial work indices in cardiac amyloidosis. Eur Heart J Cardiovasc Imaging. 2021;22(6):695–704.

Cardiovascular Magnetic Resonance: Characterization of Myocardial Involvement

10

Marianna Fontana, Ignazio Alessio Gueli, Gianluca Di Bella, and Andrea Barison

Abbreviations

AL	Light chain immunoglobulin amyloidosis
ATTR	Transthyretin amyloidosis
ATTRv	Transthyretin amyloidosis variant
CA	Cardiac amyloidosis
CMR	Cardiac magnetic resonance
DTPA	Diethylene-triamine-penta acetic acid
GRE IR	Fast gradient echo inversion recovery
LGE	Late gadolinium enhancement
LV	Left ventricle
PSIR	Phase sensitive inversion recovery
QALE	Query amyloid late enhancement
RV	Right ventricle
SSFP	Steady-state free precession
TI	Inversion time

M. Fontana
University College London, London, UK
e-mail: m.fontana@ucl.ac.uk

I. A. Gueli · A. Barison (✉)
Fondazione Toscana Gabriele Monasterio, Pisa, Italy

Scuola Superiore Sant'Anna, Pisa, Italy
e-mail: igueli@ftgm.it; abarison@ftgm.it

G. Di Bella
Department of Clinical and Experimental Medicine, University of Messina, Messina, Italy
e-mail: gianluca.dibella@unime.it

M. Emdin et al. (eds.), *Cardiac Amyloidosis*,
https://doi.org/10.1007/978-3-031-51757-0_10

10.1 Introduction

Cardiac magnetic resonance (CMR) is a multiparametric, highly reproducible, non-invasive imaging technique, with a relatively high spatial, temporal, and contrast resolution. Its versatility is made possible thanks to a great number of different sequences, each obtained by a precise combination of magnetic gradients and radio-frequency pulses, which allow the study of almost all cardiovascular diseases [1]. Indeed, CMR allows not only the quantification of biventricular volumes, mass, wall thickness, systolic- and diastolic function, intra- and extracardiac flows, but also the detection of myocardial oedema, fibrosis, and the accumulation of other intra/extracellular substances (such as fat, iron, amyloid), thus providing unique information for the etiologic, diagnostic, and prognostic definition of cardiomyopathies [2]. As compared to the wide range of information derived from CMR, there are only few contraindications, mostly related to MR-unsafe metal implants, severe renal failure (which limits the use of several gadolinium-based contrast agents), patient discomfort (claustrophobia), and tachyarrhythmias or poor breath-holding (with consequent impairment of image quality) [3].

CMR is widely regarded as the gold standard technique for the differential diagnosis of cardiomyopathies with hypertrophic phenotypes [4]. In patients with suspected or defined amyloidosis, it provides unique diagnostic and prognostic information about myocardial involvement, thanks to its capacity to characterize myocardial tissue composition *in vivo* [5]. Despite a very high diagnostic accuracy, with high specificity and good sensitivity [6, 7], CMR cannot be considered as a stand-alone gold standard diagnostic technique for the diagnosis of cardiac amyloidosis (CA), mainly because it can miss very early disease and cannot distinguish between amyloid subtypes.

A comprehensive CMR evaluation for cardiac amyloidosis includes morphologic and functional assessment of the left and right ventricles and atria using cine imaging, evaluation of native T1 signal (assessed on non-contrast T1 mapping), late gadolinium enhancement (LGE), and extracellular volume (ECV) measurement (Table 10.1). T2-mapping may be useful in selected patients, but it is usually

Table 10.1 CMR in cardiac amyloidosis

Collateral findings	Pericardial and pleural effusion, ascites, liver and spleen enlargement
Morpho-functional quantification	Hypertrophy (concentric and symmetric), preserved ejection fraction with low indexed stroke volume, atrial enlargement with hypertrophy of interatrial septum, thrombi in the left atrial appendage, thickening of valves, diastolic dysfunction
Tissue characterization	
°T1 mapping	Native T1 elevated, more sensitive to early alterations than LGE imaging
°LGE	Diffuse subendocardial LGE in a non-coronary territory distribution with apical sparing (early-intermediate phase)/transmural or intramyocardial, patchy distribution, also in the RV or in the atria; early blood darkening and myocardial nulling before the blood pool
°ECV	Elevated (>40%) indirect measure of amyloid burden

reserved to research purposes. In this chapter, we will provide an overview of the technical aspects and clinical usefulness of CMR in the management of patients with CA.

10.2 Morphological and Functional Assessment

CMR enables for a more comprehensive anatomical and functional assessment than echocardiography. Morphological and functional characterization do not require the use of contrast agents, and cine steady-state free precession (SSFP) sequences are frequently adequate to give all of the information required. The accumulation of amyloid fibrils in the interstitial spaces produces a widespread increase in myocardial wall thickness and then a pseudo-hypertrophy that is not confined to the left ventricle (LV), as is typical of other forms of cardiac hypertrophy, but can also affect the right ventricle (RV), atrial walls (e.g., interatrial septum >6 mm in up to 20% of cases) and heart valves [8]. Basal segments appear to be interested earlier in the disease course, while more advanced stages typically present diffuse biventricular and biatrial thickening. This pattern of progression is known as a base-to-apex gradient [9].

Cardiac amyloidosis may present with symmetric or asymmetric, concentric or eccentric hypertrophy, despite the typical form is concentric and symmetric hypertrophy; furthermore, right ventricular (RV) involvement is frequent, and LV-outflow obstruction has been reported in few cases [10]. LV pseudo-hypertrophy is more severe in amyloid transthyretin (ATTR) than light chain (AL) amyloidosis, with little discernible variations between the 2 subtypes [8, 11]. ATTR-CA displays more frequently an asymmetrical septal hypertrophy (sigmoid septal in 55% of cases, reverse septal in 24%), while AL-CA presents more frequently a symmetric hypertrophy (68%) [12]. It is noteworthy that up to 3% of ATTR-CA and 18% of AL-CA patients present a normal myocardial wall thickness. It may be possible to differentiate CA from other types of hypertrophic heart disease using the rapid advancement of pseudo-hypertrophy [10]. Patients with CA do not have a greater incidence of valve disease than patients of the same age, despite the possibility that cardiac valves can thicken [8, 10](Fig. 10.1).

Diastolic dysfunction gradually develops as a result of the accumulation of these abnormal proteins and the associated pseudo hypertrophy, which increases LV stiffness. Therefore, the indexed stroke volume, which is typically reduced, is a more accurate estimate of systolic function than ejection fraction. Even though CMR allows for the assessment of diastolic function, it has never been done outside of a research setting [11].

The development of diastolic dysfunction in CA may be observed indirectly by analysing and quantifying atrial volumes and may get more severe as the disease progresses with higher incidence of atrial fibrillation [13]. Indeed, in later phases, the severe reduction in the atrial contraction is often associated with signs of slow flow ("smoke") or evidence of thrombi in the left atrial appendage, that also occurs in patients in sinus rhythm.

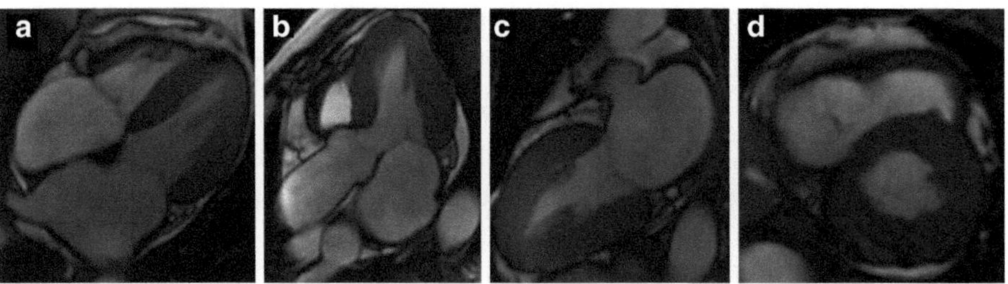

Fig. 10.1 (**Panel a**) Four chamber cine imaging with evidence of hypertrophy (concentric and symmetric), biatrial enlargement, mild pericardial effusion. (**Panel b**) Three chamber cine imaging with evidence of hypertrophy, thickening of valves, mild pericardial effusion. (**Panel c**) Two chamber cine imaging with evidence of hypertrophy and mild pericardial effusion. (**Panel d**) Short axis cine imaging with evidence of hypertrophy and mild pericardial effusion

10.3 Strain

CMR offers higher contrast resolution and image quality than echocardiography, allowing for more accurate assessment of cardiac strain, particularly in patients with difficult acoustic windows.

In cardiac amyloidosis, the strain pattern of the left ventricle typically shows a reduced longitudinal strain and the typical apical sparing [14]. This strain pattern is thought to be due to the accumulation of amyloid fibrils, which leads to stiffness and reduced ability to contract longitudinally with the typical gradient base-apex. Also the RV strain is impaired in CA patients, and a recent study by Eckstein et al. [15] showed that all global RV strain parameters showed a high diagnostic accuracy for the differential diagnosis of CA from other hypertrophic phenotypes.

Furthermore, also the left and right atrial strain patterns can show a diffuse and uniform reduction, which seems to mirror ventricular strain impairment and has been attributed to the deposition of amyloid in the atrial walls. Atrial strain reduction can be seen even in the absence of atrial enlargement, which is commonly seen in other types of cardiac diseases.

The use of strain imaging in both left and right atria can help in the early detection and monitoring of cardiac amyloidosis [16], in combination with additional clinical and radiographic characteristics. This is especially useful for patients who are not candidates for contrast agent delivery.

10.4 Diffusion Tensor Imaging

Diffusion tensor CMR (DT-CMR) is a novel, contrast-free technique that has potential to assess amyloid infiltration by examining the microstructure of the myocardium: DT-CMR has been shown to discriminate between CA and both healthy and hypertrophic cardiomyopathy hearts; moreover, it has unravelled novel abnormalities in sheetlet dynamics that differ between AL and ATTR-CA, suggesting that contractile impairment may have different underlying mechanisms depending on amyloid subtype [17]. Further efforts are needed to increase the availability and robustness of this new technique in routine clinical practice.

10.5 Late Gadolinium Enhancement

Late gadolinium enhancement (LGE) is based on the administration of gadolinium-based paramagnetic contrast media, which distributes both in the intravascular and in the extravascular extracellular space. LGE images are typically acquired 10–15 min after 0.1–0.2 mmol/Kg gadolinium chelates i.v. injection with inversion recovery T1-weighted sequences. This allows to obtain images with a high signal-to-noise ratio, highly reproducible, characterized by a high signal in the regions of diseased myocardium (LGE) and a nulled healthy myocardium. In a healthy heart, cardiomyocytes are densely packed, and the cellular components account for 75–80% of the myocardial volume, explaining the relatively small distribution volume of gadolinium chelates and a typical inversion time (TI) at 250–350 ms of normal myocardium in 1.5 T scanners. On the other hand, any increase in interstitial spaces causes an increase in LGE signal, because a higher concentration of gadolinium causes TI and T1 shortening, which is reflected by a higher signal intensity in T1-weighted sequences. As a result, LGE presence, which is expressed by a delayed wash-out of gadolinium relative to the normal myocardium, can be used to detect enlarged extracellular spaces in CA caused by extracellular amyloid deposition [18]. The presence, extent, and localization of LGE allow not only to detect cardiac amyloid deposition but also to differentiate it from ischemic heart disease (subendocardial or transmural distribution in a coronary artery territory) or non-ischemic cardiomyopathies. The typical LGE pattern in CA is variable according to disease stage, ranging from a focal and patchy intramyocardial enhancement in very early stages, to circumferential and subendocardial in intermediate stages or even diffuse transmural in more advanced stages (subendocardial-to-transmural gradient). Moreover, LGE typically spreads from the basal to the apical segments (base-apex gradient), a phenomenon known also as apical sparing and accompanied by a similar progression of myocardial hypertrophy (Fig. 10.2) [9]. LGE can be found also in the RV and has been described also in the atrial walls, interatrial septum, and cardiac valves [19–21].

To date, LGE represents the key CMR technique to image CA, being the presence of diffuse subendocardial-to-transmural LGE highly specific for CA (94%). Despite it is able to track extracellular amyloid deposition in the myocardium, this technique still presents several technical limitations. First, being CA a diffuse extracellular disease, LGE is typically not well delimited from the healthy myocardium compared to other ischaemic or non-ischaemic diseases [22, 23] and cannot provide amyloid quantification as a percentage of myocardial mass. Moreover, LGE tracks all extracellular components and is not specific for amyloid deposition [24, 25].

Second, LGE can miss very early disease where LGE is limited to small areas of basal LV segments, making it difficult to differentiate very early CA from other

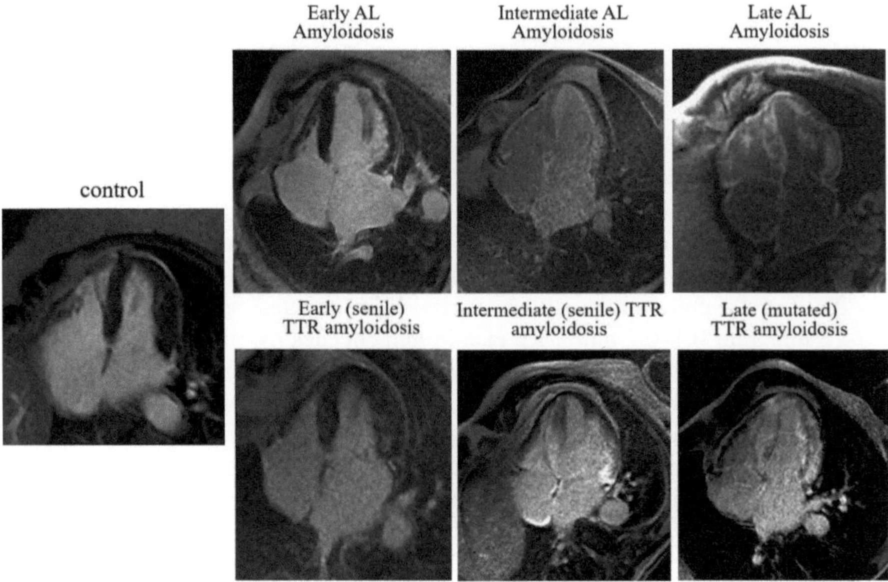

Fig. 10.2 Four chamber late enhancement imaging showing the typical pattern after contrast injection represented by diffuse enhancement, which can be focal and patchy in the early stages, circumferential and subendocardial in the intermediate stages, or even diffuse transmural in the later stages (subendocardial-to-transmural gradient). Furthermore, LGE usually spreads from the basal to apical segments (base-apex gradient). The most common pattern in AL amyloidosis is diffuse subendocardial LGE in a non-coronary territory distribution with a dark blood pool, whereas LGE in ATTR amyloidosis is typically more diffuse and even transmural

early ischaemic (subendocardial) or nonischaemic (intramyocardial) scars. On the other hand, LGE imaging may be challenging in advanced stages due to the diffuse nature of LGE and to the equalization of myocardial and blood pool nulling point. Indeed, patients with massive interstitial depositions of amyloid fibrils present a marked myocardial gadolinium uptake causing a significant post-contrast TI and T1 shortening; at the same time, they present a faster gadolinium washout from the bloodpool (due to extracellular space increase in the liver, spleen, kidneys, and other organs) causing a slight increase of bloodpool TI and T1, and appearing as a darker blood pool in LGE images. The latter phenomenon, also known as "early bloodpool darkening" is quite specific of advanced CA, particularly AL patients, while it is absent in almost all other cardiac diseases [26]. In advanced stages, this paradoxical behaviour of inversion times (significant shortening of myocardial TI, slight increase of bloodpool TI) explains why the myocardium nulls at the same time or even before the bloodpool, and why it is difficulty to choose an optimal T1 value to null the myocardium (it nulls only with very short TI, when the bloodpool too is nulled). To solve this problem, several approaches have been studied, including running a TI-scout sequence (also known as Look-Locker, i.e. a series of images with various inversion time values) to detect paradoxical TIs of the bloodpool vs the

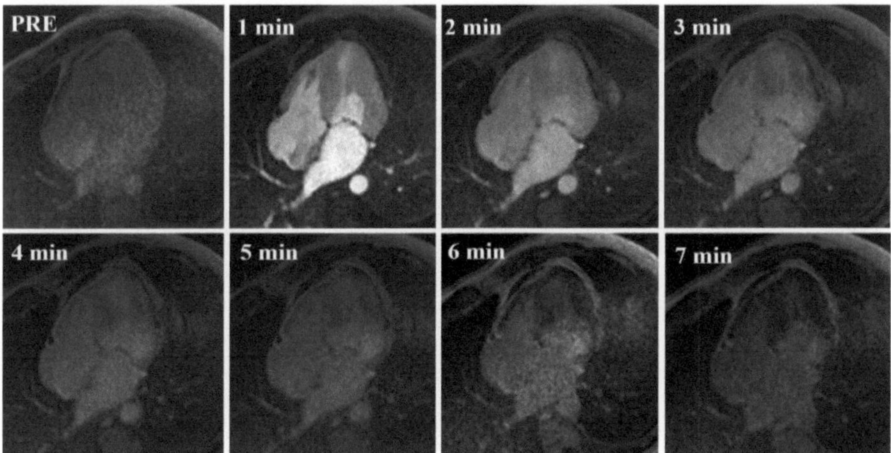

Fig. 10.3 Four chamber view early enhancement imaging, acquired every minute after gadolinium injection: an abnormal gadolinium kinetics in the basal segments of the left ventricle is apparent from the persistence of signal hyperintensity overtime, suggesting gadolinium retention due to amyloid deposition compared to the normal myocardium of the mid and apical segments (which, in turn, display a normal wash-in and wash-out gadolinium kinetics over time)

myocardium, early gadolinium enhancement sequences to track gadolinium kinetics in tissues [27] (Fig. 10.3) or Phase Sensitive Inversion Recovery (PSIR) sequences to null the tissue (blood or myocardium) with the longest T1 (least gadolinium) [23]. In particular, compared to traditional (magnitude) LGE images, PSIR LGE sequences eliminate the need to optimize null-point settings, making LGE in cardiac amyloidosis more robust and operator independent, with a near 100% accuracy for amyloid detection even when there is no healthy myocardium as a reference [28, 29]. All these characteristic alterations in inversion times responsible of the aforementioned challenges in myocardial nulling are strongly suggestive of the presence of amyloid deposits, thus supporting the diagnosis of CA.

Finally, LGE and CMR cannot distinguish between amyloid subtypes. In AL amyloidosis, the most common pattern is diffuse subendocardial LGE in a noncoronary territory distribution with a dark blood pool, while in ATTR amyloidosis LGE is typically more diffuse and even transmural [22, 23]. This different presentation is not always present and highly dependent on the disease stage, so that it is nearly impossible to reliably distinguish between the two forms of amyloidosis. A score named Query Amyloid Late Enhancement (QALE) has been proposed, which is calculated by giving a score from 0 to 6 to LGE extent (from absent to circumferential and transmural) to the basal, mid-cavity, and apical sections. Six other points are assigned when right ventricular (RV) LGE is present. A QALE score ≥ 13 identifies ATTR amyloidosis with 82% sensitivity and 76% specificity, which become 87% and 96%, respectively, if the differential diagnosis includes other variables such as age and interventricular septal thickness [30].

10.6 T1 Mapping

Over the last years, mapping techniques for a quantitative analysis of tissue changes have been developed. Their acquisition and interpretation have been standardized in recent consensus statements [31]. T1 mapping measures the longitudinal magnetization of hydrogen nuclei: each pixel in the parametric image is colour-coded, reflecting the absolute value of T1. Native (pre-contrast) T1 mapping encompasses both intracellular and extracellular changes in the myocardium: T1 times increase when myocardial edema [32], fibrosis [33], and amyloidosis [34] are present and decrease in disorders such as hemochromatosis [35] and Fabry disease [36]. Karamitsos et al. have shown that native T1 presents a higher diagnostic accuracy (sensitivity and specificity of 92% and 91%, respectively) than LGE in a population of patients with AL-CA [34]. Native T1 is increased in both AL and ATTR-CA compared with both healthy subjects and hypertrophic cardiomyopathy, with AL-CA showing slightly higher values than ATTR-CA [37] (Fig. 10.4). Moreover, in ATTR-CA patients, native T1 values have been shown to correlate with Perugini score from bone scintigraphy. In a recent study on 222 AL-CA, 214 ATTR-CA compared with 427 patients without CA, a native T1 < 1036 ms was associated with 98% negative predictive value for CA, whereas a native T1 > 1164 ms was associated with 98% positive predictive value for CA, restricting the need for contrast administration only to patients with intermediate probability (native T1 between 1036 and 1164 ms), corresponding to 58% of patients in this population [38].

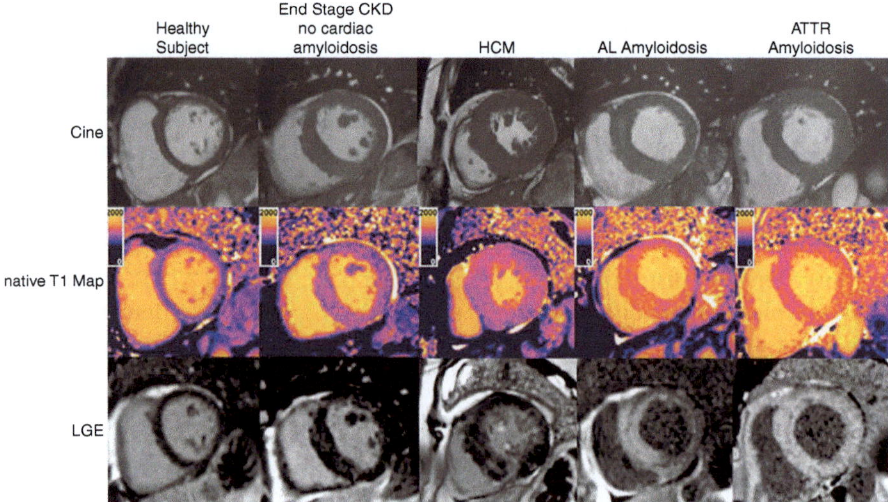

Fig. 10.4 Cardiac magnetic resonance imaging of hypertrophic phenocopies. Top row: short axis cine imaging. Middle row: native T1 is higher in AL and ATTR-CA than in healthy subjects and hypertrophic cardiomyopathy (HCM), with AL-CA having slightly higher values than ATTR-CA. Bottom row: short axis late enhancement imaging (LGE). Reprinted with permission from Baggiano et al. [38]

Moreover, myocardial radiomic phenotyping has demonstrated to enhance the diagnostic yield of T1 mapping for myocardial disease detection and classification: myocardial texture analysis by specific radiomic features outperformed mean native T1 values for the differential diagnosis between CA and other hypertrophic phenocopies [39].

10.7   T2 Mapping

T2 mapping measures the decay of transversal magnetization of hydrogen nuclei and is more specific to detect tissue water content, i.e. oedema. T2 is often elevated in cardiac amyloidosis, particularly in AL patients, and histological correlation shows that edema is part of acute cardiac amyloidosis (particularly AL) and is linked to prognosis [40].

10.8   Perfusion

Amyloid deposition affects not only myocardial interstitium, but also intramyocardial arteries, resulting in decreased myocardial perfusion. Indeed myocardial ischaemia has been described in cardiac amyloidosis, with stress myocardial blood flow mapping and myocardial perfusion reserve similar to that of patients with three vessel coronary artery disease. The reduction correlates with the degree of amyloid infiltration and prognostic indicators, emphasizing the probable significance of myocardial ischaemia as a key mechanism in the pathophysiology of cardiac amyloidosis [41].

10.9   ECV Mapping

Post-contrast T1 mapping allows to differentiate between intracellular and extracellular components by marking selectively the interstitial spaces with gadolinium chelates. The extracellular volume (ECV) can be calculated as a percentage of myocardial volume from the ratio of signal change in blood and myocardium after contrast administration, taking into account the blood contrast volume of distribution (equal to one minus haematocrit). While native T1 is a composite signal from both the extra and intracellular space, ECV is more specific for extracellular remodelling, representing to date the best parameter for quantifying amyloid compared to other CMR parameters [42]. Myocardial ECV represents the quantitative counterpart of LGE and correlates with the extent of interstitial space derangement (where gadolinium-based contrast agents accumulate): myocardial necrosis, interstitial oedema, fibrosis, and amyloidosis are the most common causes of an increased ECV [43], as demonstrated by some recent histological studies [24, 25]. Differently from LGE, ECV mapping does not require the presence of local differences in the myocardium, thus allowing the detection of diffuse myocardial changes (i.e. diffuse interstitial fibrosis) independently from disease stage: for this reason, it is of utmost importance both in earlier stages (where LGE might not be apparent) and in advanced staged (where LGE is diffuse and can hardly be distinguished from the bloodpool because of TI equalization).

Banypersad et al. have demonstrated that extracellular volume is on average significantly higher in patients with CA [44]. The normal ECV is usually in the range of 22–28%. It can grow significantly in localized scar or edema, but it nearly never exceeds 40% in diffuse fibrosis. A global increase >40% is likely to be cardiac amyloidosis (or rarely, global myocardial edema). ECV is higher in patients with ATTR (0.60 ± 0.07) than in those with AL (0.54 ± 0.07), and the opposite trend in native T1 (higher in AL, lower in ATTR) suggests that myocardial oedema may contribute to T1 increase in AL-CA, from possible light chain toxicity. Moreover, ATTR is associated with higher cell volume, suggesting that the increase in absolute left ventricular myocardial mass is not exclusively extracellular, with an additional 18% increase in the intracellular space, while in AL the increase in left ventricular mass is completely extracellular with no cellular hypertrophy [45].

10.10 Extracardiac Findings

Image interpretation and reporting should highlight effusions and other extracardiac features for a more comprehensive approach. Particularly when a hematologic condition underlies the infiltrative disorder, liver and spleen enlargement are among the most frequent extracardiac signs in individuals with AL-CA. Additionally, pleural, pericardial, or peritoneal effusions may result from heart failure related to CA, and their severity might vary [10]. Indeed the presence of effusion and ascites when systolic function is preserved is one sign of cardiac amyloidosis. Occasionally, the presence of increased gas in the bowel or dilated oesophagus from autonomic dysfunction, and fatty liver changes with hypovascular appearance can be seen. Recent research by L. Chacko et al. shows that ECV measurements taken during routine CMR scans in patients with suspected amyloidosis can detect and quantify the degree of amyloid infiltration in the liver and spleen, offering crucial indications to amyloid type and a non-invasive measure of visceral amyloid burden that can help direct and monitor treatment [46].

10.11 CMR for Prognostic Assessment

Beyond its role in the diagnostic workup of CA, CMR appears mostly important for prognostic information. Multiple CMR measures have prognostic significance in cardiac amyloidosis, including LGE presence and pattern, native T1, post-contrast T1, and multiple morphologic parameters. In some early studies on LGE patterns of cardiac amyloidosis, there were heterogeneous results due to non-standardized acquisition and analysis. The transition to more robust LGE approaches, such as PSIR, has provided more robust data on patients' prognosis, through visualization of a continuum of amyloid accumulation as determined by progression of the LGE pattern from subendocardial-to-transmural [23]. As a result, several studies now show that the LGE pattern can serve as an independent predictor of prognosis after adjustments for echocardiographic characteristics and blood biomarkers (NT-proBNP and troponin) [47], in both AL and ATTR cardiac amyloidosis. Despite its prognostic usefulness, LGE does not lend itself readily towards quantification of myocardial infiltration, owing to different patterns and signal intensities. Parametric mapping has the potential to overcome these limitations. Recent studies have shown that higher native myocardial T1 can accurately stratify worse prognosis in AL cardiac amyloidosis, but ECV has been found to be the parameter with the highest hazard ratio (as compared to LGE and native T1) in predicting patients' prognosis both in AL and ATTR cardiac amyloidosis after adjustment for known independent predictors [12, 40]. T2 mapping, a measure of myocardial edema, adds a third dimension to the tissue characterization; in patients with AL cardiac amyloidosis, it is an independent predictor of prognosis [48].

10.12 CMR for Disease Monitoring

CA is a progressive disease, which may present variable increase of LV wall thickness and mass, decline of LV systo/diastolic function, increase of LGE mirroring the progressive deposition of amyloid chains. On the other hand, several disease modifying drugs have been developed both for AL and ATTR subtypes, raising the question about the most accurate technique to monitor disease response. Besides clinical, biohumoral, and echocardiographic parameters, almost all conventional CMR parameters are all good candidate for an accurate assessment of disease progression or regression, even though they show little sensitivity to subtle diseases changes.

In addition to their diagnostic and prognostic value, native T1, T2 and ECV mapping are able to track disease severity [49], and there is early evidence that they could be sensitive markers to detect even small changes in amyloid burden over time [50]. In particular, T1 mapping (native and ECV) can indeed changes over time while wall thickness, mass, LGE, and systo/diastolic function remain unchanged, and this knowledge on myocardial remodelling might transform our knowledge of the disease. As an example, when effective chemotherapy for AL results in a full haematological response and switch-off of clonal light chains, T1 and ECV can reverse, and the time course for these events can be followed [51]. Patients with similar haematological responses may indeed be associated with quite different cardiac responses: changes in ECV independently correlate with prognosis after adjusting for known predictors, highlighting the role of CMR and T1 mapping refining treatment response in cardiac AL amyloidosis.

10.13 Use of CMR: Current Recommendations by Scientific Societies

Several scientific societies from all over the world have recently issued position papers or equivalent documents regarding amyloidosis, and most specifically cardiac amyloidosis (CA), recommending slightly different algorithms for the diagnosis of CA [52]. All documents underline the role for CMR to detect cardiac amyloidosis, even though only the German Cardiac Society (DGK) statement explicitly include a CMR-based path in the diagnostic algorithm, at the same level of myocardial scintigraphy: *"MR offers an indispensable method for the detection of cardiac amyloidosis, both in the context of classical methods (LGE) and by extension to the new mapping procedures, and should be used early in cases of unclear left-ventricular hypertrophy"* [53]. This CMR-based diagnostic path parallels the "scintigraphy-based" path and the "laboratory-based (monoclonal protein) path", even though it inevitably needs an invasive (biopsy) or non-invasive (scintigraphy and monoclonal protein assessment) to reach a definite, etiological diagnosis. Moreover, *"the decision whether to perform a multi-parametric CMR study and/or a 99mTc-phosphate scintigraphy for further non-invasive work-up of suspected cardiac amyloidosis depends (amongst others) on local availability and respective imaging expertise"*.

In all other documents, CMR has not been assigned an independent, specific role in the diagnostic algorithm, mainly because it can miss early disease and cannot distinguish between amyloid subtypes. The European Society of Cardiology (ESC) position statement indicates CMR and echocardiography as equivalent tools for invasive and non-invasive diagnosis of CA: the presence of a typical late enhancement pattern or of an increased extracellular volume allows to diagnose cardiac involvement in patients with an amyloid-positive extracardiac biopsy (invasive), or in patients with positive diphosphonate nuclear scan and negative serum/urinary immunofixation (non-invasive), respectively [54]. In particular, a diffuse subendocardial-to-transmural LGE, an abnormal gadolinium kinetics (myocardial nulling prior to or coinciding with bloodpool nulling, making it difficult to find an optimal inversion time of the myocardium), and an increased ECV (>0.40) are all diagnostic criteria of cardiac involvement in patients with suspected amyloidosis. On the other hand, a negative CMR might be used to rule out the suspicion of CA in patients with extracardiac biopsy-proven amyloidosis or with a positive monoclonal protein. Moreover, CMR (followed by cardiac or extracardiac biopsy) is indicated in case of inconclusive results, as diphosphonate scintigraphy could be negative in some ATTRv mutations (Phe84Leu, Ser97Tyr) and in rare subtypes of cardiac amyloidosis.

Similar indications are recommended by the AHA (*"Cardiac magnetic resonance imaging is not diagnostic for ATTR cardiomyopathy but can suggest the diagnosis and is useful when infiltrative cardiomyopathy, constrictive pericarditis, or myocarditis is suspected"*) [55], by the CCS/CHFS statement (*"Although findings on echocardiography and/or CMR might be highly consistent with cardiac amyloid infiltration, in isolation these tests are generally not considered confirmatory of the diagnosis, and neither test can reliably differentiate subtype"*) [56] and by the JCS guideline (*"CMR can be used to diagnose advanced CA easily, [even though] its ability to diagnose other early diseases and amyloid types is limited; [...] CMR findings should be assessed in conjunction with the results of other tests and clinical findings"*) [57]. Differently from the ESC, most other societies include an increased native T1 among the diagnostic parameters to suggest the diagnosis of CA.

Finally, similar indications have also been more recently confirmed by the joint ASNC/AHA/ASE/EANM/HFSA/ISA/SCMR/SNMMI expert consensus recommendations: *in patients with biopsy-proven systemic amyloidosis, typical CMR findings (including diffuse LGE, nulling of myocardium before or at the same inversion time as the blood pool, and extensive ECV expansion) are combined with structural findings (increased wall thickness and myocardial mass) to diagnose cardiac involvement; in the absence of documented systemic amyloidosis, typical CMR features should prompt further evaluation for cardiac amyloidosis. CMR, however, is typically unable to definitively distinguish AL from ATTR cardiac amyloidosis [and] should be combined with electrocardiographic, clinical, biomarker, and other imaging findings to maximize diagnostic accuracy* [58].

10.14 Conclusions

Cardiac amyloidosis is a progressive disease causing extracellular myocardial infiltration by light chain or transthyretin fibrils. Prompt diagnosis and treatment are critical as prognosis can be as poor as months. CMR is a key tool in the diagnosis and assessment of CA; cine sequences provide superior morphological and functional information, while LGE, T1 mapping, and ECV are used for diagnosis, localization, and quantification of myocardial amyloid infiltration and correlated with prognosis. Overall, ECV is considered the best quantitative measure of amyloid burden as it is specific for the extracellular space and is less sensitive to oedema. However, gadolinium is unsuitable for patients with significant renal impairment, where non-contrast technique (in particular native T1) may offer several advantages. Other techniques may be combined to provide further details on myocardial mechanics (strain) or tissue remodelling (T2, perfusion), and several others are on the horizon (including diffusion tensor imaging). Further studies are needed to integrate all these sequences in established diagnostic and prognostic algorithms to be used on a large scale, taking into account all other clinical parameters and imaging modalities.

References

1. Kramer CM, Barkhausen J, Bucciarelli-Ducci C, Flamm SD, Kim RJ, Nagel E. Standardized cardiovascular magnetic resonance imaging (CMR) protocols: 2020 update. J Cardiovasc Magn Reson. 2020;22:1–18. https://doi.org/10.1186/S12968-020-00607-1/FIGURES/7.
2. Merlo M, Gagno G, Baritussio A, Bauce B, Biagini E, Canepa M, et al. Clinical application of CMR in cardiomyopathies: evolving concepts and techniques a position paper of myocardial

and pericardial diseases and cardiac magnetic resonance working groups of Italian society of cardiology. Heart Fail Rev. 2023;28:77–95. https://doi.org/10.1007/s10741-022-10235-9.

3. Barison A, Baritussio A, Cipriani A, De Lazzari M, Aquaro GD, Guaricci AI, et al. Cardiovascular magnetic resonance: what clinicians should know about safety and contraindications. Int J Cardiol. 2021;331:322–8. https://doi.org/10.1016/J.IJCARD.2021.02.003.

4. Barison A, Aimo A, Todiere G, Grigoratos C, Aquaro GD, Emdin M. Cardiovascular magnetic resonance for the diagnosis and management of heart failure with preserved ejection fraction. Heart Fail Rev. 2022;27:191–205. https://doi.org/10.1007/S10741-020-09998-W/METRICS.

5. Maceira AM, Joshi J, Prasad SK, Moon JC, Perugini E, Harding I, et al. Cardiovascular magnetic resonance in cardiac amyloidosis. Circulation. 2005;111:186–93. https://doi.org/10.1161/01.CIR.0000152819.97857.9D.

6. Vogelsberg H, Mahrholdt H, Deluigi CC, Yilmaz A, Kispert EM, Greulich S, et al. Cardiovascular magnetic resonance in clinically suspected cardiac amyloidosis. Noninvasive imaging compared to endomyocardial biopsy. J Am Coll Cardiol. 2008;51:1022–30. https://doi.org/10.1016/j.jacc.2007.10.049.

7. Zhao L, Tian Z, Fang Q. Diagnostic accuracy of cardiovascular magnetic resonance for patients with suspected cardiac amyloidosis: a systematic review and meta-analysis. BMC Cardiovasc Disord. 2016;16:1–10. https://doi.org/10.1186/S12872-016-0311-6/FIGURES/5.

8. Fattori R, Rocchi G, Celletti F, Bertaccini P, Rapezzi C, Gavelli G. Contribution of magnetic resonance imaging in the differential diagnosis of cardiac amyloidosis and symmetric hypertrophic cardiomyopathy. Am Heart J. 1998;136:824–30. https://doi.org/10.1016/S0002-8703(98)70127-9.

9. Williams LK, Forero JF, Popovic ZB, Phelan D, Delgado D, Rakowski H, et al. Patterns of CMR measured longitudinal strain and its association with late gadolinium enhancement in patients with cardiac amyloidosis and its mimics. J Cardiovasc Magn Reson. 2017;19(1):61. https://doi.org/10.1186/s12968-017-0376-0.

10. Fontana M, Chung R, Hawkins PN, Moon JC. Cardiovascular magnetic resonance for amyloidosis. Heart Fail Rev. 2015;20:133–44. https://doi.org/10.1007/s10741-014-9470-7.

11. Rubinshtein R, Glockner JF, Feng DL, Araoz PA, Kirsch J, Syed IS, et al. Comparison of magnetic resonance imaging versus Doppler echocardiography for the evaluation of left ventricular diastolic function in patients with cardiac amyloidosis. Am J Cardiol. 2009;103:718–23. https://doi.org/10.1016/j.amjcard.2008.10.039.

12. Martinez-Naharro A, Treibel TA, Abdel-Gadir A, Bulluck H, Zumbo G, Knight DS, et al. Magnetic resonance in transthyretin cardiac amyloidosis. J Am Coll Cardiol. 2017;70:466–77. https://doi.org/10.1016/J.JACC.2017.05.053.

13. Di Bella G, Minutoli F, Madaffari A, Mazzeo A, Russo M, Donato R, et al. Left atrial function in cardiac amyloidosis. J Cardiovasc Med. 2016;17:113–21. https://doi.org/10.2459/JCM.0000000000000188.

14. Nardozza M, Chiodi E, Mele D. Left ventricle relative apical sparing in cardiac amyloidosis. J Cardiovasc Echogr. 2017;27:141–2. https://doi.org/10.4103/JCECHO.JCECHO_22_17.

15. Eckstein J, Körperich H, Weise Valdés E, Sciacca V, Paluszkiewicz L, Burchert W, et al. CMR-based right ventricular strain analysis in cardiac amyloidosis and its potential as a supportive diagnostic feature. Int J Cardiol Heart Vasc. 2022;44:44. https://doi.org/10.1016/J.IJCHA.2022.101167.

16. Qu Y-Y, Buckert D, Ma G-S, Rasche V. Quantitative assessment of left and right atrial strains using cardiovascular magnetic resonance based tissue tracking. Front Cardiovasc Med. 2021;8:633. https://doi.org/10.3389/FCVM.2021.690240.

17. Khalique Z, Ferreira PF, Scott AD, Nielles-Vallespin S, Martinez-Naharro A, Fontana M, et al. Diffusion tensor cardiovascular magnetic resonance in cardiac amyloidosis. Circ Cardiovasc Imaging. 2020;13:9901. https://doi.org/10.1161/CIRCIMAGING.119.009901.

18. Doltra A, Amundsen B, Gebker R, Fleck E, Kelle S. Emerging concepts for myocardial late gadolinium enhancement MRI. Curr Cardiol Rev. 2013;9:185–90. https://doi.org/10.2174/1573403x113099990030.

19. Kristen AV, Scherer K, Kammerer R, Andre F, Buss SJ, Bauer R, et al. Comparison of different types of cardiac amyloidosis by cardiac magnetic resonance imaging. Amyloid. 2015;00:1–10. https://doi.org/10.3109/13506129.2015.1020153.
20. Austin BA, Tang WHW, Rodriguez ER, Tan C, Flamm SD, Taylor DO, et al. Delayed hyperenhancement magnetic resonance imaging provides incremental diagnostic and prognostic utility in suspected cardiac amyloidosis. JACC Cardiovasc Imaging. 2009;2:1369–77. https://doi.org/10.1016/j.jcmg.2009.08.008.
21. Kwong RY, Heydari B, Abbasi S, Stell K, Al-Mallah M, Wu H, et al. Characterization of cardiac amyloidosis by atrial late gadolinium enhancement using contrast enhanced cardiac magnetic resonance imaging and correlation with left atrial conduit and contractile function. Am J Cardiol. 2016;116:622–9. https://doi.org/10.1016/j.amjcard.2015.05.021.Characterization.
22. Fontana M, Corovic A, Scully P, Moon JC. Myocardial amyloidosis: the exemplar interstitial disease. JACC Cardiovasc Imaging. 2019;12:2345–56. https://doi.org/10.1016/j.jcmg.2019.06.023.
23. Fontana M, Pica S, Reant P, Abdel-gadir A, Treibel TA, Banypersad SM, et al. Prognostic value of late gadolinium enhancement cardiovascular magnetic resonance in cardiac amyloidosis. Circulation. 2015;132(16):1570–9. https://doi.org/10.1161/CIRCULATIONAHA.115.016567.
24. Morioka M, Takashio S, Nakashima N, Nishi M, Fujiyama A, Hirakawa K, et al. Correlation between cardiac images, biomarkers, and amyloid load in wild-type transthyretin amyloid cardiomyopathy. J Am Heart Assoc. 2022;11:e024717. https://doi.org/10.1161/JAHA.121.024717.
25. Pucci A, Aimo A, Musetti V, Barison A, Vergaro G, Genovesi D, et al. Amyloid deposits and fibrosis on left ventricular endomyocardial biopsy correlate with extracellular volume in cardiac amyloidosis. J Am Heart Assoc. 2021;10:10. https://doi.org/10.1161/JAHA.120.020358.
26. Martini N, Aimo A, Barison A, Della Latta D, Vergaro G, Aquaro GD, et al. Deep learning to diagnose cardiac amyloidosis from cardiovascular magnetic resonance. J Cardiovasc Magn Reson. 2020;22:1–11. https://doi.org/10.1186/S12968-020-00690-4/FIGURES/6.
27. Emdin M, Aquaro GD, Pugliese NR, Del Franco A, Todiere G, Perfetto F, et al. Myocardial gadolinium kinetics evaluation at Mri for the diagnosis of cardiac amyloidosis. J Am Coll Cardiol. 2013;61:E1237. https://doi.org/10.1016/s0735-1097(13)61237-1.
28. Everett RJ, Stirrat CG, Semple SIR, Newby DE, Dweck MR, Mirsadraee S. Assessment of myocardial fi brosis with T1 mapping MRI. Clin Radiol. 2016;71:768–78. https://doi.org/10.1016/j.crad.2016.02.013.
29. Tseng W-YI, Su M-YM, Tseng Y-HE. Introduction to cardiovascular magnetic resonance: technical principles and clinical applications. Acta Cardiol Sin. 2016;32:129–44.
30. Dungu JN, Valencia O, Pinney JH, Gibbs SDJ, Rowczenio D, Gilbertson JA, et al. CMR-based differentiation of AL and ATTR cardiac amyloidosis. JACC Cardiovasc Imaging. 2014;7:133–42. https://doi.org/10.1016/j.jcmg.2013.08.015.
31. Messroghli DR, Moon JC, Ferreira VM, Grosse-Wortmann L, He T, Kellman P, et al. Clinical recommendations for cardiovascular magnetic resonance mapping of T1, T2, T2* and extracellular volume: a consensus statement by the Society for Cardiovascular Magnetic Resonance (SCMR) endorsed by the European Association for Cardiovascular Imaging (EACVI). J Cardiovasc Magn Reson. 2017;19:75. https://doi.org/10.1186/S12968-017-0389-8.
32. Germain P, El Ghannudi S, Jeung M-Y, Ohlmann P, Epailly E, Roy C, et al. Native T1 mapping of the heart—a pictorial review. Clin Med Insights Cardiol. 2014;8:1–11. https://doi.org/10.4137/CMC.S19005.
33. Puntmann VO, Voigt T, Chen Z, Mayr M, Karim R, Rhode K, et al. Native T1 mapping in differentiation of normal myocardium from diffuse disease in hypertrophic and dilated cardiomyopathy. JACC Cardiovasc Imaging. 2013;6:475–84. https://doi.org/10.1016/j.jcmg.2012.08.019.
34. Karamitsos TD, Piechnik SK, Banypersad SM, Fontana M, Ntusi NB, Ferreira VM, et al. Noncontrast T1 mapping for the diagnosis of cardiac amyloidosis. JACC Cardiovasc Imaging. 2013;6:488–97. https://doi.org/10.1016/j.jcmg.2012.11.013.
35. Feng Y, He T, Carpenter J-P, Jabbour A, Alam MH, Gatehouse PD, et al. In vivo comparison of myocardial T1 with T2 and T2* in thalassaemia major. J Magn Reson Imaging. 2013;38:588–93. https://doi.org/10.1002/jmri.24010.

36. Sado DM, White SK, Piechnik SK, Banypersad SM, Treibel T, Captur G, et al. Identification and assessment of Anderson-Fabry disease by cardiovascular magnetic resonance noncontrast myocardial T1 mapping. Circ Cardiovasc Imaging. 2013;6:392–8. https://doi.org/10.1161/CIRCIMAGING.112.000070.

37. Fontana M, Banypersad SM, Treibel TA, Maestrini V, Sado DM, White SK, et al. Native T1 mapping in transthyretin amyloidosis. JACC Cardiovasc Imaging. 2014;7:157–65. https://doi.org/10.1016/J.JCMG.2013.10.008.

38. Baggiano A, Boldrini M, Martinez-Naharro A, Kotecha T, Petrie A, Rezk T, et al. Noncontrast magnetic resonance for the diagnosis of cardiac amyloidosis. JACC Cardiovasc Imaging. 2020;13:69–80. https://doi.org/10.1016/J.JCMG.2019.03.026.

39. Antonopoulos AS, Boutsikou M, Simantiris S, Angelopoulos A, Lazaros G, Panagiotopoulos I, et al. Machine learning of native T1 mapping radiomics for classification of hypertrophic cardiomyopathy phenotypes. Sci Rep. 2021;11:1–11. https://doi.org/10.1038/s41598-021-02971-z.

40. Banypersad SM, Fontana M, Maestrini V, Sado DM, Captur G, Petrie A, et al. T1 mapping and survival in systemic light-chain amyloidosis. Eur Heart J. 2015;36:244–51. https://doi.org/10.1093/eurheartj/ehu444.

41. Kotecha T, Martinez-Naharro A, Brown J, Little C, Knight D, Steriotis A, et al. 19 myocardial perfusion mapping in cardiac amyloidosis- unearthing the spectrum from infiltration to ischaemia. Heart. 2019;105:A17–7. https://doi.org/10.1136/HEARTJNL-2019-BSCMR.19.

42. Pan JA, Kerwin MJ, Salerno M. Native T1 mapping, extracellular volume mapping, and late gadolinium enhancement in cardiac amyloidosis: a meta-analysis. JACC Cardiovasc Imaging. 2020;13:1299–310. https://doi.org/10.1016/J.JCMG.2020.03.010.

43. Ugander M, Oki AJ, Hsu LY, Kellman P, Greiser A, Aletras AH, et al. Extracellular volume imaging by magnetic resonance imaging provides insights into overt and sub-clinical myocardial pathology. Eur Heart J. 2012;33:1268–78. https://doi.org/10.1093/EURHEARTJ/EHR481.

44. Banypersad SM, Sado DM, Flett AS, Gibbs SDJ, Pinney JH, Maestrini V, et al. Quantification of myocardial extracellular volume fraction in systemic AL amyloidosis: an equilibrium contrast cardiovascular magnetic resonance study. Circ Cardiovasc Imaging. 2013;6:34–9. https://doi.org/10.1161/CIRCIMAGING.112.978627.

45. Fontana M, Banypersad SM, Treibel TA, Abdel-Gadir A, Maestrini V, Lane T, et al. Differential myocyte responses in patients with cardiac transthyretin amyloidosis and light-chain amyloidosis: a cardiac MR imaging study. Radiology. 2015;277:388–97. https://doi.org/10.1148/RADIOL.2015141744.

46. Chacko L, Boldrini M, Martone R, Law S, Martinez-Naharrro A, Hutt DF, et al. Cardiac magnetic resonance–derived extracellular volume mapping for the quantification of hepatic and splenic amyloid. Circ Cardiovasc Imaging. 2021;14:314–24. https://doi.org/10.1161/CIRCIMAGING.121.012506.

47. Raina S, Lensing SY, Nairooz RS, Pothineni NVK, Hakeem A, Bhatti S, et al. Prognostic value of late gadolinium enhancement CMR in systemic amyloidosis. JACC Cardiovasc Imaging. 2016;9:1267–77. https://doi.org/10.1016/J.JCMG.2016.01.036.

48. Kotecha T, Martinez-Naharro A, Treibel TA, Francis R, Nordin S, Abdel-Gadir A, et al. Myocardial edema and prognosis in amyloidosis. J Am Coll Cardiol. 2018;71:2919–31. https://doi.org/10.1016/J.JACC.2018.03.536.

49. Barison A, Aquaro GD, Pugliese NR, Cappelli F, Chiappino S, Vergaro G, et al. Measurement of myocardial amyloid deposition in systemic amyloidosis: insights from cardiovascular magnetic resonance imaging. J Intern Med. 2015;277:605–14. https://doi.org/10.1111/joim.12324.

50. Martinez-Naharro A, Abdel-Gadir A, Treibel TA, Zumbo G, Knight DS, Rosmini S, et al. CMR-verified regression of cardiac AL amyloid after chemotherapy. JACC Cardiovasc Imaging. 2018;11:152–4. https://doi.org/10.1016/J.JCMG.2017.02.012.

51. Martinez-Naharro A, Patel R, Kotecha T, Karia N, Ioannou A, Petrie A, et al. Cardiovascular magnetic resonance in light-chain amyloidosis to guide treatment. Eur Heart J. 2022;43:4722–35. https://doi.org/10.1093/EURHEARTJ/EHAC363.

52. Rapezzi C, Aimo A, Serenelli M, Barison A, Vergaro G, Passino C, et al. Critical comparison of documents from scientific societies on cardiac amyloidosis: JACC state-of-the-art review. J Am Coll Cardiol. 2022;79:1288–303. https://doi.org/10.1016/J.JACC.2022.01.036.
53. Yilmaz A, Bauersachs J, Bengel F, Büchel R, Kindermann I, Klingel K, et al. Diagnosis and treatment of cardiac amyloidosis: position statement of the German cardiac society (DGK). Clin Res Cardiol. 2021;110:479. https://doi.org/10.1007/S00392-020-01799-3.
54. Garcia-Pavia P, Rapezzi C, Adler Y, Arad M, Basso C, Brucato A, et al. Diagnosis and treatment of cardiac amyloidosis: a position statement of the ESC working group on myocardial and pericardial diseases. Eur Heart J. 2021;42:1554–68. https://doi.org/10.1093/EURHEARTJ/EHAB072.
55. Kittleson MM, Maurer MS, Ambardekar AV, Bullock-Palmer RP, Chang PP, Eisen HJ, et al. Cardiac amyloidosis: evolving diagnosis and management: a scientific statement from the American Heart Association. Circulation. 2020;142:E7–22. https://doi.org/10.1161/CIR.0000000000000792.
56. Fine NM, Davis MK, Anderson K, Delgado DH, Giraldeau G, Kitchlu A, et al. Canadian cardiovascular society/Canadian heart failure society joint position statement on the evaluation and management of patients with cardiac amyloidosis. Can J Cardiol. 2020;36:322–34. https://doi.org/10.1016/J.CJCA.2019.12.034.
57. Kitaoka H, Izumi C, Izumiya Y, Inomata T, Ueda M, Kubo T, et al. JCS 2020 guideline on diagnosis and treatment of cardiac amyloidosis. Circ J. 2020;84:1610–71. https://doi.org/10.1253/CIRCJ.CJ-20-0110.
58. Dorbala S, Ando Y, Bokhari S, Dispenzieri A, Falk RH, Ferrari VA, et al. ASNC/AHA/ASE/EANM/HFSA/ISA/SCMR/SNMMI expert consensus recommendations for multimodality imaging in cardiac amyloidosis: part 1 of 2—evidence base and standardized methods of imaging. Circ Cardiovasc Imaging. 2021;14:E000029. https://doi.org/10.1161/HCI.0000000000000029.

Biomarkers: Monoclonal Protein and Indicators of Cardiac Damage

11

Vincenzo Castiglione, Maria Franzini, Silvia Masotti, Chiara Arzilli, Michele Emdin, and Giuseppe Vergaro

Abbreviations

(e)GFR	(estimated) glomerular filtration rate
(hs-)TnT	(high-sensitivity) troponin T/I
AL	Amyloid light chain
AS	Aortic stenosis
ASCT	Autologous stem cell transplant
ATTR	Amyloid transthyretin (ATTRv, variant form; ATTRwt, wild-type form)
AUC	Area under the curve
BNP	B-type natriuretic peptide
CA	Cardiac amyloidosis
dFLC	Difference between involved and uninvolved free light chains
ECOG	Eastern Cooperative Oncology Group
FLC	Free light chain
HF	Heart failure

V. Castiglione (✉) · M. Emdin · G. Vergaro
Fondazione Toscana Gabriele Monasterio, Pisa, Italy

Health Science Interdisciplinary Center, Scuola Superiore Sant'Anna, Pisa, Italy
e-mail: vcastiglione@ftgm.it; emdin@ftgm.it; vergaro@ftgm.it

M. Franzini
Department of Translational Research and New Technologies in Medicine and Surgery, University of Pisa, Pisa, Italy
e-mail: maria.franzini@unipi.it

S. Masotti · C. Arzilli
Fondazione Toscana Gabriele Monasterio, Pisa, Italy
e-mail: silvia.masotti@alumni.sssup.it; carzilli@monasterio.it

iFLC	"Involved" free light chains
NAC	National Amyloidosis Centre
NP	Natriuretic peptide
NT-proBNP	N-terminal pro-B-type natriuretic peptide
NYHA	New York Heart Association
TTR	Transthyretin
uFLC	"Uninvolved" free light chains

Cardiac amyloidosis (CA) is a group of systemic disorders characterized by the deposition of abnormal protein fibrils in the heart, leading to progressive heart failure (HF) and poor prognosis. Early detection, accurate diagnosis, and effective risk stratification are critical for guiding treatment decisions and improving patient outcomes. Circulating biomarkers reflect the pathophysiology of amyloidosis (Fig. 11.1), and some of them have emerged as valuable tools in the management of

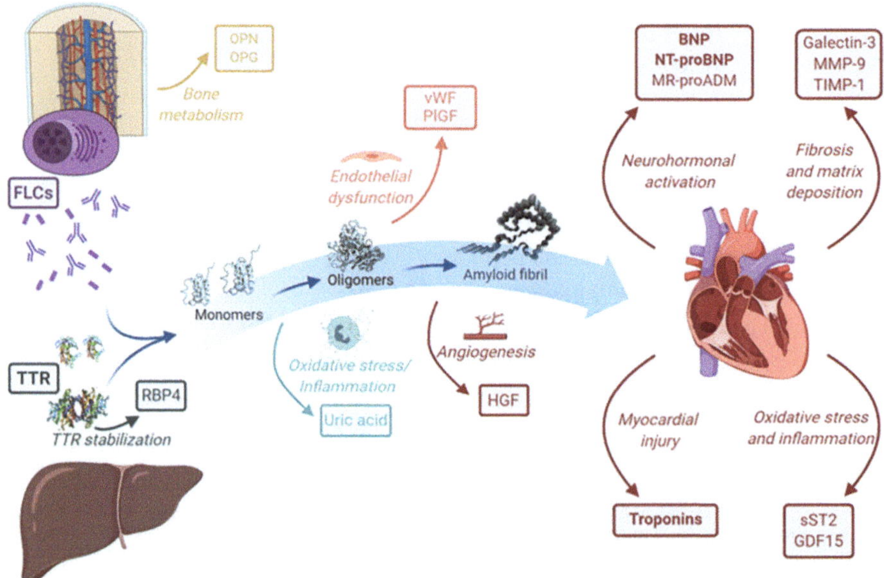

Fig. 11.1 Circulating biomarkers reflect the pathophysiology of cardiac amyloidosis. The amyloidogenic cascade is the pathophysiological process leading to progressive tissue amyloid fibril deposition starting from misfolded monomers. Along this process, multiple pathways are activated, each reflected by the increase of a distinct biomarker. Nonetheless, only a limited number of biomarkers have been incorporated into clinical practice, namely amyloidogenic precursors such as free light chains (FLCs), as well as biomarkers indicating cardiac involvement, such as natriuretic peptides and troponins. *BNP* B-type natriuretic peptide, *GDF15* growth differentiation factor-15, *HGF* hepatocyte growth factor, *MMP-9* matrix metalloproteinase-9, *MR-proADM* mid-regional pro-adrenomedullin, *NT-proBNP* N-terminal pro-B-type natriuretic peptide, *OPG* osteoprotegerin, *OPN* osteopontin, *PlGF* placental growth factor, *RBP4* retinol-binding protein 4, *sST2* soluble suppression of tumorigenicity-2, *TIMP-1* tissue inhibitor of metalloproteinase-1, *TTR* transthyretin, *vWF* von Willebrand factor. Reproduced with permission from Castiglione et al. [18]

CA, providing insights into organ involvement, disease progression, and response to therapy. This review paper aims to explore the role of biomarkers in CA, focusing on two major subtypes: biomarkers related to monoclonal protein and indicators of cardiac damage, namely natriuretic peptides (NPs) and troponins.

11.1 Amyloidogenic Precursors of AL Amyloidosis

Free light chains (FLCs) are the amyloidogenic precursors of amyloid light chain (AL) amyloidosis. FLCs are extensively used in clinical practice for the diagnosis, risk stratification, and treatment monitoring of AL amyloidosis. Transthyretin (TTR) dosage might also have a role to monitor therapeutic response to novel disease-modifying therapies in transthyretin (ATTR) amyloidosis, as discussed in the following chapter.

In healthy individuals, a small quantity of FLCs can be detected in the bloodstream, secreted by plasma cells in slightly higher amounts than heavy chains. κ FLCs primarily exist as monomers, while λ FLCs tend to form dimers. The daily production of FLCs is modest (0.5–1 g/die), with a half-life of 2–4 h. FLCs are typically not detected in urine because they are filtered, reabsorbed, and metabolized by the kidneys. When there is an uncontrolled proliferation of a plasma cell clone, the production of FLCs increases, affecting their levels in the bloodstream and the κ/λ ratio. If the production surpasses the renal reabsorption capacity, FLCs can be identified in the urine as Bence-Jones proteins [1].

FLCs play a role in tissue damage in AL amyloidosis through two mechanisms. First, the amyloidogenic precursors can directly harm cardiomyocytes. In fact, FLCs themselves can promote apoptosis, oxidative stress, mitochondrial dysfunction, impaired calcium handling and contractility, abnormal autophagy, and lysosomal dysfunction. These harmful effects have been observed in both animal models and human cardiomyocytes and fibroblasts. Second, the deposition of amyloid fibrils disrupts the structure of tissues and compromises organ function [2].

FLCs are typically measured using immunochemical methods, which distinguish them from complete antibodies, hence form the overall pool of light chains. There are several commercially available FLC assays, such as Freelite®, N Latex FLC, Diazyme, Seralite®, and Sebia FLC assays, which utilize either polyclonal or monoclonal antibodies. These assays exhibit comparable diagnostic accuracy [3], albeit the International Myeloma Working Group guidelines for serum FLC analysis currently recommend the use of polyclonal assays for clinical use [1]. Moreover, it is crucial to use the same assay for follow-up evaluations in the same patient due to modest agreement between different assays [2, 3].

FLCs serve as important diagnostic tools for all plasma cell disorders, including AL amyloidosis. The combination of FLC quantification, κ/λ ratio, and serum and urine immunofixation provides a precise screening and diagnostic tool for AL amyloidosis. In fact, the κ/λ ratio is altered in over 90% of AL amyloidosis patients while remaining normal in over 50% of individuals with monoclonal gammopathy of unknown significance [1, 4]. Notably, renal function significantly influences the

FLC concentration and can lead to false positive outcomes in individuals with chronic kidney disease. As the glomerular filtration rate (GFR) decreases, there is a noticeable preference for the removal of lambda free light chains by the reticuloendothelial system. This phenomenon, combined with the increased physiological production of kappa free light chains, progressively expands the reference range for polyclonal assays [3, 5, 6]. To address this issue, some researchers utilizing the Freelite® assay have proposed a distinct FLC ratio cutoff for subjects with an estimated GFR (eGFR) of less than 60 mL/min/1.73 m² [5]. Furthermore, a recent study involving a cohort of over 75,000 individuals, also employing the Freelite® assay, suggested revised reference intervals for FLC and FLC ratio for subjects with an eGFR of 45–59, 30–44, and less than 30 mL/min/1.73 m² [6].

The clonal light chains are referred to as "involved" FLCs (iFLCs), while the remaining light chains are classified as "uninvolved" FLCs (uFLCs). The difference between the concentrations of uFLCs and iFLCs, known as dFLC, allows for the assessment of the extent of clonal light chain production responsible for AL amyloidosis [7]. This measurement, along with N-terminal pro-B-type natriuretic peptide (NT-proBNP) and troponin T (TnT), is incorporated into the widely used Mayo2012 prognostic scores for AL amyloidosis [8].

Furthermore, dFLC plays a crucial role in monitoring organ response to therapy in AL amyloidosis as it accurately reflects the quantity of FLCs generated by the monoclonal plasma cells. According to a revised consensus paper from 2012, hematologic response to chemotherapy is classified as follows (Table 11.1): (i) complete response, characterized by negative results in serum and urine immunofixation tests together with either a normal FLC ratio or a uFLC concentration greater that the iFLC concentration with or without an abnormal FLC ratio; (ii) very good partial response, indicated by a decrease in dFLC to <40 mg/L; (iii) partial response, marked by a reduction in dFLC >50%; and (iv) no response. Conversely, haematological disease progression or relapse is defined as follows: (i) in cases of previous complete response, the presence of any detectable monoclonal protein or abnormal κ/λ ratio (FLCs must double); (ii) in cases of previous partial or stable response, a 50% increase in serum M protein levels to values >0.5 g/dL or a 50% increase in urine M protein levels to values >200 mg/day (a monoclonal peak must be visible in electrophoresis); (iii) a 50% increase in FLC up to values >10 mg/dL. The disease is considered stable in the absence of treatment response or disease progression [9, 10].

FLC quantification and urine and serum immunofixation are also crucial in diagnosing ATTR amyloidosis. Specifically, a high-grade cardiac uptake at scintigraphy with bone tracers allows to establish a "non-biopsy" diagnosis of ATTR-CA only after ruling out the presence of a monoclonal gammopathy. Otherwise, a histological demonstration of ATTR amyloid deposits is mandatory [11]. A recent study has suggested that the performance of bone scintigraphy-based non-biopsy diagnostic criteria for ATTR-CA can be further improved by incorporating the revised cutoff values for FLC ratio in patients with impaired renal function [12].

Table 11.1 Haematologic and cardiac response and progression criteria for AL amyloidosis

Response category	Criteria
Haematologic response and progression criteria	
Complete	Both criteria must be met: • Absence of amyloidogenic light chains (either free and/or as part of a complete immunoglobulin) defined by negative immunofixation electrophoresis of both serum and urine • Either a FLC ratio within the reference range or an uninvolved FLC concentration greater than the involved FLC concentration, with or without an abnormal FLC ratio
Very good partial	dFLC decrease to <40 mg/L
Partial	dFLC reduction >50% compared to baseline
Stable/no response	Less than a partial response
Progression	• From complete response, any detectable monoclonal protein or abnormal FLC ratio (light chain must double) • From partial or stable response, 50% increase in serum M protein to >0.5 g/dL or 50% increase in urine M protein to >200 mg/day (a visible peak must be present) • FLC increase of 50% to >10 mg/dL
Cardiac response and progression criteria	
Response	NT-proBNP decrease >30% and > 300 ng/L (>30% and > 50 ng/L respectively for BNP) in patients with baseline NT-proBNP ≥650 ng/L (≥150 ng/L for BNP) Alternatively: • Cardiac complete response (CarCR): Nadir NT-proBNP ≤350 ng/L or BNP ≤80 ng/L • Cardiac very good partial response: >60% reduction in NT-proBNP/BNP from baseline level not meeting CarCR • Cardiac partial response: 31%–60% reduction in NT-proBNP from baseline level not meeting CarCR • Cardiac no response: ≤30% reduction in NT-proBNP from baseline level
Progression	• NT-proBNP increase >30% and > 300 ng/L (>30% and > 70 ng/L respectively for BNP) from nadir not precipitated by infection, elevated creatinine, or cardiac arrhythmia • Troponin T/I increase ≥33% from nadir • Left ventricular ejection fraction decrease ≥10% from best value

BNP B-type natriuretic peptide, *dFLC* difference between involved and uninvolved FLC, *FLC* free light chain, *NT-proBNP* N-terminal fraction of pro–B-type natriuretic peptide

11.2 Biomarkers of Cardiac Damage in Light Chain Amyloidosis

11.2.1 Screening and Diagnosis

A screening biomarker should be sensitive enough to identify subjects, among the general population or within particular cohorts, who may deserve further diagnostic testing to detect early-stage disease. The screening of AL amyloidosis is most effectively accomplished by biomarkers that reflect the underlying hematologic disease, particularly the FLCs. NPs and troponins have been demonstrated as effective screening tools for various cardiac disease in the general population, including HF [13]. Notably, NPs and troponins are significantly increased in CA, but no study to date has investigated the role of circulating biomarkers as screening tools for CA in the general population or in subgroups at risk. Nonetheless, cardiac biomarkers are employed as "red flags" to support the diagnosis of CA [14], especially among cohorts with high prevalence of the disease (e.g. patients with HF with preserved ejection fraction [12%], aortic stenosis [AS, 8%], history of surgery for carpal tunnel syndrome [7%]) [15]. Small studies have shown that troponins are able to discriminate patients with CA from subjects with HF and cardiac hypertrophy of different aetiology [16, 17], but large cohort analyses are lacking [18].

NP levels tend to increase prior to the manifestation of symptoms or echocardiographic evidence of cardiac involvement, potentially serving as predictors for the progression to clinically overt AL-CA [19–21]. Numerous studies have demonstrated the high accuracy of both NT-proBNP and B-type NP (BNP) in identifying cardiac involvement among patients with systemic AL amyloidosis [19, 22]. Although renal function, especially in the case of NT-proBNP, influences serum NP levels due to kidney clearance, these biomarkers still exhibit good diagnostic accuracy for AL-CA even when the GFR is reduced [23]. Furthermore, age, obesity, and atrial arrhythmias should be considered when interpreting NP levels in this context [13]. The current haematologic consensus criteria state that an end-diastolic interventricular septal thickness > 12 mm, in the absence of other causes, and a NT-proBNP >332 ng/L, in the absence of end-stage renal disease or atrial fibrillation, are indicative of cardiac involvement in AL amyloidosis [9, 24]. However, it is important to note that the threshold of 332 ng/L for NT-proBNP was primarily validated for prognostic purposes (specifically, it was the upper reference limit of normal for women aged >50 years using the assay employed in the study that validated NT-proBNP as a predictor of outcome within the Mayo2004 score [25]), and its diagnostic performance for AL-CA has been a subject of debate in recent years. A study conducted by the UK National Amyloidosis Centre (NAC) on 378 Mayo I stage patients (NT-proBNP <332 ng/L, high-sensitivity TnT [hs-TnT] <55 ng/L) revealed that although no patient showed cardiac involvement according to echocardiogram, 28% exhibited evidence of cardiac involvement through cardiac magnetic resonance [21], thereby challenging the sensitivity of the NT-proBNP <332 ng/L cutoff. In a French cohort, a diagnostic score (ranging from 0 to 3 points) that combined hs-TnT (>35 ng/L), global longitudinal strain (≥−17%), and apical sparing (≥0.90) outperformed the haematologic consensus criteria in identifying cardiac involvement (score > 1 vs. consensus criteria: area under the curve [AUC] 0.98 vs. 0.75, $p < 0.001$) [26]. In a multicentric study conducted by Vergaro et al., the haematologic consensus criteria demonstrated lower specificity compared to a single hs-TnT cutoff of 86 ng/L (specificity 85% vs. 98%), as they identified a greater proportion of CA patients (109 [42%] vs. 44 [17%]) at the expense of a higher percentage of false positives (17 [7%] vs. 2 [1%]) [27]. As indicated by these and other smaller studies, troponins are emerging as effective diagnostic tools for AL-CA [16, 26, 27]. In the study by Vergaro et al., NT-proBNP <180 ng/L and hs-TnT <14 ng/L were identified as reliable rule-out cutoffs for cardiac involvement among individuals with clinical suspicion of the disease due to an underlying plasma cell disorder (97% sensitivity). Conversely, the rule-in cutoff of hs-TnT ≥86 ng/L proved effective in diagnosing cardiac involvement, as previously mentioned. Importantly, these biomarkers enhanced the diagnostic accuracy when added to the AL score, a validated echocardiographic score used to determine cardiac involvement in individuals with systemic AL amyloidosis [27].

11.2.2 Risk Stratification

NT-proBNP and TnT hold significant prognostic value in AL amyloidosis [19, 28] (Table 11.2), which resulted in their inclusion in the initial version of the Mayo

Table 11.2 Biomarker-based staging systems for AL and ATTR amyloidosis

Amyloidosis	Model	Biomarker, cut-off	Stages
AL	Mayo2004 [25]	• NT-proBNP, 332 ng/L • TnT, 35 ng/L (or TnI, 100 ng/L)	I: Both biomarkers < cut-offs II: 1 biomarker > cut-off III: 2 biomarkers > cut-offs
	Mayo3b (Mayo2004/ European) [29]	Mayo2004 stage III is divided in 2 groups according to: • NT-proBNP, 8500 ng/L	IIIa: NT-proBNP < cut-off IIIb: NT-proBNP > cut-off
	Mayo2012 [8]	• NT-proBNP, 1800 ng/L • TnT, 25 ng/L • dFLC, 180 mg/L	I: 3 biomarkers < cut-offs II: 1 biomarker > cut-off III: 2 biomarkers > cut-offs IV: 3 biomarkers > cut-offs
	Boston University staging system [30]	• BNP, 81 ng/L • TnT, 35 ng/L (or TnI, 100 ng/L)	I: 2 biomarkers < cut-offs II: 1 biomarker > cut-off III: 2 biomarkers > cut-offs
	Dispenzieri et al. [31]	• hs-TnT, 14 ng/L (lower cut-off) or 54 ng/L (higher cut-off)	I: hs-TnT < lower cut-off II: hs-TnT between lower and higher cut-offs III: hs-TnT > higher cut-off
	Dispenzieri et al. [32]	• NT-proBNP, 2257 ng/L • TnT, 30 ng/L • dFLC, 116 mg/L • sST2, >30 ng/mL	0: All biomarkers < cut-offs I: 1 biomarker > cut-off II: 2 biomarkers > cut-offs III: 3 biomarkers > cut-offs IV: 4 biomarkers > cut-offs

(continued)

Table 11.2 (continued)

Amyloidosis	Model	Biomarker, cut-off	Stages
ATTR	Kristen et al. [43]	• NT-proBNP, 2584 ng/L (or BNP, 195 ng/L) • TnT, 50 ng/L (or TnI, 580 ng/L)	A: 2 biomarkers > cut-offs B: 2 biomarkers < cut-offs C: 1 biomarker > cut-off
	Grogan et al. [46]	• NT-proBNP, 3000 ng/L • TnT, 50 ng/L	I: Both biomarkers < the cut-offs II: 1 biomarker > the cut-off III: Both biomarkers > the cut-offs
	NAC ATTR staging system [47]	• NT-proBNP, 3000 ng/L • eGFR, 45 mL/min/1.73 m [2]	I: Both biomarkers < the cut-offs II: 1 biomarker > the cut-off III: Both biomarkers > the cut-offs
	Revised NAC ATTR staging system [49]	NAC stage I is divided in 2 groups according to: • NT-proBNP, 500 ng/L (1000 ng/L in AF) • Daily dose of furosemide or equivalent, 0.75 mg/kg	Ia: Both biomarkers < the cut-offs Ib: At least 1 biomarker > the cut-offs
	Cheng et al. [50]	• Mayo or NAC score (0–2 points) • Daily dose of furosemide or equivalent: 0 mg/kg (0 points), >0–0.5 mg/kg (1 point), >0.5–1 mg/kg (2 points), >1 mg/kg (3 points) • NYHA class I-IV (1–4 points)	Score 1–3 Score 4–6 Score 7–9

AF atrial fibrillation, *AL* amyloid light-chain amyloidosis, *ATTR* transthyretin amyloidosis, *BNP* B-type natriuretic peptide, *dFLC* difference between concentrations of involved and uninvolved free light-chains, *eGFR* estimated glomerular filtration rate, *NAC* National Amyloidosis Centre, *NT-proBNP* N-terminal fraction of pro–B-type natriuretic peptide, *NYHA* New York Heart Association, *sST2 (hs-)TnT* (high-sensitivity) troponin T

staging system (Mayo2004). In the validation study, patients were classified into three stages based on NT-proBNP (332 ng/L) and either TnT (35 ng/L) or TnI (100 ng/L) levels. Using NT-proBNP and TnT, 33% of patients were categorized as stage I, 30% as stage II, and 37% as stage III, with median survivals of 26.4, 10.5, and 3.5 months, respectively [25]. A revised version of the Mayo2004 (Mayo3b or Mayo2004/European) subdivides stage III into IIIA and IIIB (median survival <3 months) based on an NT-proBNP cutoff of 8500 ng/L [29]. The Boston University staging system is another variation of Mayo2004, incorporating BNP (cutoff of 81 ng/L) instead of NT-proBNP (98% agreement between the two scores) [30].

Notably, NT-proBNP and BNP maintain independent prognostic value in patients with a eGFR between 60 and 15 mL/min/1.73 m^2, while only BNP can assess risk in subjects with a eGFR <15 mL/min/1.73 m^2 [23]. A three-staged risk stratification tool based solely on hs-TnT values (cutoff values of 14 and 54 ng/L) has also been validated, exhibiting similar discriminative power to the Mayo2004 [31]. The identification of the independent prognostic value of dFLC in AL amyloidosis led to the development of the Mayo2012 score, which assigns 1 point for each biomarker above the reference limit according to serum NT-proBNP (1800 ng/L), TnT (25 ng/L), and dFLC (180 mg/L), resulting in median survivals of 94.1, 40.3, 14, and 5.8 months for stages I, II, III, and IV, respectively [8]. sST2, a decoy receptor, inhibits the beneficial effects of interleukin-33 on the myocardium, leading to adverse outcomes in HF. In AL amyloidosis, sST2 (cutoff of 30 ng/mL) enhances the prognostic value of the Mayo2004 and Mayo2012 criteria for 1- and 5-year survival. Galectin-3, a marker of myocardial fibrosis, was only a univariate predictor in the same study [32].

11.2.3 Treatment Management

The treatment of AL amyloidosis relies on the administration of different chemotherapy protocols, sometimes in combination with autologous stem cell transplant (ASCT) [33]. Additionally, recent studies have shown promising outcomes with monoclonal antibodies that remove amyloid deposits from affected organs [34]. There has been limited research exploring the potential of cardiac biomarkers in guiding treatment decisions for AL amyloidosis. A study on patients with AL amyloidosis who underwent ASCT revealed that individuals with a baseline TnT ≥60 ng/L had a higher mortality rate within 100 days compared to those with TnT <60 ng/L [35]. This threshold was further confirmed in another study, which also demonstrated poorer survival at 10 months among ASCT recipients with a baseline NT-proBNP ≥5000 ng/L [36]. Consequently, TnT cutoff of 60 ng/L and NT-proBNP of 5000 ng/L were recommended as exclusion criteria for ASCT. To select the appropriate treatment approach in AL amyloidosis, a three-stage classification system has been proposed, which takes into account biomarker levels, age, renal function, and functional status. "Fit patients" (NT-proBNP <5000 ng/dL, TnT <60 ng/dL, age <70 years, creatinine <1.8 mg/dL) are considered suitable candidates for high-dose melphalan and ASCT. "Intermediate-fit patients" (NT-proBNP ≤8500 ng/L, Eastern Cooperative Oncology Group [ECOG] 2, New York Heart Association [NYHA] class I-II) may benefit from various chemotherapy regimens but should avoid ASCT. "Frail patients" (NT-proBNP >8500 ng/L, systolic blood pressure <100 mmHg, significant coagulopathy, ECOG 4, NYHA class III-IV) have limited therapeutic options [33].

Cardiac biomarkers have also been employed to define organ response to chemotherapy (Table 11.1). Specifically, cardiac response is indicated by a >30% or a >300 ng/L NT-proBNP reduction (>30% and >50 ng/L, respectively for BNP) after treatment in patients with baseline NT-proBNP ≥650 ng/L (≥150 ng/L for BNP).

Conversely, a >30% or a >300 ng/L increase in NT-proBNP (>30% and >70 ng/L, respectively for BNP) from nadir not precipitated by infection, elevated creatinine, or cardiac arrhythmia, as well as a >33% increase in TnT/I or a left ventricular ejection fraction reduction $\geq$10% from best value are indicative of progression of cardiac involvement [10, 37]. More recently, some authors have proposed a classification system for cardiac response, similar to that used to define haematologic response: (i) cardiac complete response, defined as nadir NT-proBNP $\leq$350 ng/L or BNP $\leq$80 ng/L; (ii) cardiac very good partial response, defined as >60% reduction in NT-proBNP/BNP from baseline level not meeting complete response; (iii) cardiac partial response, defined as 31–60% reduction in NT-proBNP from baseline level not meeting cardiac complete response; (iv) cardiac no response, defined as $\leq$30% reduction in NT-proBNP from baseline level [38].

11.3 Biomarkers of Cardiac Damage in Transthyretin Amyloidosis

11.3.1 Screening and Diagnosis

NPs and troponin levels are typically lower in patients with ATTR amyloidosis compared to those with AL amyloidosis, possibly due to lower cytotoxicity of amyloidogenic precursors. Nevertheless, cardiac biomarkers play a crucial role as "red flags" in suspecting ATTR-CA [18]. Although no studies have evaluated these biomarkers as screening tools for ATTR-CA, it has been demonstrated that NPs and troponins are significantly elevated in patients with AS and concurrent CA, in comparison to patients with isolated AS who undergo aortic valve replacement [39]. Nitsche et al. have even included a hs-TnT >20 ng/L, along with other clinical, electrocardiographic, and echographic parameters, as part of a scoring system for the discrimination of lone AS from dual pathology AS-CA, the latter consisting of almost exclusively of ATTR-CA patients (47 out of 48) [40].

As for the diagnostic value of cardiac biomarkers, a recent multicentric study by Vergaro et al. (Fig. 11.2) reported that NT-proBNP and hs-TnT, either alone or combined, hold a strong diagnostic value in cohort of 343 patients with suspected CA (AUC for NT-proBNP 0.721; AUC for hs-TnT 0.810; AUC for biomarker combination 0.821). These results were confirmed in an external validation cohort of 806 patients with suspected CA from the NAC (AUC for NT-proBNP 0.830; AUC for hs-TnT 0.841; AUC for biomarker combination 0.843). The addition of these biomarkers even improved the diagnostic performance of previously validated echocardiographic score, namely the AL and IWT scores. In this study, the authors also identified NT-proBNP <180 ng/L and hs-TnT <14 ng/L to be reliable rule-out thresholds for CA (100% sensitivity), whereas hs-TnT $\geq$86 ng/L emerged as an effective rule-in cutoff for CA (95% specificity) in both the derivation and validation cohorts. The same cutoffs performed well also in several subgroups including patients with increased left ventricular wall thickness (i.e. interventricular septal or posterior wall thickness $\geq$12 mm; IWT cohort) or patients with suspicion of

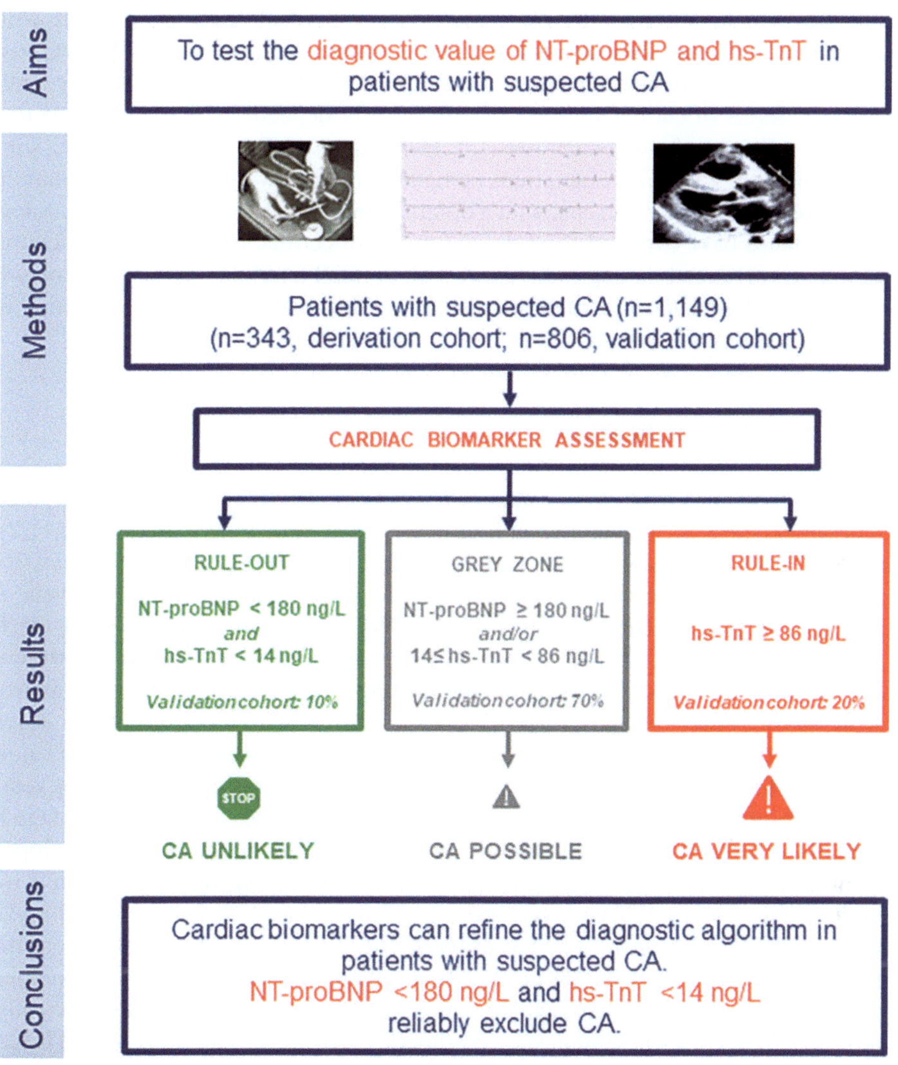

Fig. 11.2 N-terminal pro-B-type natriuretic peptide and high-sensitivity troponin T to diagnose cardiac amyloidosis. Cardiac biomarkers hold diagnostic value in cardiac amyloidosis (CA). The diagnosis can be reliably excluded when N-terminal pro-B-type natriuretic peptide (NT-proBNP) is <180 ng/L and high-sensitivity troponin T (hs-TnT) is <14 ng/L. Reproduced with permission from Vergaro et al. [27]

ATTR-CA, namely those from the IWT cohort without plasma cell disorders. Notably, NT-proBNP and hs-TnT cutoffs retained their rule-out and rule-in performance also in cohorts with CA prevalence of 20%, 10%, 5%, and 1% derived from the original cohort through bootstrap analysis, confirming their potential application also in non-referral settings with lower prevalence of CA [27].

After adjustment for left ventricular mass and renal function, patients with ATTRv amyloidosis show lower NP levels compared to those with ATTRwt, possibly related to differences in age and renal function. Additionally, in ATTRv amyloidosis, levels of cardiac biomarkers vary greatly depending on the presence and severity of cardiac involvement [41–43]. For example, NP levels are higher in subjects with non-V30M *TTR* mutations compared to those with V30M *TTR* mutation, since the latter usually presents with a dominant neuropathic phenotype [43]. A few small studies have explored the potential utility of cardiac biomarkers in detecting cardiac involvement among individuals with familial amyloid polyneuropathy [44, 45]. These studies have yielded promising findings, although further validation in larger populations is necessary.

11.3.2 Risk Stratification

NPs and troponins hold strong prognostic value in ATTR amyloidosis [18]. These biomarkers have been integrated in four main risk stratification scores (Table 11.2). In the Transthyretin Amyloidosis Outcome Survey (THAOS), elevated NPs and troponins were found to be associated with worse survival. Based on the levels of BNP/NT-proBNP (BNP 195 ng/L; NT-proBNP 2584 ng/L) and TnT/TnI (TnT, 50 ng/L; TnI, 580 ng/L), patients were categorized into three groups (a, both biomarkers above threshold; b, both biomarkers under threshold; c, none of the above) with varying outcomes [43]. Another classification system proposed by the Mayo Clinic team identified three stages for ATTRwt amyloidosis based on specific cutoff values of TnT (50 ng/L) and NT-proBNP (3000 ng/L). The survival rates at 4 years were 57%, 42%, and 18% for stage I (both biomarker values below cutoff), stage II (one above), and stage III (both above), respectively [46]. Gillmore et al. developed a three-stage classification system (known as "NAC ATTR staging system") for both ATTRwt and ATTRv amyloidosis, which relies on NT-proBNP (3000 ng/L) and eGFR (45 mL/min/1.73 m^2) as criteria. The distribution of patients across the stages was 45% in stage I, 38% in stage II, and 16% in stage III, with corresponding median survival of 69.2, 46.7, and 24.1 months [47]. In an external validation study, the NAC ATTR staging system showed superior prognostic accuracy for ATTR-CA compared to a classification system based on NT-proBNP and TnI [48]. Additionally, Gillmore et al. examined the impact of genotype on biomarker levels and prognosis. Patients with the V122I *TTR* variant, the most common genetic mutation associated with ATTRv-CA, exhibited a worse prognosis across all three stages compared to those with ATTRwt-CA [47]. Recently, the same authors proposed a modified version of the NAC ATTR staging system aimed at improving patient stratification for early-stage CA by dividing stage I into Ia and Ib based on furosemide equivalent diuretic requirement of <0.75 mg/kg and NT-proBNP ≤500 ng/L (≤1000 ng/L in the presence of atrial fibrillation). Notably, stage Ia ATTR-CA patients, while facing significant cardiovascular morbidity during follow-up, exhibited estimated survival rates comparable to those of controls from the UK general population [49]. Additionally, a study from the US has provided further insights by reporting that furosemide equivalent dose (expressed in categories: 0 mg/kg, >0–0.5 mg/kg, >0.5–1 mg/kg, and >1–2 mg/kg) and NYHA class provide incremental value to both the NAC ATTR staging system (AUC change from 0.711 to 0.816) and the Mayo Clinic staging system (AUC change from 0.693 to 0.798) [50].

11.3.3 Treatment Management

No studies have investigated the use of cardiac biomarkers to guide treatment selection for ATTR-CA. However, there is preliminary evidence regarding the impact of new disease-modifying therapies on cardiac biomarkers although the results are somewhat controversial. For instance, phase I/II trials on diflunisal (a TTR stabilizer) [51, 52] or epigallocatechin gallate (an inhibitor of oligomer aggregation) [53] in ATTR amyloidosis have shown an increase in cardiac biomarkers during follow-up. Similarly, a phase II trial investigating tafamidis 20 mg in ATTRwt amyloidosis demonstrated a moderate increase in TnT/I after 12 months, while NT-proBNP remained stable, along with echocardiographic parameters [54]. In the subsequent phase III trial, the Transthyretin Amyloidosis Cardiomyopathy Clinical Trial (ATTR-ACT), tafamidis proved to have a prognostic benefit in ATTR amyloidosis, but there was an increase in NT-proBNP at 12 and 30 months. However, the increase was smaller among patients on tafamidis compared to controls (least-squares mean difference, −735.14 [95% confidence interval, −1249.16 to −221.13] at 12 months and −2180.54 [95% confidence interval, −3326.14 to −1034.95] at 30 months) [55]. Moreover, the NT-proBNP increase was less significant with a higher tafamidis dose (80 mg) compared to a lower dose (20 mg; $p = 0.047$) or placebo ($p < 0.001$) [56]. Other smaller single-centre studies have reported either a reduction or stabilization of NPs and troponins following the introduction of tafamidis at commercially available doses (tafamidis free acid 61 mg or tafamidis meglumine 80 mg) [57–59], which aligns with the stabilizing effect of this drug on the disease course.

As for RNA-targeting therapies, the APOLLO trial, which examined the efficacy of patisiran (a siRNA) compared to placebo in patients with familial amyloid polyneuropathy, stands out as the sole phase III trial that exhibited a notable reduction in NT-proBNP levels during the follow-up period in patients with ATTR amyloidosis [60]. Notably, a considerable proportion of patients in the study had troponin I values below the limit of detection for the used assay (<0.1 µg/L), thus preventing any analysis on impact of patisiran on troponin I levels [60]. Additionally, a small-scale study investigating the effects of inotersen (an antisense oligonucleotide) revealed a decrease in BNP levels after 12 months of treatment in the majority of patients with variant ATTRv amyloidosis, but not in most patients with ATTRwt amyloidosis [61].

11.4 Conclusions and Future Perspectives

The use of biomarkers in CA has demonstrated significant value in various aspects of disease management. For AL amyloidosis, the quantification of FLCs, along with the κ/λ ratio and serum and urine immunofixation, is crucial for accurate diagnosis. Additionally, the assessment of dFLC plays a pivotal role in risk stratification and monitoring hematologic response to therapy. NPs and troponins have established themselves as important tools in detecting cardiac involvement, risk stratification, and monitoring organ response to therapy in AL amyloidosis. Moreover, in the case of ATTR amyloidosis, cardiac biomarkers are emerging as effective tools for aiding diagnosis and stratifying prognosis.

To improve the management of CA, it is crucial to address several unmet needs and explore potential directions. Firstly, there should be a concerted effort to integrate high-sensitivity troponin assays into the diagnostic algorithm of CA, particularly in non-tertiary referral centres. The use of natriuretic peptides and troponins, not only as red flags but also as rule-out tools, has the potential to greatly benefit the management of patients with suspected CA by avoiding unnecessary and costly diagnostic exams, especially in resource-limited settings. Furthermore, there is a pressing need for more studies that investigate the usefulness of biomarkers for screening of CA, both in the general population and within high-risk subgroups, such as patients with plasma cell disorders or individuals carrying *TTR* mutations. Such biomarkers should be employed to expedite diagnosis and access to life-saving treatments. Additionally, it is crucial to develop novel disease-specific biomarkers, ideally capable to forecast the onset of ATTRwt amyloidosis. Indeed, this condition remains challenging to predict due to the limited understanding of the underlying etiological mechanisms. Lastly, with the recent availability of disease-modifying therapies for ATTR amyloidosis, it is imperative to establish biomarkers for selecting and monitoring therapy in ATTR-CA, thus enabling personalized treatment strategies.

In conclusion, by addressing these unmet needs and exploring future perspectives regarding the use of biomarkers, significant advancements could be achieved in early detection, accurate diagnosis, and effective management of CA, ultimately leading to improved patient outcomes.

References

1. Dispenzieri A, Kyle R, Merlini G, Miguel JS, Ludwig H, Hajek R, et al. International myeloma working group guidelines for serum-free light chain analysis in multiple myeloma and related disorders. Leukemia. 2009;23:215–24.
2. Camerini L, Aimo A, Pucci A, Castiglione V, Musetti V, Masotti S, et al. Serum and tissue light-chains as disease biomarkers and targets for treatment in AL amyloidosis. Vessel Plus. 2022:6.
3. Caponi L, Romiti N, Koni E, Fiore AD, Paolicchi A, Franzini M. Inter-assay variability in automated serum free light chain assays and their use in the clinical laboratory. Crit Rev Clin Lab Sci. 2020;57:73–85.

4. Rajkumar SV, Dimopoulos MA, Palumbo A, Blade J, Merlini G, Mateos MV, et al. International myeloma working group updated criteria for the diagnosis of multiple myeloma. Lancet. 2014;15:e538.
5. Hutchison CA, Plant T, Drayson M, Cockwell P, Kountouri M, Basnayake K, et al. Serum free light chain measurement aids the diagnosis of myeloma in patients with severe renal failure. BMC Nephrol. 2008;9:11.
6. Long TE, Indridason OS, Palsson R, Rognvaldsson S, Love TJ, Thorsteinsdottir S, et al. Defining new reference intervals for serum free light chains in individuals with chronic kidney disease: results of the iStopMM study. Blood Cancer J. 2022;12:1–8.
7. Kumar S, Dispenzieri A, Katzmann JA, Larson DR, Colby CL, Lacy MQ, et al. Serum immunoglobulin free light-chain measurement in primary amyloidosis: prognostic value and correlations with clinical features. Blood. 2010;116:5126–9.
8. Kumar S, Dispenzieri A, Lacy MQ, Hayman SR, Buadi FK, Colby C, et al. J OURNAL OF C LINICAL O NCOLOGY revised prognostic staging system for light chain amyloidosis incorporating cardiac biomarkers and serum free light chain measurements. J Clin Oncol Off J Am Soc Clin Oncol. 2015;30:989–95.
9. Gertz MA, Comenzo R, Falk RH, Fermand JP, Hazenberg BP, Hawkins PN, et al. Definition of organ involvement and treatment response in immunoglobulin light chain amyloidosis (AL). Am J Hematol. 2005;79:319–28.
10. Palladini G, Dispenzieri A, Gertz MA, Kumar S, Wechalekar A, Hawkins PN, et al. New criteria for response to treatment in immunoglobulin light chain amyloidosis based on free light chain measurement and cardiac biomarkers: impact on survival outcomes. J Clin Oncol. 2012;30:4541–9.
11. Garcia-Pavia P, Rapezzi C, Adler Y, Arad M, Basso C, Brucato A, et al. Diagnosis and treatment of cardiac amyloidosis: a position statement of the ESC working group on myocardial and pericardial diseases. Eur Heart J. 2021;42:1554–68.
12. Rauf MU, Hawkins PN, Cappelli F, Perfetto F, Zampieri M, Argiro A, et al. Tc-99m labelled bone scintigraphy in suspected cardiac amyloidosis. Eur Heart J. 2023;44:2187–98.
13. Castiglione V, Aimo A, Vergaro G, Saccaro L, Passino C, Emdin M. Biomarkers for the diagnosis and management of heart failure. Heart Fail Rev. 2021;27:625–43.
14. Vergaro G, Aimo A, Barison A, Genovesi D, Buda G, Passino C, et al. Keys to early diagnosis of cardiac amyloidosis: red flags from clinical, laboratory and imaging findings. Eur J Prev Cardiol. 2020;27:1806–15.
15. Aimo A, Merlo M, Porcari A, Georgiopoulos G, Pagura L, Vergaro G, et al. Redefining the epidemiology of cardiac amyloidosis. A systematic review and meta-analysis of screening studies. Eur J Heart Fail. 2022;24:2342–51.
16. Takashio S, Yamamuro M, Izumiya Y, Hirakawa K, Marume K, Yamamoto M, et al. Diagnostic utility of cardiac troponin T level in patients with cardiac amyloidosis. ESC Heart Fail. 2018;5:27–35.
17. Hu K, Liu D, Salinger T, Oder D, Knop S, Ertl G, et al. Value of cardiac biomarker measurement in the differential diagnosis of infiltrative cardiomyopathy patients with preserved left ventricular systolic function. J Thorac Dis. 2018;10:4966–75.
18. Castiglione V, Franzini M, Aimo A, Carecci A, Lombardi CM, Passino C, et al. Use of biomarkers to diagnose and manage cardiac amyloidosis. Eur J Heart Fail. 2021;23:217–30.
19. Palladini G, Campana C, Klersy C, Balduini A, Vadacca G, Perfetti V, et al. Serum N-terminal pro-brain natriuretic peptide is a sensitive marker of myocardial dysfunction in AL amyloidosis. Circulation. 2003;107:2440–5.
20. Wechalekar AD, Gillmore JD, Wassef N, Lachmann HJ, Whelan C, Hawkins PN. Abnormal N-terminal fragment of brain natriuretic peptide in patients with light chain amyloidosis without cardiac involvement at presentation is a risk factor for development of cardiac amyloidosis. Haematologica. 2011;96:1079–80.

21. Sharpley FA, Fontana M, Martinez-Naharro A, Manwani R, Mahmood S, Sachchithanantham S, et al. Cardiac biomarkers are prognostic in systemic light chain amyloidosis with no cardiac involvement by standard criteria. Haematologica. 2020;105:1405–13.
22. Kimishima Y, Yoshihisa A, Kiko T, Yokokawa T, Miyata-Tatsumi M, Misaka T, et al. Utility of B-type natriuretic peptide for detecting cardiac involvement in immunoglobulin amyloidosis. Int Heart J. 2019;60:1106–12.
23. Palladini G, Foli A, Milani P, Russo P, Albertini R, Lavatelli F, et al. Best use of cardiac biomarkers in patients with AL amyloidosis and renal failure. Am J Hematol. 2012;87:465–71.
24. Grogan M, Dispenzieri A, Gertz MA. Light-chain cardiac amyloidosis: strategies to promote early diagnosis and cardiac response. Heart Br Card Soc. 2017;103:1065–72.
25. Dispenzieri A, Gertz MA, Kyle RA, Lacy MQ, Burritt MF, Therneau TM, et al. Serum cardiac troponins and N-terminal pro-brain natriuretic peptide: a staging system for primary systemic amyloidosis. J Clin Oncol. 2004;22:3751–7.
26. Nicol M, Baudet M, Brun S, Harel S, Royer B, Vignon M, et al. Diagnostic score of cardiac involvement in AL amyloidosis. Eur Heart J Cardiovasc Imaging. 2020;21:542–8.
27. Vergaro G, Castiglione V, Aimo A, Prontera C, Masotti S, Musetti V, et al. N-terminal pro-B-type natriuretic peptide and high-sensitivity troponin T hold diagnostic value in cardiac amyloidosis. Eur J Heart Fail. 2023;25:335–46.
28. Dispenzieri A, Kyle RA, Gertz MA, Therneau TM, Miller WL, Chandrasekaran K, et al. Survival in patients with primary systemic amyloidosis and raised serum cardiac troponins. Lancet. 2003;361:1787–9.
29. Wechalekar AD, Schonland SO, Kastritis E, Gillmore JD, Dimopoulos MA, Lane T, et al. A European collaborative study of treatment outcomes in 346 patients with cardiac stage III AL amyloidosis. Blood. 2013;121:3420–7.
30. Tomlinson R, Matigian N, Mollee P. Validation of the Boston University staging system in AL amyloidosis. Amyloid. 2019;26:125–7.
31. Dispenzieri A, Gertz MA, Kumar SK, Lacy MQ, Kyle RA, Saenger AK, et al. High sensitivity cardiac troponin T in patients with immunoglobulin light chain amyloidosis. Heart Br Card Soc. 2014;100:383–8.
32. Dispenzieri A, Gertz MA, Saenger A, Kumar SK, Lacy MQ, Buadi FK, et al. Soluble suppression of tumorigenicity 2 (sST2), but not galactin-3, adds to prognostication in patients with systemic AL amyloidosis independent of NT-proBNP and troponin T. Am J Hematol. 2015;90:8–12.
33. Aimo A, Buda G, Fontana M, Barison A, Vergaro G, Emdin M, et al. Therapies for cardiac light chain amyloidosis: an update. Int J Cardiol. 2018;271:152–60.
34. Gertz MA, Cohen AD, Comenzo RL, Kastritis E, Landau HJ, Libby EN, et al. Birtamimab plus standard of care in light chain amyloidosis: the phase 3 randomized placebo-controlled VITAL trial. Blood. 2023;142:1208–18.
35. Gertz M, Lacy M, Dispenzieri A, Hayman S, Kumar S, Buadi F, et al. Troponin T level as an exclusion criterion for stem cell transplantation in light-chain amyloidosis. Leuk Lymphoma. 2008;49:36–41.
36. Gertz MA, Lacy MQ, Dispenzieri A, Kumar SK, Dingli D, Leung N, et al. Refinement in patient selection to reduce treatment-related mortality from autologous stem cell transplantation in amyloidosis. Bone Marrow Transplant. 2012;48:557–61.
37. Palladini G, Milani P, Merlini G. Management of AL amyloidosis in 2020. Blood. 2020;136:2620–7.
38. Muchtar E, Dispenzieri A, Wisniowski B, Palladini G, Milani P, Merlini G, et al. Graded cardiac response criteria for patients with systemic light chain amyloidosis. J Clin Oncol Off J Am Soc Clin Oncol. 2023;41:1393–403.
39. Cannata F, Chiarito M, Pinto G, Villaschi A, Sanz-Sánchez J, Fazzari F, et al. Transcatheter aortic valve replacement in aortic stenosis and cardiac amyloidosis: a systematic review and meta-analysis. ESC Heart Fail. 2022;9:3188–97.

40. Nitsche C, Scully PR, Patel KP, Kammerlander AA, Koschutnik M, Dona C, et al. Prevalence and outcomes of concomitant aortic stenosis and cardiac amyloidosis. J Am Coll Cardiol. 2021;77:128–39.
41. Perfetto F, Bergesio F, Grifoni E, Fabbri A, Ciuti G, Frusconi S, et al. Different NT-proBNP circulating levels for different types of cardiac amyloidosis. J Cardiovasc Med. 2016;17:810–7.
42. Usuku H, Obayashi K, Shono M, Oshima T, Tasaki M, Yasuda H, et al. Usefulness of plasma B-type natriuretic peptide as a prognostic marker of cardiac function in senile systemic amyloidosis and in familial amyloidotic polyneuropathy. Amyloid. 2013;20:251–5.
43. Kristen AV, Maurer MS, Rapezzi C, Mundayat R, Suhr OB. Impact of genotype and phenotype on cardiac biomarkers in patients with transthyretin amyloidosis—Report from the Transthyretin Amyloidosis Outcome Survey (THAOS). 2017;1–17.
44. Damy T, Deux JF, Moutereau S, Guendouz S, Mohty D, Rappeneau S, et al. Role of natriuretic peptide to predict cardiac abnormalities in patients with hereditary transthyretin amyloidosis. Amyloid. 2013;6129:212–20.
45. Suhr OB, Anan I, Backman C, Karlsson A, Lindqvist P, Mörner S, et al. Do troponin and B-natriuretic peptide detect cardiomyopathy in transthyretin amyloidosis? J Intern Med. 2008;263:294–301.
46. Grogan M, Scott CG, Kyle RA, Zeldenrust SR, Gertz MA, Lin G, et al. Natural history of wild-type transthyretin cardiac amyloidosis and risk stratification using a novel staging system. J Am Coll Cardiol. 2016;68:1014–20.
47. Gillmore JD, Damy T, Fontana M, Hutchinson M, Lachmann HJ, Martinez-naharro A, et al. A new staging system for cardiac transthyretin amyloidosis. Eur Heart J. 2017;44:1–8.
48. Cappelli F, Martone R, Gabriele M, Taborchi G, Morini S, Vignini E, et al. Biomarkers and prediction of prognosis in transthyretin-related cardiac amyloidosis: direct comparison of two staging systems. Can J Cardiol. 2020;36:424–31.
49. Law S, Bezard M, Petrie A, Chacko L, Cohen OC, Ravichandran S, et al. Characteristics and natural history of early-stage cardiac transthyretin amyloidosis. Eur Heart J. 2022;43:2622–32.
50. Cheng RK, Levy WC, Vasbinder A, Teruya S, De Los SJ, Leedy D, et al. Diuretic dose and NYHA functional class are independent predictors of mortality in patients with transthyretin cardiac amyloidosis. JACC CardioOncol. 2020;2:414–24.
51. Castaño A, Helmke S, Alvarez J, Delisle S, Maurer MS. Diflunisal for ATTR cardiac amyloidosis. Congest Heart Fail. 2012;18:315–9.
52. Sekijima Y, Tojo K, Morita H, Koyama J, Ikeda S, ichi. Safety and efficacy of long-term diflunisal administration in hereditary transthyretin (ATTR) amyloidosis. Amyloid Int J Exp Clin Investig. 2015;22:79–83.
53. Kristen AV, Lehrke S, Buss S, Mereles D, Steen H, Ehlermann P, et al. Green tea halts progression of cardiac transthyretin amyloidosis: an observational report. Clin Res Cardiol. 2012;101:805–13.
54. Maurer MS, Grogan DR, Judge DP, Mundayat R, Packman J, Lombardo I, et al. Tafamidis in transthyretin amyloid cardiomyopathy: effects on transthyretin stabilization and clinical outcomes. Circ Heart Fail. 2015;8:519–26.
55. Maurer MS, Schwartz JH, Gundapancni B, Elliott PM, Merlini G, Waddington-Cruz M, et al. Tafamidis treatment for patients with transthyretin amyloid cardiomyopathy. N Engl J Med. 2018;379:1007–16.
56. Damy T, Garcia-Pavia P, Hanna M, Judge DP, Merlini G, Gundapaneni B, et al. Efficacy and safety of tafamidis doses in the tafamidis in transthyretin cardiomyopathy clinical trial (ATTR-ACT) and long-term extension study. Eur J Heart Fail. 2021;23:277–85.
57. Takashio S, Morioka M, Ishii M, Morikawa K, Hirakawa K, Hanatani S, et al. Clinical characteristics, outcome, and therapeutic effect of tafamidis in wild-type transthyretin amyloid cardiomyopathy. ESC Heart Fail. 2023;10:2319–29.
58. Ochi Y, Kubo T, Baba Y, Sugiura K, Miyagawa K, Noguchi T, et al. Early experience of tafamidis treatment in Japanese patients with wild-type transthyretin cardiac amyloidosis from the Kochi amyloidosis cohort. Circ J. 2022;86:1121–8.

59. Oghina S, Josse C, Bézard M, Kharoubi M, Delbarre MA, Eyharts D, et al. Prognostic value of N-terminal pro-brain natriuretic peptide and high-sensitivity troponin T levels in the natural history of transthyretin amyloid cardiomyopathy and their evolution after tafamidis treatment. J Clin Med. 2021;10:4868.
60. Solomon SD, Adams D, Kristen A, Grogan M, González-Duarte A, Maurer MS, et al. Effects of Patisiran, an RNA interference therapeutic, on cardiac parameters in patients with hereditary transthyretin-mediated amyloidosis: analysis of the APOLLO study. Circulation. 2019;139:431–43.
61. Benson MD, Dasgupta NR, Rissing SM, Smith J, Feigenbaum H. Safety and efficacy of a TTR specific antisense oligonucleotide in patients with transthyretin amyloid cardiomyopathy. Amyloid. 2017;24:219–25.

Maria Franzini, Chiara Sanguinetti, Veronica Musetti, Vincenzo Castiglione, Alberto Aimo, Giuseppe Vergaro, and Michele Emdin

Transthyretin (TTR), also named prealbumin, is a protein found in plasma and cerebrospinal fluid, mainly synthesized by the liver and choroid plexus [1]. TTR is a homotetrameric protein composed of 4 identical subunits rich in β-sheets structures. In the assembling of the TTR tetramers, two cylindrical hydrophobic channels are generated at dimer–dimer interface that can accommodate one T4 molecule each but, because of negative co-operativity between the two sites, only one site can be occupied [2]. In addition to T4, TTR can also accommodate two retinol-binding proteins 4 (RBP4) on its external surface (Fig. 12.1) [3]. The main physiological functions of TTR are to stabilize and transport both T4 and the retinol-RBP4 complexes through the circulation and the cerebrospinal fluid [1]. Furthermore, new

Maria Franzini and Chiara Sanguinetti contributed equally with all other contributors.

M. Franzini (✉) · C. Sanguinetti
Department Translational Research and New Technologies in Medicine and Surgery, University of Pisa, Pisa, Italy
e-mail: maria.franzini@unipi.it; chiara.sanguinetti@phd.unipi.it

V. Musetti
Health Science Interdisciplinary Center, Scuola Superiore, S. Anna, Pisa, Italy
e-mail: veronica.musetti@santannapisa.it

V. Castiglione · A. Aimo · G. Vergaro · M. Emdin
Health Science Interdisciplinary Center, Scuola Superiore Sant'Anna, Pisa, Italy

Fondazione Toscana G. Monasterio, Pisa, Italy
e-mail: vcastiglione@ftgm.it; aimoalb@ftgm.it; vergaro@ftgm.it; emdin@ftgm.it

M. Emdin et al. (eds.), *Cardiac Amyloidosis*, https://doi.org/10.1007/978-3-031-51757-0_12

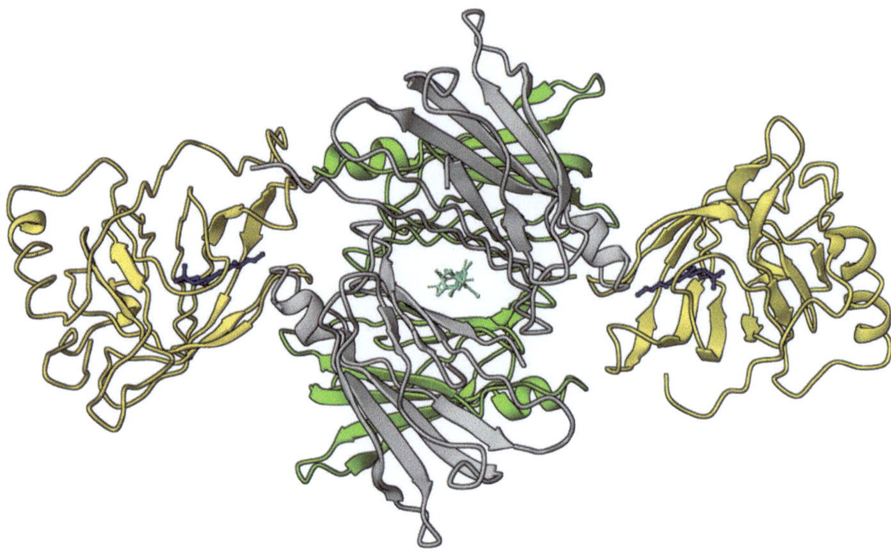

Fig. 12.1 Structure of the TTR-holoRPB4$_2$-T4 complex. Ribbon structure of the TTR tetramer in association with its ligands. Transthyretin (TTR) monomers: gray and green. Retinol binding protein (RPB4): yellow. Retinol: blue. T4: sky blue. The figure has been produced using www.rcsb.org web site

Table 12.1 Reference values for TTR expressed in g/L and divided by age-group and gender

	Age classes				
	Newborns	1–7	7–20	20–60	> 60
Man	0.07–0.17	0.12–0.27	0.13–0.41	0.20–0.45	0.16–0.40
Women	0.08–0.17	0.12–0.28	0.13–0.38	0.20–0.45	0.14–0.37

Ranges correspond to 2.5–97.5 th percentiles. Data from [5]

functions for TTR as a regulator of cell proliferation, by IGF1-R pathway, and energetic metabolism are emerging [4].

TTR plasma concentration rises after birth, reaching the concentration of 0.2–0.4 g/L in adults, then it decreases after 60 years of age, so it must be kept in mind that the reference values change with age both in males and females being higher in males (Table 12.1) [5, 6]. Plasma TTR has a relative short half-life (~2 days) [7].

TTR plasma levels can increase after kidney failure or drugs intake like anti-inflammatory (steroid and not steroid) or oral contraceptives. Instead, liver diseases, hyperthyroidism, hyperglycemia, dialysis, and malnutrition are associated with a decrease of TTR plasma levels [8, 9]. Finally, TTR synthesis is negatively regulated during inflammatory process, so TTR quantification should be combined with that of the C-reactive protein to be correctly interpreted [5].

Plasma TTR quantification is clinically available since 1970s when it was proposed as a marker of nutritional state [10], although its specificity in this field is still a matter of debate [8]. In the last years, TTR, both as wild-type or mutated protein, has achieved a renewed interest in a completely different clinical field, i.e., those related to amyloidosis. Amyloidosis is a protein misfolding disorder caused by extracellular deposition of a β-sheet rich protein in insoluble fibrils, and TTR is one of the 30 precursor proteins that have been identified to induce a clinically relevant form of amyloidosis [11].

A few studies on patients affected by TTR amyloidosis (ATTR) showed that plasma TTR concentrations allowed to stratify the risk of short-term mortality (2.8 years) [12]. Patients with TTR amyloidosis have indeed reduced values of TTR plasma concentration [12, 13]. However, plasma TTR has not entered yet in the diagnostic algorithms for TTR amyloidosis which include only the laboratory biomarkers of organ damage [14].

In comparison with immunoglobulin light chain (AL) amyloidosis, ATTR has a longer survival rate with a median survival of 75 months [15], but therapeutic options have been limited until very recently. Treatment of ATTR amyloidosis will be extensively discussed in Chap. 19. This field is rapidly evolving, and the use of plasma TTR levels to assess response and adherence to therapy is still under evaluation. To date, 3 main pharmacological strategies are available for ATTR amyloidosis for which a disease-modifying impact has been shown [16, 17]: (i) block of TTR liver synthesis, (ii) stabilization of TTR tetramers, and (iii) disruption of deposited amyloid fibrils. The first two strategies are also expected to modify TTR plasma levels and are the only one for which FDA approved drugs are available.

Therapies inhibiting TTR liver synthesis are based on small interfering RNA (siRNA) or antisense oligonucleotide (ASO) targeting both mutated and wild-type TTR [18]. The siRNA patisiran and vutrisiran and the ASO inotersen have been approved for the treatment of patients with ATTR variant polyneuropathy, while the ASO eplontersen is still under approval.

The formulation of patisiran includes the siRNA (ALN-18328) encapsulated into lipid nanoparticles, the recommended dosing regimen is 0.3 mg/kg administered every 3 weeks by intravenous infusion. In phase II [19] and III studies [20], patisiran reduced plasma TTR levels within 6 weeks allowing a median reduction of 81% over 18 months of treatment. This data were confirmed by pharmacokinetic–pharmacodynamic (PK/PD) model linking plasma ALN-18328 levels to the inhibition of hepatic TTR synthesis [21]. Vutrisiran (ALN-TTRsc02) administration induces a dramatic and persistent plasma TTR reduction in a dose-dependent manner, with a mean-maximum TTR reduction of 57–97%, maintained for about 90 days at doses ≥25 mg [22]. The recommended dosing regimen of vutrisiran is 25 mg every 3 months by subcutaneous administrations.

As observed for the siRNA-based drugs, also the ASO inotersen induces the reduction of TTR plasma levels in a dose-dependent manner. On the basis of a multiple-dose trial, the weekly subcutaneous injection of 300 mg was chosen as dosing-regimen [23]. In the phase III clinical study, a median plasma TTR reduction of 79% was observed starting from the 13th week after the treatment initiation [24].

The ASO eplontersen showed to be more potent than inotersen in reducing TTR gene expression, indeed 45 mg every 4 weeks allowed a mean reduction of plasma

TTR levels of 86%, at the 12th week after starting the treatment [25]. Eplontersen is still under evaluation in a phase 3 clinical study [26].

A further approach for TTR-gene silencing is based on genome editing with CRISPR-Cas9 system. This technology has been investigated in a phase I study with patients receiving a single dose of 0.1, 0.3, 0.7, or 1 mg/kg of the lipid nanoparticle CRISPR–Cas9 system (NTLA-2001); after 28 days from the intravenous injection of the drug, plasma levels were reduced of 52%, 87%, 86%, and 93%, respectively [27, 28]. This knockdown strategy is expected to be permanent after a single injection.

The quantification of plasma TTR concentration as a surrogate of TTR stabilization has been investigated in ATTR patients undergoing therapy based on the specific tetramer-stabilizing agents tafamidis or acoramidis (AG10). Indeed, both treatments are associated with the progressive increase of plasma TTR up to the reference values in those patients with low baseline TTR levels [13, 29–31]. Therefore, the evaluation of plasma TTR levels could be of importance both for prognostic assessment and as biomarker of response to therapy.

To date, two automated analytical methods are available for the quantification of TTR plasma concentrations. Both are immunoassays based on the aggregation of specific antibodies and antigens into large complexes which are detected by nephelometry or turbidimetry technique. These methods have been shown to be equivalent for the quantification of TTR [32], but neither of them is able of distinguishing the different forms of TTR possibly present in the circulation (e.g., tetramers bound or unbound to T4 or RBP4) nor to discriminate between the wild type from the mutated TTR proteins. In suitable experimental conditions, the nephelometric assay has been tested as a tool to characterize the propensity of TTR tetramers to disaggregate or their sensitivity to the stabilizing action of pharmacological agents. Briefly, this method consists in inducing the denaturation of TTR tetramers with urea and then fixing with glutaraldehyde the residual fraction of tetramers that will be subsequently quantified by the nephelometric assay. The quantification of TTR before and after treatment with urea, in the presence or absence of a stabilizing agent, could allow the estimation of the drug efficacy [13, 33, 34]. However, this modification of the nephelometric assay has never been translated from research to clinical diagnostics. Moreover, there has never been an evaluation of the analytical and diagnostic characteristics of this method in terms of specificity, sensitivity, and reproducibility.

As regards the characterization of the familial forms of TTR, genetic analysis is necessary to identify the exact mutation associated with clinical phenotype [35]. Nonetheless, it is also possible to distinguish the mutated TTR proteins based on the specific charge and mass variations caused by the mutation. Electrophoretic separation based on the isoelectric point (isoelectric focusing), and mass spectrometry analysis, respectively, are used for these purposes [36]. Electrophoretic techniques allow the analysis of multiple samples simultaneously and have a 100% specificity, and it has been possible to identify a specific migration pattern for many mutations [37, 38].

Several mass spectrometry methods have been proposed for the identification of TTR variants, for example, MALDI-TOF (matrix-assisted laser desorption/

ionization—time of flight) [39–41], ESI (electrospray ionization) [42–44], and SELDI-TOF (surface-enhanced laser desorption/ionization—time of flight) [45, 46]. All methods were found to be able to identify the variants of TTR, but the complex sample preparation, as well as the need for sophisticated equipment, limited their application. A new simplified MALDI-TOF mass spectrometry method has been recently proposed; it overcomes the pre-purification stage of the sample and allows to obtain results in about 30 min [47]. This method has been tested on 15 different TTR mutations and has shown a 91% specificity as it fails to distinguish mutations that result in a mass-to-charge ratio change from the wild-type protein of less than 0.99 m/z [47]. Future studies will test the validity of this method as a preliminary screening test for molecular investigation.

Several studies showed that both the physiological ligands of TTR, RPB4, and T4 prevent its misfolding and amyloid fibril formation in in vitro experimental models [48, 49] suggesting yet another structure–function relationship to this protein–protein complex. The binding of T4 and RPB4 to TTR is independent of each other, similarly their stabilizing effect on the tetrameric form of TTR is also independent as well as additive [48]. Notably, the pathway of dissociation of TTR has been proposed to begin with the scission of tetramers along the dimer/dimer interface where the two possible T4 binding sites are located [50, 51]. Interestingly, it has been shown that the dissociation of TTR tetramers could be prevented by the presence of a ligand in one of the two T4 binding sites [50, 51]. These studies laid the foundation for the development of the TTR-stabilizing drug category that to date include the molecules tafamidis [33, 52], acoramidis (AG10) [13, 53], and diflunisal [54, 55].

The two binding sites for RPB4 are located on opposite surfaces of TTR, and each one involves three monomers; in humans, the two RPB4 proteins bind in a two-fold symmetry axis [56]. The interaction between RPB4 and TTR is modulated by retinol, as holo-RPB4 shows higher affinity for TTR (Kd 0.2 μM) than apo-RPB4 (Kd 1.2 μM) [57, 58]. The influence of retinol in the formation and stabilization of TTR-RPB4 complexes has been deeply investigated by Hyung and collaborators [59]. Authors showed that holo-RBP4 conferred the maximum stability to TTR while reducing the concentration of the free tetramers which are at the beginning of the amyloidogenic cascade.

For its part, TTR affects the plasma concentration of RPB4 by preventing its glomerular filtration but TTR variants favoring the dissociation of tetramers result in fewer circulating TTR/RPB4 complexes and increased urinary excretion of RPB4. Indeed, ATTR V1221I amyloidosis patient showed lower plasma RPB4 levels than controls [60]. RPB4 is actively reabsorbed in renal proximal tubule, thus it can be quantified in urine only as a consequence of tubular injury for which is actually considered a sensitive biomarker [61].

Plasma levels of RBP and, as a consequence of retinol, can be affected also by therapies inhibiting TTR liver synthesis [19, 23, 25]. Thus, a long-term surveillance of patients receiving TTR-silencing therapies is needed to clarify the possible adverse effects related to the reduced availability of RPB4 and retinol.

To date, almost all studies about the dynamics of TTR stability have been conducted in vitro using a recombinant TTR protein in the absence of apo/holoRPB4 or

T4. Thus, the dynamics of the TTR/holoRPB4/T4 complex within a physiological context has not been studied yet in detail, indeed we still do not know which conditions favor the increase of free TTR tetramers and their destabilization in vivo. There is some evidence suggesting that the degradation forms of TTR (trimers, dimers) are also present in plasma [54]. Furthermore, Schonhoft and collaborators reported of peptide-based probes that label TTR oligomers in plasma of TTR hereditary amyloidosis patients exhibiting a neuropathic phenotype [62]. The characterization of circulating forms of TTR is limited by the lack of suitable analytical method. A native polyacrylamide gel electrophoresis (PAGE) approach has been developed by our research group and applied both to ATTR amyloidosis patients and sex and age-matched healthy subjects. This method was designed to obtain an electrophoretic separation of TTR forms based on their molecular weights. Preliminary data showed that the most represented TTR forms in patients and controls were TTR dimers or trimers (37–50 kDa), TTR tetramers complexed with RBP4 in a 1:1 (75 kDa) or 1:2 ratio (100 kDa), and high molecular weight aggregates (>150 kDa). RBP4 was detectable only in association with TTR tetramers in a 1:1 or 1:2 ratio. Free TTR tetramers (55 kDa) were detectable only in ATTR amyloidosis patients (Fig. 12.2). After the initiation of tafamidis, a progressive increase

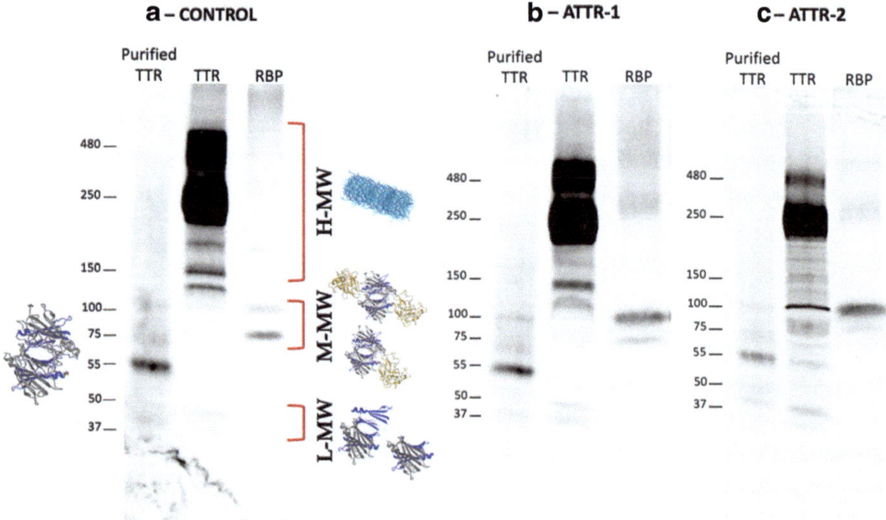

Fig. 12.2 Plasma TTR fractional analysis. Native polyacrylamide gel electrophoresis associated with western blot for the detection of transthyretin (TTR) or retinol binding protein 4 (RBP) in lithium-heparin plasma samples of a representative control subject (**a**) and two representative ATTR amyloidosis patients (**b**, **c**). A commercial preparation of TTR purified from plasma was used as reference for the electrophoretic mobility of free tetramers (55 kDa). In all samples, TTR aggregates (>150 kDa), TTR complexed with 2 or 1 RBP (100 and 75 kDa, respectively), and degradation form of TTR (<50 kDa, trimers and dimers) were observed. Free tetramers were also detectable, especially in some ATTR amyloidosis patients. *L-MW* low molecular weights, TTR dimers and trimers, *M-MW* medium molecular weights, TTR complexed with 1 or 2 RBP, *H-MW* high molecular weights, TTR aggregates

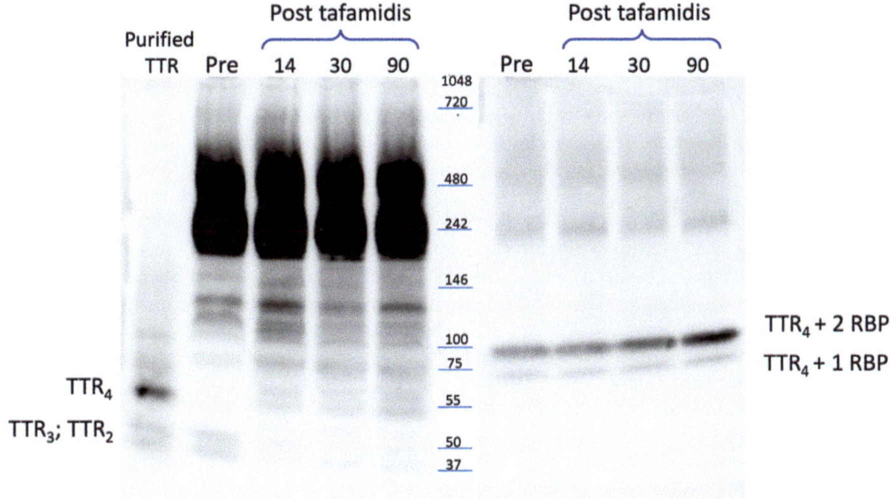

Fig. 12.3 Plasma TTR fractional analysis. Native polyacrylamide gel electrophoresis associated with western blot for the detection of transthyretin (left) or retinol binding protein 4 (right) in lithium-heparin plasma samples of a representative ATTR amyloidosis patients undergoing tafamidis treatment. *Pre* baseline sample, *Post tafamidis* plasma samples collected after 14, 30, and 90 days of treatment, *TTR$_4$* TTR tetramers, *TTR$_3$* TTR trimers, *TTR$_2$* dimers, *RBP* retinol binding protein 4

of the intensity of the band corresponding to TTR tetramers, free or complexed to RBP, was observed in patients with ATTR. Interestingly dimers and trimers, detectable at baseline, were progressively lost during tafamidis treatment (Fig. 12.3). These results agree with the stabilizing action on TTR tetramers of tafamidis and support the use of native PAGE as a tool to directly test the effects of stabilizing drugs in ATTR amyloidosis patients.

Native PAGE may increase our knowledge on the pattern of aggregate or disaggregate TTR-related structures in healthy subjects and ATTR amyloidosis patients and set the bases for their use as circulating biomarkers.

References

1. Sanguinetti C, Minniti M, Susini V, Caponi L, Panichella G, Castiglione V, et al. The journey of human transthyretin: synthesis, structure stability, and catabolism. Biomedicines. 2022;10:1906.
2. Ferguson RN, Edelhoch H, Saroff HA, Robbins J, Cahnmann HJ. Negative cooperativity in the binding of thyroxine to human serum prealbumin. Biochemistry. 1975;14:282–9.
3. Naylor HM, Newcomer ME. The structure of human retinol-binding protein (RBP) with its carrier protein transthyretin reveals an interaction with the carboxy terminus of RBP. Biochemistry. 1999;38:2647–53.
4. Magalhães J, Eira J, Liz MA. The role of transthyretin in cell biology: impact on human pathophysiology. Cell Mol Life Sci. 2021;78:6105–17.
5. Ritchie RF, Palomaki GE, Neveux LM, Navolotskaia O, Ledue TB, Craig WY. Reference distributions for the negative acute-phase serum proteins, albumin, transferrin and transthyre-

tin: a practical, simple and clinically relevant approach in a large cohort. J Clin Lab Anal. 1999;13:273–9.

6. Raynaud-Simon A, Lafont S, Berr C, Dartigues JF, Baulieu EE, Le Bouc Y. Plasma insulin-like growth factor I levels in the elderly: relation to plasma dehydroepiandrosterone sulfate levels, nutritional status, health and mortality. Gerontology. 2001;47:198–206.

7. Ingenbleek Y, Young V. Transthyretin (prealbumin) in health and disease: nutritional implications. Annu Rev Nutr. 1994;14:495–533.

8. Dellière S, Cynober L. Is transthyretin a good marker of nutritional status? Clin Nutr. 2017;36:364–70.

9. Myron Johnson A, Merlini G, Sheldon J, Ichihara K, Scientific Division Committee on Plasma Proteins (C-PP), International Federation of Clinical Chemistry and Laboratory Medicine (IFCC). Clinical indications for plasma protein assays: transthyretin (prealbumin) in inflammation and malnutrition. Clin Chem Lab Med. 2007;45:419–26.

10. Ingenbleek Y, De Visscher M, De Nayer P. Measurement of prealbumin as index of protein-calorie malnutrition. Lancet. 1972;2:106–9.

11. Falk RH, Comenzo RL, Skinner M. The systemic amyloidoses. N Engl J Med. 1997;337:898–909.

12. Scirpa R, Cittadini E, Mazzocchi L, Tini G, Sclafani M, Russo D, et al. Risk stratification in transthyretin-related cardiac amyloidosis. Front Cardiovasc Med. 2023;10:1151803.

13. Judge DP, Heitner SB, Falk RH, Maurer MS, Shah SJ, Witteles RM, et al. Transthyretin stabilization by AG10 in symptomatic transthyretin amyloid cardiomyopathy. J Am Coll Cardiol. 2019;74:285–95.

14. Castiglione V, Franzini M, Aimo A, Carecci A, Lombardi CM, Passino C, et al. Use of biomarkers to diagnose and manage cardiac amyloidosis. Eur J Heart Fail. 2021;23:217–30.

15. Ng B, Connors LH, Davidoff R, Skinner M, Falk RH. Senile systemic amyloidosis presenting with heart failure: a comparison with light chain-associated amyloidosis. Arch Intern Med. 2005;165:1425–9.

16. Emdin M, Aimo A, Rapezzi C, Fontana M, Perfetto F, Seferović PM, et al. Treatment of cardiac transthyretin amyloidosis: an update. Eur Heart J. 2019;40:3699–706.

17. Ruberg FL, Grogan M, Hanna M, Kelly JW, Maurer MS. Transthyretin amyloid cardiomyopathy: JACC state-of-the-art review. J Am Coll Cardiol. 2019;73:2872–91.

18. Aimo A, Castiglione V, Rapezzi C, Franzini M, Panichella G, Vergaro G, et al. RNA-targeting and gene editing therapies for transthyretin amyloidosis. Nat Rev Cardiol. 2022;19:655–67.

19. Suhr OB, Coelho T, Buades J, Pouget J, Conceicao I, Berk J, et al. Efficacy and safety of patisiran for familial amyloidotic polyneuropathy: a phase II multi-dose study. Orphanet J Rare Dis. 2015;10:109.

20. Adams D, Gonzalez-Duarte A, O'Riordan WD, Yang C-C, Ueda M, Kristen AV, et al. Patisiran, an RNAi therapeutic, for hereditary transthyretin amyloidosis. N Engl J Med. 2018;379:11–21.

21. Goel V, Gosselin NH, Jomphe C, Zhang X, Marier J-F, Robbie GJ. Population pharmacokinetic-pharmacodynamic model of serum transthyretin following Patisiran administration. Nucleic Acid Ther. 2020;30:143–52.

22. Habtemariam BA, Karsten V, Attarwala H, Goel V, Melch M, Clausen VA, et al. Single-dose pharmacokinetics and pharmacodynamics of transthyretin targeting N-acetylgalactosamine-small interfering ribonucleic acid conjugate, vutrisiran, in healthy subjects. Clin Pharmacol Ther. 2021;109:372–82.

23. Ackermann EJ, Guo S, Benson MD, Booten S, Freier S, Hughes SG, et al. Suppressing transthyretin production in mice, monkeys and humans using 2nd-generation antisense oligonucleotides. Amyloid. 2016;23:148–57.

24. Benson MD, Waddington-Cruz M, Berk JL, Polydefkis M, Dyck PJ, Wang AK, et al. Inotersen treatment for patients with hereditary transthyretin amyloidosis. N Engl J Med. 2018;379:22–31.

25. Viney NJ, Guo S, Tai L-J, Baker BF, Aghajan M, Jung SW, et al. Ligand conjugated antisense oligonucleotide for the treatment of transthyretin amyloidosis: preclinical and phase 1 data. ESC Heart Fail. 2021;8:652–61.

26. Ionis Pharmaceuticals, Inc. A Phase 3 Global, Open-Label, Randomized Study to Evaluate the Efficacy and Safety of ION-682884 in Patients With Hereditary Transthyretin-Mediated Amyloid Polyneuropathy [Internet]. clinicaltrials.gov; 2023 mag. Report No.: NCT04136184. Recuperato da: https://clinicaltrials.gov/study/NCT04136184
27. Gillmore JD, Gane E, Taubel J, Kao J, Fontana M, Maitland ML, et al. CRISPR-Cas9 in vivo gene editing for transthyretin amyloidosis. N Engl J Med. 2021;385:493–502.
28. Intellia and Regeneron Announce Updated Phase 1 Data Demonstrating a Single Dose of NTLA-2001, an Investigational CRISPR Therapy for Transthyretin (ATTR) Amyloidosis, Resulted in Rapid, Deep and Sustained Reduction in Disease-Causing Protein—Intellia Therapeutics [Internet]. [citato 31 luglio 2023]. Recuperato da: https://ir.intelliatx.com/news-releases/news-release-details/intellia-and-regeneron-announce-updated-phase-1-data
29. Hanson JLS, Arvanitis M, Koch CM, Berk JL, Ruberg FL, Prokaeva T, et al. Use of serum transthyretin as a prognostic indicator and predictor of outcome in cardiac amyloid disease associated with wild-type transthyretin. Circ Heart Fail. 2018;11:e004000.
30. Falk RH, Haddad M, Walker CR, Dorbala S, Cuddy SAM. Effect of tafamidis on serum transthyretin levels in non-trial patients with transthyretin amyloid cardiomyopathy. JACC CardioOncol. 2021;3:580–6.
31. Fox JC, Hellawell JL, Rao S, O'Reilly T, Lumpkin R, Jernelius J, et al. First-in-human study of AG10, a novel, oral, specific, selective, and potent transthyretin stabilizer for the treatment of transthyretin amyloidosis: a phase 1 safety, tolerability, pharmacokinetic, and pharmacodynamic study in healthy adult volunteers. Clin Pharmacol Drug Dev. 2020;9:115–29.
32. Thuillier F, Demarquilly C, Szymanowicz A, Gaillard C, Boniface M, Braidy C, et al. Nephelometry or turbidimetry for the determination of albumin, ApoA, CRP, haptoglobin, IgM and transthyretin: which choice? Ann Biol Clin (Paris). 2008;66:63–78.
33. Bulawa CE, Connelly S, Devit M, Wang L, Weigel C, Fleming JA, et al. Tafamidis, a potent and selective transthyretin kinetic stabilizer that inhibits the amyloid cascade. Proc Natl Acad Sci USA. 2012;109:9629–34.
34. Gamez J, Salvadó M, Reig N, Suñé P, Casasnovas C, Rojas-Garcia R, et al. Transthyretin stabilization activity of the catechol-O-methyltransferase inhibitor tolcapone (SOM0226) in hereditary ATTR amyloidosis patients and asymptomatic carriers: proof-of-concept study. Amyloid. 2019;26:74–84.
35. Gopal DM, Ruberg FL, Siddiqi OK. Impact of genetic testing in transthyretin (ATTR) cardiac amyloidosis. Curr Heart Fail Rep. 2019;16:180–8.
36. Benson MD, Yazaki M, Magy N. Laboratory assessment of transthyretin amyloidosis. Clin Chem Lab Med. 2002;40:1262–5.
37. Altland K, Banzhoff A. Separation by hybrid isoelectric focusing of normal human transthyretin (prealbumin) and a variant with a methionine for valine substitution associated with familial amyloidotic polyneuropathy. Electrophoresis. 1986;7:529–33.
38. Connors LH, Ericsson T, Skare J, Jones LA, Lewis WD, Skinner M. A simple screening test for variant transthyretins associated with familial transthyretin amyloidosis using isoelectric focusing. Biochim Biophys Acta. 1998;1407:185–92.
39. Tachibana N, Tokuda T, Yoshida K, Taketomi T, Nakazato M, Li YF, et al. Usefulness of MALDI/TOF mass spectrometry of immunoprecipitated serum variant transthyretin in the diagnosis of familial amyloid polyneuropathy. Amyloid. 1999;6:282–8.
40. Terazaki H, Ando Y, Misumi S, Nakamura M, Ando E, Matsunaga N, et al. A novel compound heterozygote (FAP ATTR Arg104His/ATTR Val30Met) with high serum transthyretin (TTR) and retinol binding protein (RBP) levels. Biochem Biophys Res Commun. 1999;264:365–70.
41. Théberge R, Connors L, Skinner M, Skare J, Costello CE. Characterization of transthyretin mutants from serum using immunoprecipitation, HPLC/electrospray ionization and matrix-assisted laser desorption/ionization mass spectrometry. Anal Chem. 1999;71:452–9.
42. Ando Y, Ohlsson PI, Suhr O, Nyhlin N, Yamashita T, Holmgren G, et al. A new simple and rapid screening method for variant transthyretin-related amyloidosis. Biochem Biophys Res Commun. 1996;228:480–3.

43. Kishikawa M, Nakanishi T, Miyazaki A, Shimizu A, Nakazato M, Kangawa K, et al. Simple detection of abnormal serum transthyretin from patients with familial amyloidotic polyneuropathy by high-performance liquid chromatography/electrospray ionization mass spectrometry using material precipitated with specific antiserum. J Mass Spectrom. 1996;31:112–4.
44. Ranløv I, Ando Y, Ohlsson PI, Holmgren G, Ranløv PJ, Suhr OB. Rapid screening for amyloid-related variant forms of transthyretin is possible by electrospray ionization mass spectrometry. Eur J Clin Investig. 1997;27:956–9.
45. Tasaki M, Ueda M, Obayashi K, Motokawa H, Kinoshita Y, Suenaga G, et al. Rapid detection of wild-type and mutated transthyretins. Ann Clin Biochem. 2016;53:508–10.
46. Ueda M, Misumi Y, Mizuguchi M, Nakamura M, Yamashita T, Sekijima Y, et al. SELDI-TOF mass spectrometry evaluation of variant transthyretins for diagnosis and pathogenesis of familial amyloidotic polyneuropathy. Clin Chem. 2009;55:1223–7.
47. Nomura T, Ueda M, Tasaki M, Misumi Y, Masuda T, Inoue Y, et al. New simple and quick method to analyze serum variant transthyretins: direct MALDI method for the screening of hereditary transthyretin amyloidosis. Orphanet J Rare Dis. 2019;14:116.
48. White JT, Kelly JW. Support for the multigenic hypothesis of amyloidosis: the binding stoichiometry of retinol-binding protein, vitamin A, and thyroid hormone influences transthyretin amyloidogenicity in vitro. Proc Natl Acad Sci USA. 2001;98:13019–24.
49. Ferreira N, Saraiva MJ, Almeida MR. Uncovering the neuroprotective mechanisms of curcumin on transthyretin amyloidosis. Int J Mol Sci. 2019;20:1287.
50. Foss TR, Kelker MS, Wiseman RL, Wilson IA, Kelly JW. Kinetic stabilization of the native state by protein engineering: implications for inhibition of transthyretin amyloidogenesis. J Mol Biol. 2005;347:841–54.
51. Foss TR, Wiseman RL, Kelly JW. The pathway by which the tetrameric protein transthyretin dissociates. Biochemistry. 2005;44:15525–33.
52. Tess DA, Maurer TS, Li Z, Bulawa C, Fleming J, Moody AT. Relationship of binding-site occupancy, transthyretin stabilisation and disease modification in patients with tafamidis-treated transthyretin amyloid cardiomyopathy. Amyloid. 2023;30:208–19.
53. Miller M, Pal A, Albusairi W, Joo H, Pappas B, Haque Tuhin MT, et al. Enthalpy-driven stabilization of transthyretin by AG10 mimics a naturally occurring genetic variant that protects from transthyretin amyloidosis. J Med Chem. 2018;61:7862–76.
54. Sekijima Y, Dendle MA, Kelly JW. Orally administered diflunisal stabilizes transthyretin against dissociation required for amyloidogenesis. Amyloid. 2006;13:236–49.
55. Kingsbury JS, Laue TM, Klimtchuk ES, Théberge R, Costello CE, Connors LH. The modulation of transthyretin tetramer stability by cysteine 10 adducts and the drug diflunisal. Direct analysis by fluorescence-detected analytical ultracentrifugation. J Biol Chem. 2008;283:11887–96.
56. Monaco HL, Rizzi M, Coda A. Structure of a complex of two plasma proteins: transthyretin and retinol-binding protein. Science. 1995;268:1039–41.
57. Malpeli G, Folli C, Berni R. Retinoid binding to retinol-binding protein and the interference with the interaction with transthyretin. Biochim Biophys Acta. 1996;1294:48–54.
58. Goodman DS. Plasma retinol-binding protein. Ann N Y Acad Sci. 1980;348:378–90.
59. Hyung S-J, Deroo S, Robinson CV. Retinol and retinol-binding protein stabilize transthyretin via formation of retinol transport complex. ACS Chem Biol. 2010;5:1137–46.
60. Arvanitis M, Koch CM, Chan GG, Torres-Arancivia C, LaValley MP, Jacobson DR, et al. Identification of transthyretin cardiac amyloidosis using serum retinol-binding protein 4 and a clinical prediction model. JAMA Cardiol. 2017;2:305–13.
61. Ratajczyk K, Konieczny A, Czekaj A, Piotrów P, Fiutowski M, Krakowska K, et al. The clinical significance of urinary retinol-binding protein 4: a review. Int J Environ Res Public Health. 2022;19:9878.
62. Schonhoft JD, Monteiro C, Plate L, Eisele YS, Kelly JM, Boland D, et al. Peptide probes detect misfolded transthyretin oligomers in plasma of hereditary amyloidosis patients. Sci Transl Med. 2017;9:eaam7621.

Cardiac Scintigraphy with Bone-Avid Tracers: Old and New Applications

Shilpa Vijayakumar and Sharmila Dorbala

13.1 Background

The field of cardiac amyloidosis (CA) has grown tremendously over the past decade due to advances in noninvasive imaging techniques and new targeted therapies [1, 2]. Until recently, the only reliable method of specifically diagnosing the two main forms of CA, amyloid light-chain (AL-CA) or transthyretin (ATTR-CA), was biopsy with typing of the amyloid by immunohistochemistry or mass spectrometry. While biopsy remains the standard of care for diagnosing AL-CA, data from a large global registry indicate that biopsy is being replaced by noninvasive diagnosis using technetium-99m-labeled bone-avid radiotracer cardiac scintigraphy for ATTR-CA. This chapter provides an overview of the current and novel applications of bone-avid radiotracer cardiac scintigraphy in ATTR-CA.

13.2 Evolution of Cardiac Scintigraphy with Technetium-99m-Labeled Bone-Avid Radiotracers

Myocardial uptake of technetium-99m-labeled bone-avid radiotracers on bone scans has long been recognized to represent CA [3–8]. However, interest in this diagnostic method faded due to reports of inconsistent sensitivity [9]. In hindsight, reports of lower sensitivities were likely due to the studies including patients with

S. Vijayakumar · S. Dorbala (✉)
Division of Cardiovascular Imaging, Department of Radiology, Brigham and Women's Hospital, Boston, MA, USA

Cardiac Amyloidosis Program, Division of Cardiology, Department of Medicine, Brigham and Women's Hospital, Boston, MA, USA
e-mail: svijayakumar@bwh.harvard.edu; sdorbala@bwh.harvard.edu

M. Emdin et al. (eds.), *Cardiac Amyloidosis*,
https://doi.org/10.1007/978-3-031-51757-0_13

both AL and ATTR-CA. In the early 2000s, researchers first recognized that [99mTc]-3,3-diphosphono-1,2-propanodicarboxylic acid had far greater avidity for ATTR-CA than AL-CA [10, 11]. With this newfound knowledge, subsequent studies focused on patients with suspected ATTR-CA, rather than all forms of CA, and have confirmed its high specificity for ATTR-CA. Tc-99m-labeled bone-avid radiotracer cardiac imaging is now an accepted standard for noninvasive diagnosis of ATTR-CA. The imaging technique has evolved from purely planar imaging methods of the 1980s to SPECT and now quantitative SPECT/CT cardiac scintigraphy. Conventional scan interpretation focused on visual grades comparing tracer uptake in the myocardium to that of the bone in the form of heart-to-whole body or heart-to-rib ratio measures based on planar imaging. SPECT-based visual grading provides the advantage of better delineation of blood pool from myocardial activity. Novel SPECT/CT-based methods are providing semiquantitative standardized uptake value (SUV) measures, which are promising for disease monitoring.

13.3 Mechanism of Myocardial Uptake of Bone-Avid Tracers in ATTR-CA

The molecular basis of myocardial uptake of Tc-99m-labeled bone-avid radiotracers is not entirely understood. It has been speculated that these bone-avid tracers might bind to the calcium deposits in amyloid-infiltrated myocardial tissue. Tc-99m-PYP was originally validated to detect irreversibly damaged myocardium, such as in acute myocardial infarction, with uptake correlating temporally and topographically to calcium accumulation in animal models [12]. In the evaluation of endomyocardial biopsies of both ATTR-CA and AL-CA, compared to AL-CA, ATTR-CA contained a greater density of microcalcifications, which may explain the predilection of these tracers for ATTR-CA [13]. However, more recent evidence argues against this theory. [18]Fluorine-labeled sodium fluoride, a positron emission tomography (PET) tracer known to consistently detect cardiovascular microcalcification [14, 15], did not show reliable myocardial uptake in ATTR-CA or AL-CA [16, 17]. In addition, not all 99m-labeled bone-avid radiotracers show avidity for ATTR-CA, and Tc-99m methylene diphosphonate is not recommended due to low sensitivity compared to 99mTc-PYP/DPD/HMDP [18].

13.4 Diagnostic Accuracy of 99mTc-PYP/DPD/HMDP for ATTR-CA

Numerous studies have shown high specificity and diagnostic accuracy of Tc-99m-PYP/DPD/HMDP for ATTR-CA [10, 11, 19–23]. A large, multicenter, pivotal study by Gillmore et al. analyzed bone scintigraphy, including Tc-99m-PYP/DPD/HMDP, from 1217 patients with suspected CA [23]. This study showed that after exclusion of AL amyloidosis, grade 2 or grade 3 myocardial radiotracer uptake had a specificity and positive predictive value for ATTR-CA of 100%. Importantly, this study also noted that over 20% of patients with AL-CA also demonstrated grade 2 or grade 3 myocardial radiotracer uptake, underscoring the importance of AL-CA exclusion prior to diagnosis of ATTR-CA using bone scintigraphy [23]. A combination of urine and serum protein immunofixation assay and serum free light chains has a sensitivity of 99% for diagnosing AL-CA, and thus, it is the recommended method of AL-CA assessment [24].

Although nearly 100% specific, grade 2/3 myocardial uptake on bone-avid tracer cardiac scintigraphy is only ~70% specific for the diagnosis of cardiac amyloidosis. Inclusion of grades 1, 2, and 3 as cardiac amyloidosis improved the sensitivity to 99%, but at the expense of a decrease in specificity for ATTR-CA to 78%. This decrease in specificity is primarily due to AL-CA. Hence, grades 2/3 were considered positive, while grades 0/1 were considered negative. The true significance of a visual grade 1, which was previously interpreted as a negative study, is currently being determined. A recent multinational retrospective analysis by Rauf et al. assessed over 3000 patients with known or suspected CA referred to specialist centers and found that the majority of patients with a grade 1 scan, in the absence of a monoclonal gammopathy, had early ATTR-CA, and the majority of patients with a grade 1 scan and monoclonal gammopathy had advanced AL-CA [25].

Early diagnosis of AL-CA is crucial due to its high mortality rate in the absence of therapy. Thus, all patients suspected of having CA should undergo an AL assessment promptly. If the evaluation shows abnormalities, urgent evaluation by a hematologist is necessary to rule out AL-CA. However, certain older adults with renal dysfunction may manifest an isolated elevation of free kappa light chains, as kappa light chains are renally excreted. This scenario poses a potential diagnostic dilemma for a noninvasive diagnosis of ATTR-CA. To address this issue, a new algorithm has recently been developed for diagnosing ATTR-CA. The algorithm utilizes estimated glomerular filtration rate (eGFR)-specific cutoffs for normal serum free light chain ratio, allowing for a higher "normal" kappa/lambda ratio in patients with reduced eGFR. This approach maintains the high specificity of bone scintigraphy-based non-biopsy diagnostic criteria while reducing the need for unnecessary biopsies in patients who might otherwise be misclassified as having a monoclonal gammopathy (Fig. 13.1).

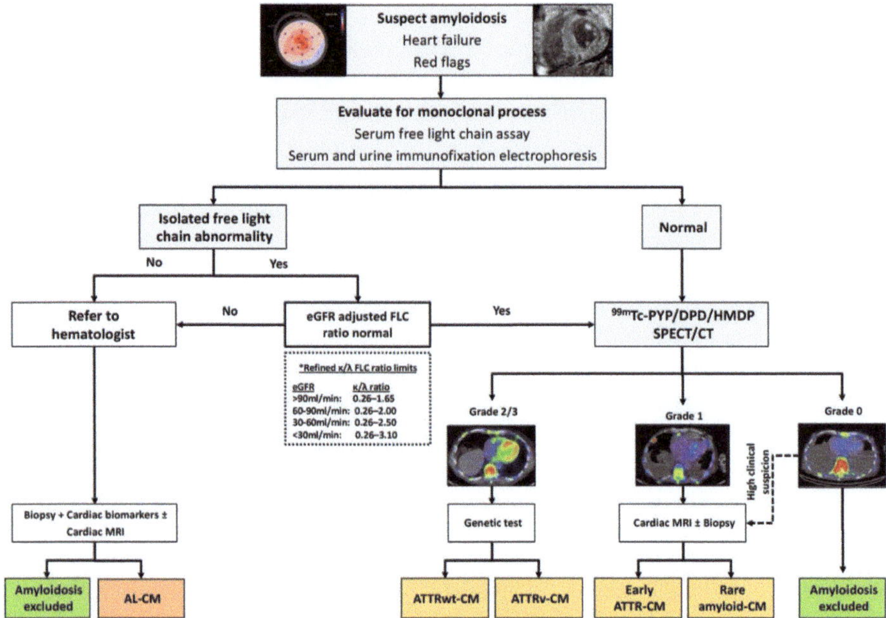

Fig. 13.1 Diagnostic algorithm for cardiac amyloidosis. Modified with permission from Gillmore et al. [23]

13.5 Diagnostic Criteria for ATTR-CA

Diagnostic criteria for ATTR-CA are listed in Table 13.1. ATTR-CA can be diagnosed by histological confirmation or by imaging. Endomyocardial proof of amyloid by Congo red staining with confirmation of transthyretin type by immunohistochemistry or mass spectrometry makes a diagnosis of ATTR-CA. A systemic biopsy proof of ATTR amyloidosis in combination with typical cardiac imaging findings is also an accepted means for diagnosis of ATTR-CA. A noninvasive diagnosis without biopsy is the accepted standard for diagnosis of ATTR-CA and is supported by the American Society of Nuclear Cardiology and multiple societies, including the European Society of Cardiology (ESC) [26].

Table 13.1 Expert consensus recommendations for diagnosis of cardiac amyloidosis. Adapted from Dorbala S, Ando Y, Bokhari S et al. ASNC/AHA/ASE/EANM/HFSA/ISA/SCMR/SNMMI expert consensus recommendations for multimodality imaging in cardiac amyloidosis: Part 2 of 2-Diagnostic criteria and appropriate utilization. Journal of nuclear cardiology: Official publication of the American Society of Nuclear Cardiology 2019;26:2065–2123

Criteria for diagnosis	Subtype
Histological diagnosis of cardiac amyloidosis: Endomyocardial biopsy[a]	
1. Endomyocardial biopsy positive for cardiac amyloidosis with Congo red staining with apple-green birefringence under polarized light; typing by immunohistochemistry and/or mass spectrometry at specialized centers	AL, ATTR, other subtypes
Histological diagnosis of cardiac amyloidosis: Extracardiac biopsy	
1. ATTR cardiac amyloidosis is diagnosed when below criteria are met: (a) Extracardiac biopsy-proven ATTR amyloidosis **AND** (b) Typical cardiac imaging features (as defined below)	ATTR
2. AL cardiac amyloidosis is diagnosed when below criteria are met: (a) Extracardiac biopsy-proven AL amyloidosis **AND** (b) Typical cardiac imaging features (as defined below) **OR** (c) Abnormal cardiac biomarkers: Abnormal age-adjusted NTpro-BNP or abnormal troponin T/I/Hs-troponin with all other causes for these changes excluded	AL
Clinical diagnosis of ATTR cardiac amyloidosis: ^{99m}Tc-PYP, DPD, HMDP	
1. ATTR cardiac amyloidosis is diagnosed when below criteria are met: (a) 99mTc-PYP, DPD, HMDP grade 2 or 3 myocardial uptake of radiotracer **AND** (b) Absence of a clonal plasma cell process as assessed by serum FLCs and serum and urine immunofixation **AND** (c) Typical cardiac imaging features (as defined below)	ATTR
Typical imaging features of cardiac amyloidosis	
Typical cardiac echo or CMR or PET features: **ANY** of the below imaging features with all other causes for these cardiac manifestations, including hypertension, reasonably excluded	
1. Echo (a) LV wall thickness > 12 mm (b) Relative apical sparing of global LS ratio (average of apical LS/average of combined mid + basal LS > 1) (c) ≥grade 2 diastolic dysfunction[b]	ATTR/AL
2. CMR (a) LV wall thickness > ULN for sex on SSFP cine CMR (b) Global ECV > 0.40 (c) Diffuse LGE[b] (d) Abnormal gadolinium kinetics typical for amyloidosis, myocardial nulling prior to blood pool nulling	ATTR/AL
3. PET: 18F-florbetapir[b] or 18F-florbetaben PET[b,c] (a) Target-to-background (LV myocardium to blood pool) ratio > 1.5 (b) Retention index > 0.030 min^{-1}	ATTR/AL

Abbreviations: *AL* amyloidogenic light chain, *ATTR* amyloidogenic transthyretin, *ECV* extracellular volume, *LGE* late gadolinium enhancement, *LS* longitudinal strain, *LV* left ventricular, *SSFP* steady-state free precession, *ULN* upper limit of normal, per reference [38] at mid-cavity level ULN for women/men was 7 mm/9 mm (long axis) and 7 mm/8 mm (short axis)

[a] Endomyocardial biopsy should be considered in cases of equivocal 99mTc-PYP, DPD, and HMDP scan. When 99mTc-PYP, DPD, and HMDP are positive in the context of any abnormal evaluation for serum/urine immunofixation or serum free light-chain assay, or MGUS, this should not be seen as diagnostic for ATTR cardiac amyloidosis. In these instances, referral to a specialist amyloid center for further evaluation and consideration of biopsy is recommended

[b] Off-label use of FDA-approved commercial products

[c] 18F-flutemetamol not studied systematically in the heart. 11C-Pittsburgh B compound is not FDA approved and not available to sites without a cyclotron in proximity

13.6 Imaging Protocols for Tc-99m-PYP/DPD/HMDP Cardiac Scintigraphy

The American Society of Nuclear Cardiology (ASNC) [27, 28] has developed recommendations for optimal image acquisition for Tc-99m-PYP/DPD/HMDP (Table 13.1). Per these recommendations, no specific patient preparation is required for imaging. Images are acquired 2–3 h after radiotracer injection to imaging to allow for blood pool activity to clear. Single-photon emission computed tomography (SPECT), and ideally SPECT/CT, is recommended in all cases. Planar imaging alone is not recommended. SPECT, and ideally SPECT/CT, will help differentiate radiotracer uptake in the myocardium from that in the blood pool [27]. After image acquisition, SPECT images are reviewed in axial, coronal, and sagittal projections. Current approaches to interpretation are largely based on visual grading (known as the Perugini score). In this visual grading system (Fig. 13.2), myocardial uptake is compared with rib uptake and characterized as:

- Grade 0: No myocardial uptake and normal rib uptake.
- Grade 1: Myocardial uptake less than rib uptake.
- Grade 2: Myocardial uptake equal to rib uptake.
- Grade 3: Myocardial uptake greater than rib uptake.

A semiquantitative approach, known as the heart-to-contralateral lung (H/CL) ratio or heart-to-whole body ratio (H/WB), has also been described [27]. An H/CL ratio $\geq$1.5 at 1-h imaging in the absence of AL amyloidosis has been shown to accurately differentiate AL-CA from ATTR-CA [29]. However, this ratio has not been validated to diagnose ATTR-CA in patients with suspected CA. Also, there are many limitations to this method, including incorrect positioning or sizing of ROI, inclusion of blood pool activity, inclusion of adjacent lung in the heart ROI, and inclusion of right ventricle in the lung ROI. Given these limitations and given that this method does not provide significant added benefit over visual grading, many centers do not perform this semiquantitative analysis and only report visual grading score.

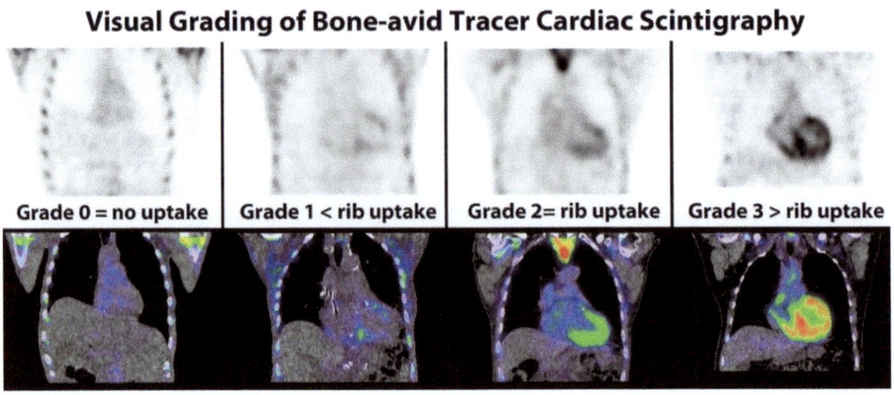

Fig. 13.2 Visual grading of cardiac uptake of bone tracers

13.7   Current Applications of Bone Scintigraphy

A comprehensive meta-analysis has summarized the published literature on bone-avid tracer cardiac scintigraphy [30] (Fig. 13.3).

13.7.1 Diagnosis of ATTR-CA in Patients with Heart Failure

Myocardial amyloid deposits are prevalent in older adults with heart failure at autopsy and detected by imaging in older adults with heart failure hospitalization, those with HFpEF with and without thick ventricles. In an autopsy study of patients with heart failure with preserved ejection fraction (HFpEF), left ventricular ATTR amyloid deposition was found in an age-dependent manner, with over 20% of specimens showing ATTR amyloid deposition in patients over 80 years of age [31]. Thus, Tc-99m-DPD cardiac scintigraphy was used in the diagnostic workup of hospitalized older adults with HFpEF and increased left ventricular wall thickness of ≥12 mm, and ATTR-CA was subsequently diagnosed in 13–19% of these patients [32, 33]. AbouEzzeddine et al. [34] evaluated community-dwelling patients with HFpEF and left ventricular wall thickness >12 mm; in that study, 18 of 286 patients (6.3%) who underwent Tc-99-PYP imaging were diagnosed with ATTR-CA, with higher prevalence in men (10.1%; 95% CI, 5.7–16.1%) than

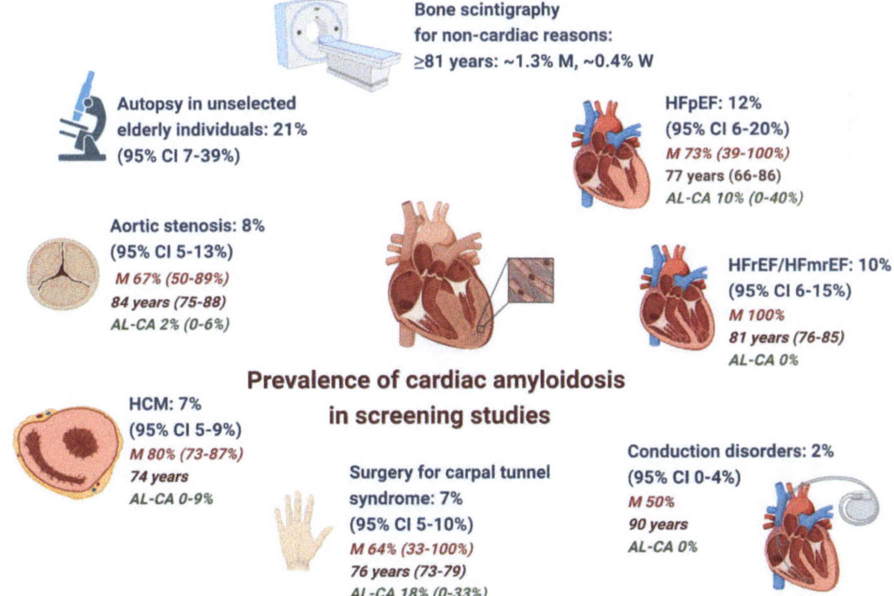

Fig. 13.3 Meta-analysis of studies on the prevalence of cardiac amyloidosis in different settings. Reproduced with permission from Aimo et al. [30]

in women (2.2%; 95% CI, 0.4–6.3%, $P = 0.002$). Another study screening patients with HFpEF without left ventricular thickening found a 5% prevalence of ATTR-CA in this cohort [35].

13.7.2 Diagnosis of ATTR-CA in Patients with Heart Failure and Severe Aortic Valve Stenosis

ATTR-CA has also been increasingly identified in older patients with severe aortic valve stenosis. In numerous studies of Tc-99m-PYP and Tc-99m-DPD prospectively used in all patients with severe aortic valve stenosis who underwent transcatheter aortic valve replacement (TAVR), the prevalence of ATTR-CA was approximately 16%, with higher prevalence in those presenting with low-flow low-gradient severe aortic stenosis [36, 37]. Patients with concomitant CA and severe aortic stenosis had worse initial presentation by functional capacity, cardiac remodeling, and biomarker and lower rates of survival if untreated compared with patients with severe aortic stenosis without CA [38]. After TAVR, the presence of CA was not found to have significant effect on mortality [39, 40]. In contrast, the presence of wild-type ATTR-CA was associated with poorer outcome after surgical aortic valve replacement (SAVR), although this was in a very small sample size of six participants [41].

13.7.3 Screening of At-Risk Patients for Early Detection of ATTR-CA: Carpal Tunnel Syndrome

Given the ease of diagnosis with bone-avid tracer cardiac scintigraphy, it has also been used to screen higher risk populations for ATTR-CA, providing new insight into the true prevalence of disease in these populations. Musculoskeletal manifestations of carpal tunnel syndrome, biceps tendon rupture, and lumbar spinal stenosis are risk markers for ATTR-CA, and ATTR amyloid deposits have been reported in the tendons and other soft tissue. Carpal tunnel syndrome often precedes cardiac ATTR-CA manifestations by 5–10 years [42, 43]. In a cohort of 98 patients undergoing carpal tunnel release surgery, 10 (10.2%) had a positive biopsy for amyloid, and of these, 2 were found to have cardiac involvement using Tc-99m-PYP [44]. Several other studies have confirmed similar findings [45–49].

13.7.4 Temporal Trends in Detection of ATTR-CA Due to Use of Bone-Avid Tracer Cardiac Scintigraphy

Advancements in bone scintigraphy for the diagnosis of ATTR-CA have simplified the diagnosis of ATTR-CA and dramatically increased disease detection. In a large, observational, retrospective study using data from the National Amyloidosis Centre in London of 2995 patients with suspected ATTR-CA, of which 1967 were diagnosed with ATTR-CA over the past 20 years, there has been a progressive increase in referrals for suspected ATTR-CA, which has been accompanied by a far greater number of ATTR-CA diagnoses ($n = 35$ in the first period of 2002–2006, compared to $n = 968$ in the last period of 2017–2021) [50]. Of these diagnoses, none were wild-type ATTR-CA between 2002 and 2006, compared to 642 out of 968 (66%) diagnosed with wild type in the last period of 2017–2021. Over time, the use of bone scintigraphy for diagnosis of ATTR-CA has steadily increased, and the use of endomyocardial biopsy has decreased. Notably, the severity of cardiac disease at diagnosis has also progressively decreased. At diagnosis, patients with ATTR-CA over time have had better functional capacity, assessed by New York Heart Association (NYHA) class, better 6-min walk test, and higher blood pressure. In fact, when using a UK National Amyloidosis Centre (NAC) staging system [51] based on N-terminal pro-B-type natriuretic peptide (NT-proBNP) and estimated glomerular filtration rate, where stage I represents mild disease, stage II represents moderate disease, and stage III represents severe disease, between the years of 2002 and 2016, an average of 42% of ATTR-CA was diagnosed at stage I NAC, compared to an average of 56% from 2017 to 2021 [50].

Similarly, in another study using data from 2007 to 2020 from the Transthyretin Amyloidosis Outcomes Survey (THAOS) registry, a global, multicenter, longitudinal observational survey, of the 1069 patients with wild-type ATTR-CA and 525 patients with hereditary ATTR-CA analyzed, the diagnosis of wild-type ATTR-CA increased from 2 in 2005 to >100 per year from 2016 onwards, with the most pronounced increase in the United States compared to other global sites [52]. Diagnosis of wild-type ATTR-CA by bone scintigraphy has markedly increased since 2011, and diagnosis with tissue biopsy has steadily declined since 2014. In this study, the proportion of wild-type ATTR-CA patients with NYHA class III/IV, indicative of marked limitations due to symptoms, decreased from 46% in 2012 to 16% in 2019 [52].

Importantly, 95% of patients enrolled in the THAOS registry were male, and only 5% were female. Although wild-type ATTR-CA has been previously been thought to disproportionately affect males [34], in recent databases, fewer sex differences in disease prevalence were noted. Screening studies have shown similar sex prevalence, but studies assessing diagnosis of ATTR-CA in patients with symptoms show a male predominance. In a large in-hospital Japanese database, over half (53.7%) of the patients with wild-type ATTR-CA were female. In another study using Medicare beneficiaries from 2000 to 2012, an overall increase in prevalence of CA was reported (18–55 per 100,000 person-years). Of the individual patients with newly diagnosed ATTR-CA from 2000 to 2012, 50% were women [53]. The discrepancy between sexes in incidence and prevalence of ATTR-CA previously reported may have been due to biological differences in left ventricular wall thickness between men and women. A left ventricular wall thickness ≥ 12 mm in the setting of other typical clinical features raises suspicion of CA. However, normal values of LV wall thickness are lower in women, and using the same cutoff values for both sexes may lead to underdiagnosis of disease in women. Indexed left ventricular wall thickness values, especially by height, have been shown to reflect cardiac involvement more accurately in both sexes [30]. Some studies assessing 99m-labeled bone-avid radiotracer imaging found similar proportions of men and women with positive scan results [32].

Despite disease incidence and prevalence remaining constant, bone scintigraphy has dramatically improved diagnosis of ATTR-CA, particularly wild-type ATTR-CA. As a result, patients are also being diagnosed much earlier in the course of the disease, allowing opportunity to implement therapies in a timely manner to slow disease progression, improve functional capacity and quality of life, and extend survival. There is also now information to suggest that women may have been particularly underdiagnosed in the past and are now being increasingly diagnosed.

13.8 Novel Applications of Bone Scintigraphy: Assessment of Response to Therapy

With the increasing availability of TTR-stabilizing and -silencing therapies and the emerging novel amyloid-depleting therapies, there is a great need for imaging methods to monitor myocardial changes in amyloid burden using bone-avid tracer scintigraphy. Current techniques for assessing radiotracer uptake, mainly by visual grading and semiquantitative metrics, can diagnose ATTR-CA with high specificity. In ATTR-CA, the burden of CA has also correlated with myocardial radiotracer uptake using bone scintigraphy in most cases (except in Ser777Tyr hereditary ATTR-CA) [54]. However, visual grading and semiquantitative measurements are inadequate to analyze amyloid burden, disease progression, and response to therapy. Thus, quantitative methods for assessing myocardial radiotracer uptake are needed. Recent advances in SPECT technology with CT-based attenuation correction, quantification using SUV metrics, and improved geometry of the SPECT scanners allow for robust quantification of SPECT radiotracers. These advances make semiquantitative approaches using continuous metrics feasible for detection of early disease and disease progression.

Quantitative metrics were assessed in a study by Dorbala et al. of 72 patients who underwent 99mTc-pyrophosphate SPECT/CT using a novel general-purpose cadmium-zinc-telluride-based SPECT/CT scanner [55]. The metrics assessed were standardized uptake value (SUV)max and SUVmean, defined as the maximum and mean decay-corrected activity concentration of 99mTc-pyrophosphate divided by injected activity per unit body weight within the volume of interest (VOI), cardiac amyloid activity (CAA), product of the VOI volume and SUVmean, and percentage injected dose (%ID), defined as the absolute 99mTc-pyrophosphate activity concentration in the VOI multiplied by the VOI volume, normalized to injected dose. These four metrics were accurate (area under ROC curve more than 0.96 for each), tracked 99mTc-PYP visual grade, correlated moderately to LV mass by echocardiography ($r = 0.485$ for %ID) and strongly to ECV ($r = 0.873$, SUV_{max}), and demonstrated excellent intraobserver repeatability. These metrics may also be complementary to visual grading alone, since some patients with grade 0 and grade 1 visual uptake had similar quantitative values to patients diagnosed with ATTR-CA [55]. Several other investigators, using single center and small cohorts, have also evaluated SUV measures of bone-avid tracer cardiac scintigraphy.

Assessment of treatment response is a major application of quantitative metrics. In a study determining the effect of patisiran on CA load, CMR metrics and Tc-99m-DPD scintigraphy were evaluated at baseline and 1 year post-therapy [56]. Percent injected dose of Tc-99m-DPD showed a median reduction in cardiac uptake by bone scintigraphy of 19.6% [56] in the patisiran cohort; however, median ECV did not change significantly (baseline ECV 46% vs. posttreatment ECV 48%). These findings may reflect the biologic effect of patisiran on facilitating natural resorption of amyloid, with molecular imaging identifying a change prior to changes in ECV. However, the mechanism of binding of Tc-99m-DPD to myocardial amyloid is not well known. Also, the tracer kinetics with distribution to the bone, soft tissue, and heart compartments may differ based on changes to any of these compartments with therapy. Thus, this reduction in uptake may also represent increased altered tracer distribution [56] or concomitant onset of myocardial fibrosis.

In another study on 40 wild-type ATTR-CA patients who underwent Tc-99m-DPD SPECT/CT imaging with determination of SUV retention index, calculated as (SUVpeak cardiac/SUVpeak vertebral) x SUV peak paraspinal muscle, there was a significant decrease in SUV retention index after tafamidis therapy [57]. This study demonstrated that in the overall cohort, there were no significant changes in cardiac function with tafamidis therapy. But the cohort of patients with a greater median improvement in Tc-99m-DPD retention index (after a median of 7 months of tafamidis) demonstrated a significant improvement in LVEF. These findings raise the possibility of changes in Tc-99m-DPD identifying subjects who are more likely to improve functionally after TTR-stabilizing therapy.

13.9 Limitations

Although cardiac scintigraphy has significantly improved the diagnosis of ATTR-CA in appropriately selected patients, some important limitations of this method must be understood. First, the overall sensitivity of bone scintigraphy-based non-biopsy diagnostic criteria for the diagnosis of ATTR-CA is modest (~60%), owed largely to the presence of incidental monoclonal gammopathy [25]. Thus, up to 40% of patients with ATTR-CA may continue to require biopsy proof of amyloid type in order for a definitive diagnosis. This method is also unable to detect early ATTR-CA, some forms of hereditary ATTR-CA, AL-CA, and other rare forms of CA. In these situations, imaging with positron emission tomography (PET) with amyloid-specific radiotracers may be of added value.

13.10 Conclusion/Summary

In appropriately selected patients with clinical symptoms, typical echocardiographic or CMR features, and exclusion of AL-CA, cardiac scintigraphy allows for the definitive diagnosis of ATTR-CA without the need for endomyocardial biopsy. Developments in cardiac scintigraphy-based imaging of ATTR-CA, coupled with the significant growth of therapeutic options, have significantly advanced the field of CA. In addition, with ease of non-biopsy diagnosis, it allows for early diagnosis and screening of higher risk populations and providing insight into the true prevalence of ATTR-CA. Novel techniques of quantification will further facilitate early diagnosis of disease and monitoring of disease progression and response to treatment, and ultimately inform therapeutics and shape clinical care for CA.FundingThis work was supported by the National Institutes of Health grant to Dorbala: K24 HL157648.

Conflicts of Interest SD: Consulting fees: Pfizer, GE Healthcare; investigator-initiated grant: Pfizer, Attralus, GE Healthcare, Philips.

References

1. Maurer MS, Schwartz JH, Gundapaneni B, Elliott PM, Merlini G, Waddington-Cruz M, et al. Tafamidis treatment for patients with transthyretin amyloid cardiomyopathy. N Engl J Med. 2018;379(11):1007–16.
2. Adams D, Gonzalez-Duarte A, O'Riordan WD, Yang CC, Ueda M, Kristen AV, et al. Patisiran, an RNAi therapeutic, for hereditary transthyretin amyloidosis. N Engl J Med. 2018;379(1):11–21.
3. Ali A, Turner DA, Rosenbush SW, Fordham EW. Bone Scintigram in cardiac amyloidosis: a case report. Clin Nucl Med. 1981;6(3):105–8.
4. Schiff S, Bateman T, Moffatt R, Davidson R, Berman D. Diagnostic considerations in cardiomyopathy: unique scintigraphic pattern of diffuse biventricular technetium-99m-pyrophosphate uptake in amyloid heart disease. Am Heart J. 1982;103(4, Part 1):562–3.
5. Sobol SM, Brown JM, Bunker SR, Patel J, Lull RJ. Noninvasive diagnosis of cardiac amyloidosis by technetium-99m-pyrophosphate myocardial scintigraphy. Am Heart J. 1982;103(4, Part 1):563–6.
6. Li CK, Rabinovitch MA, Juni JE, Thrall JH, Pitt B, Das SK, et al. Scintigraphic characterization of amyloid cardiomyopathy. Clin Nucl Med. 1985;10(3):156–9.
7. Janssen S, van Rijswijk MH, Albertus Piers D, de Jong GMT. Soft-tissue uptake of 99mTc-diphosphonate in systemic AL amyloidosis. Eur J Nucl Med. 1984;9(12):538–41.
8. Falk RH, Lee VW, Rubinow A, Hood WB, Cohen AS. Sensitivity of technetium-99m-pyrophosphate scintigraphy in diagnosing cardiac amyloidosis. Am J Cardiol. 1983;51(5):826–30.
9. Gertz MA, Brown ML, Hauser MF, Kyle RA. Utility of technetium Tc 99m pyrophosphate bone scanning in cardiac amyloidosis. Arch Intern Med. 1987;147(6):1039–44.
10. Perugini E, Guidalotti PL, Salvi F, Cooke RMT, Pettinato C, Riva L, et al. Noninvasive etiologic diagnosis of cardiac amyloidosis using ^{99m}Tc-3,3-Diphosphono-1,2-Propanodicarboxylic acid scintigraphy. J Am Coll Cardiol. 2005;46(6):1076–84.
11. Rapezzi C, Quarta CC, Guidalotti PL, Longhi S, Pettinato C, Leone O, et al. Usefulness and limitations of 99mTc-3,3-diphosphono-1,2-propanodicarboxylic acid scintigraphy in the aetiological diagnosis of amyloidotic cardiomyopathy. Eur J Nucl Med Mol Imaging. 2011;38(3):470–8.
12. Buja LM, Parkey RW, Dees JH, Stokely EM, Harris RA, Bonte FJ, Willerson JT. Morphologic correlates of technetium-99m stannous pyrophosphate imaging of acute myocardial infarcts in dogs. Circulation. 1975;52(4):596–607.
13. Stats MA, Stone JR. Varying levels of small microcalcifications and macrophages in ATTR and AL cardiac amyloidosis: implications for utilizing nuclear medicine studies to subtype amyloidosis. Cardiovasc Pathol. 2016;25(5):413–7.

14. Dweck MR, Jenkins WSA, Vesey AT, Pringle MAH, Chin CWL, Malley TS, et al. 18F-sodium fluoride uptake is a marker of active calcification and disease progression in patients with aortic stenosis. Circ Cardiovasc Imaging. 2014;7(2):371–8.

15. Ishiwata Y, Kaneta T, Nawata S, Hino-Shishikura A, Yoshida K, Inoue T. Quantification of temporal changes in calcium score in active atherosclerotic plaque in major vessels by 18F-sodium fluoride PET/CT. Eur J Nucl Med Mol Imaging. 2017;44(9):1529–37.

16. Martineau P, Finnerty V, Giraldeau G, Authier S, Harel F, Pelletier-Galarneau M. Examining the sensitivity of 18F-NaF PET for the imaging of cardiac amyloidosis. J Nucl Cardiol. 2021;28(1):209–18.

17. Morgenstern R, Yeh R, Castano A, Maurer MS, Bokhari S. (18)fluorine sodium fluoride positron emission tomography, a potential biomarker of transthyretin cardiac amyloidosis. J Nucl Cardiol. 2018;25(5):1559–67.

18. Lee VW, Caldarone AG, Falk RH, Rubinow A, Cohen AS. Amyloidosis of heart and liver: comparison of Tc-99m pyrophosphate and Tc-99m methylene diphosphonate for detection. Radiology. 1983;148(1):239–42.

19. Bokhari S, Castaño A, Pozniakoff T, Deslisle S, Latif F, Maurer MS. ^{99m}Tc-pyrophosphate scintigraphy for differentiating light-chain cardiac amyloidosis from the transthyretin-related familial and senile cardiac amyloidoses. Circ Cardiovasc Imaging. 2013;6(2):195–201.

20. Quarta CC, Guidalotti PL, Longhi S, Pettinato C, Leone O, Ferlini A, et al. Defining the diagnosis in Echocardiographically suspected senile systemic amyloidosis. JACC Cardiovasc Imaging. 2012;5(7):755–8.

21. Glaudemans AW, van Rheenen RW, van den Berg MP, Noordzij W, Koole M, Blokzijl H, et al. Bone scintigraphy with (99m)technetium-hydroxymethylene diphosphonate allows early diagnosis of cardiac involvement in patients with transthyretin-derived systemic amyloidosis. Amyloid. 2014;21(1):35–44.

22. Fontana M, Banypersad SM, Treibel TA, Maestrini V, Sado DM, White SK, et al. Native T1 mapping in transthyretin amyloidosis. JACC Cardiovasc Imaging. 2014;7(2):157–65.

23. Gillmore JD, Maurer MS, Falk RH, et al. Nonbiopsy diagnosis of cardiac transthyretin amyloidosis. Circulation. 2016;133(24):2404–12.

24. Palladini G, Russo P, Bosoni T, Verga L, Sarais G, Lavatelli F, et al. Identification of amyloidogenic light chains requires the combination of serum-free light chain assay with immunofixation of serum and urine. Clin Chem. 2009;55(3):499–504.

25. Rauf MU, Hawkins PN, Cappelli F, Perfetto F, Zampieri M, Argiro A, et al. Tc-99m labelled bone scintigraphy in suspected cardiac amyloidosis. Eur Heart J. 2023;44(24):2187–98.

26. Garcia-Pavia P, Rapezzi C, Adler Y, Arad M, Basso C, Brucato A, et al. Diagnosis and treatment of cardiac amyloidosis. A position statement of the European Society of Cardiology Working Group on myocardial and pericardial diseases. Eur J Heart Fail. 2021;23(4):512–26.

27. Dorbala S, Ando Y, Bokhari S, Dispenzieri A, Falk RH, Ferrari VA, et al. ASNC/AHA/ASE/EANM/HFSA/ISA/SCMR/SNMMI expert consensus recommendations for multimodality imaging in cardiac amyloidosis: part 1 of 2-evidence base and standardized methods of imaging. Circ Cardiovasc Imaging. 2021;14(7):e000029.

28. Dorbala S, Ando Y, Bokhari S, Dispenzieri A, Falk RH, Ferrari VA, et al. ASNC/AHA/ASE/EANM/HFSA/ISA/SCMR/SNMMI expert consensus recommendations for multimodality imaging in cardiac amyloidosis: part 2 of 2—diagnostic criteria and appropriate utilization. Circ Cardiovasc Imaging. 2021;14(7):e000030.

29. Castano A, Haq M, Narotsky DL, Goldsmith J, Weinberg RL, Morgenstern R, et al. Multicenter study of planar technetium 99m pyrophosphate cardiac imaging: predicting survival for patients with ATTR cardiac amyloidosis. JAMA Cardiol. 2016;1(8):880–9.

30. Aimo A, Merlo M, Porcari A, et al. Redefining the epidemiology of cardiac amyloidosis. A systematic review and meta-analysis of screening studies. Eur J Heart Fail. 2022;24(12):2342–51.

31. Mohammed SF, Mirzoyev SA, Edwards WD, Dogan A, Grogan DR, Dunlay SM, et al. Left ventricular amyloid deposition in patients with heart failure and preserved ejection fraction. JACC Heart Fail. 2014;2(2):113–22.

32. González-López E, Gallego-Delgado M, Guzzo-Merello G, de Haro-del Moral FJ, Cobo-Marcos M, Robles C, et al. Wild-type transthyretin amyloidosis as a cause of heart failure with preserved ejection fraction. Eur Heart J. 2015;36(38):2585–94.
33. Bennani Smires Y, Victor G, Ribes D, Berry M, Cognet T, Méjean S, et al. Pilot study for left ventricular imaging phenotype of patients over 65 years old with heart failure and preserved ejection fraction: the high prevalence of amyloid cardiomyopathy. Int J Cardiovasc Imaging. 2016;32(9):1403–13.
34. AbouEzzeddine OF, Davies DR, Scott CG, Fayyaz AU, Askew JW, McKie PM, et al. Prevalence of transthyretin amyloid cardiomyopathy in heart failure with preserved ejection fraction. JAMA Cardiol. 2021;6(11):1267–74.
35. Devesa A, Camblor Blasco A, Pello Lázaro AM, Askari E, Lapeña G, Gómez Talavera S, et al. Prevalence of transthyretin amyloidosis in patients with heart failure and no left ventricular hypertrophy. ESC Heart Fail. 2021;8(4):2856–65.
36. Castaño A, Narotsky DL, Hamid N, Khalique OK, Morgenstern R, DeLuca A, et al. Unveiling transthyretin cardiac amyloidosis and its predictors among elderly patients with severe aortic stenosis undergoing transcatheter aortic valve replacement. Eur Heart J. 2017;38(38):2879–87.
37. Scully PR, Patel KP, Treibel TA, Thornton GD, Hughes RK, Chadalavada S, et al. Prevalence and outcome of dual aortic stenosis and cardiac amyloid pathology in patients referred for transcatheter aortic valve implantation. Eur Heart J. 2020;41(29):2759–67.
38. Nitsche C, Scully PR, Patel KP, Kammerlander AA, Koschutnik M, Dona C, et al. Prevalence and outcomes of concomitant aortic stenosis and cardiac amyloidosis. J Am Coll Cardiol. 2021;77(2):128–39.
39. Nitsche C, Aschauer S, Kammerlander AA, Schneider M, Poschner T, Duca F, et al. Light-chain and transthyretin cardiac amyloidosis in severe aortic stenosis: prevalence, screening possibilities, and outcome. Eur J Heart Fail. 2020;22(10):1852–62.
40. Rosenblum H, Masri A, Narotsky DL, Goldsmith J, Hamid N, Hahn RT, et al. Unveiling outcomes in coexisting severe aortic stenosis and transthyretin cardiac amyloidosis. Eur J Heart Fail. 2021;23(2):250–8.
41. Treibel TA, Fontana M, Gilbertson JA, Castelletti S, White SK, Scully PR, et al. Occult transthyretin cardiac amyloid in severe calcific aortic stenosis: prevalence and prognosis in patients undergoing surgical aortic valve replacement. Circ Cardiovasc Imaging. 2016;9(8):e005066.
42. Gioeva Z, Urban P, Rüdiger Meliss R, Haag J, Axmann H-D, Siebert F, et al. ATTR amyloid in the carpal tunnel ligament is frequently of wildtype transthyretin origin. Amyloid. 2013;20(1):1–6.
43. Kyle RA, Eilers SG, Linscheid RL, Gaffey TA. Amyloid localized to Tenosynovium at carpal tunnel release: natural history of 124 cases. Am J Clin Pathol. 1989;91(4):393–7.
44. Sperry BW, Reyes BA, Ikram A, Donnelly JP, Phelan D, Jaber WA, et al. Tenosynovial and cardiac amyloidosis in patients undergoing carpal tunnel release. J Am Coll Cardiol. 2018;72(17):2040–50.
45. Fosbol EL, Rorth R, Leicht BP, Schou M, Maurer MS, Kristensen SL, et al. Association of Carpal Tunnel Syndrome with Amyloidosis, heart failure, and adverse cardiovascular outcomes. J Am Coll Cardiol. 2019;74(1):15–23.
46. Milandri A, Farioli A, Gagliardi C, Longhi S, Salvi F, Curti S, et al. Carpal tunnel syndrome in cardiac amyloidosis: implications for early diagnosis and prognostic role across the spectrum of aetiologies. Eur J Heart Fail. 2020;22(3):507–15.
47. Zegri-Reiriz I, de Haro-Del Moral FJ, Dominguez F, Salas C, de la Cuadra P, Plaza A, et al. Prevalence of cardiac amyloidosis in patients with carpal tunnel syndrome. J Cardiovasc Transl Res. 2019;12(6):507–13.
48. Westin O, Fosbol EL, Maurer MS, Leicht BP, Hasbak P, Mylin AK, et al. Screening for cardiac amyloidosis 5 to 15 years after surgery for bilateral carpal tunnel syndrome. J Am Coll Cardiol. 2022;80(10):967–77.
49. Ladefoged B, Clemmensen T, Dybro A, Hartig-Andreasen C, Kirkeby L, Gormsen LC, et al. Identification of wild-type transthyretin cardiac amyloidosis in patients with carpal tunnel syndrome surgery (CACTuS). ESC Heart Fail. 2023;10(1):234–44.

50. Ioannou A, Patel RK, Razvi Y, Porcari A, Sinagra G, Venneri L, et al. Impact of earlier diagnosis in cardiac ATTR amyloidosis over the course of 20 years. Circulation. 2022;146(22):1657–70.
51. Gillmore JD, Damy T, Fontana M, Hutchinson M, Lachmann HJ, Martinez-Naharro A, et al. A new staging system for cardiac transthyretin amyloidosis. Eur Heart J. 2018;39(30):2799–806.
52. Nativi-Nicolau J, Siu A, Dispenzieri A, Maurer MS, Rapezzi C, Kristen AV, et al. Temporal trends of wild-type transthyretin amyloid cardiomyopathy in the transthyretin amyloidosis outcomes survey. JACC CardioOncol. 2021;3(4):537–46.
53. Gilstrap LG, Dominici F, Wang Y, El-Sady MS, Singh A, Carli MFD, et al. Epidemiology of Cardiac Amyloidosis–Associated Heart Failure Hospitalizations Among Fee-for-Service Medicare Beneficiaries in the United States. Circ Heart Fail. 2019;12(6):e005407.
54. Ioannou A, Patel RK, Razvi Y, Porcari A, Knight D, Martinez-Naharro A, et al. Multi-imaging characterization of cardiac phenotype in different types of amyloidosis. J Am Coll Cardiol Img. 2023;16(4):464–77.
55. Dorbala S, Park MA, Cuddy S, Singh V, Sullivan K, Kim S, et al. Absolute quantitation of cardiac (99m)Tc-pyrophosphate using cadmium-zinc-telluride-based SPECT/CT. J Nucl Med. 2021;62(5):716–22.
56. Fontana M, Martinez-Naharro A, Chacko L, Rowczenio D, Gilbertson JA, Whelan CJ, et al. Reduction in CMR derived extracellular volume with Patisiran indicates cardiac amyloid regression. J Am Coll Cardiol Img. 2021;14(1):189–99.
57. Rettl R, Wollenweber T, Duca F, Binder C, Cherouny B, Dachs TM, et al. Monitoring tafamidis treatment with quantitative SPECT/CT in transthyretin amyloid cardiomyopathy. Eur Heart J Cardiovasc Imaging. 2023;24(8):1019–30.

Dario Genovesi and Assuero Giorgetti

A definite diagnosis of transthyretin cardiac amyloidosis (ATTR-CA) can be made without histological confirmation when the following elements coexist: a clinical and imaging suspicion of CA, a moderate-to-high cardiac uptake of bone tracers (^{99m}Tc-PYP, ^{99m}Tc-DPD, ^{99m}Tc-HMDP) on planar scintigraphy, and no evidence of a monoclonal protein [1–3]. When bone tracer scintigraphy is mildly positive or negative and/or a monoclonal component is present, the diagnosis of ATTR-CA requires further instrumental investigations and a histological confirmation by biopsy examination. Furthermore, the diagnosis of AL-CA always requires a biopsy in the heart or another clinically affected organ [4]. Over the past 15 years, the development of new positron-emission tomography (PET) radiopharmaceuticals for the search for amyloid deposits has disclosed new perspectives for the noninvasive diagnosis of AL-CA.

PET is a nuclear medicine technique that allows assessing the accumulation of specific radioactive molecules in vivo by using the principle of particle annihilation. PET radiopharmaceuticals typically consist of a biologically active molecule, called a tracer or ligand, labeled with a short-lived radioactive isotope, such as fluorine-18 (^{18}F) or carbon-11 (^{11}C). Once the radiopharmaceutical is injected into the body, the molecule is taken up by the target tissue, where it emits positrons, which are positively charged particles. After its emission, a positron rapidly collides with an electron producing a particle named positronium that is annihilated in a fraction of second emitting energy in the form of two 511 keV photons that fly at the speed of light along the same line, but in opposite directions. The detection in the same time window of the two photons derived from the same annihilation event is the physical principle at the basis of PET imaging [5]. PET acquisition is now combined with

D. Genovesi (✉) · A. Giorgetti
Nuclear Medicine Unit, Fondazione Toscana "Gabriele Monasterio", Pisa, Italy
e-mail: dario.genovesi@ftgm.it; asso@ftgm.it

M. Emdin et al. (eds.), *Cardiac Amyloidosis*,
https://doi.org/10.1007/978-3-031-51757-0_14

morphological images by X-ray computed tomography to more accurately localize the areas of radiopharmaceutical accumulation and to use tissue attenuation map to correct PET findings according to the degree of X-ray attenuation by tissues [6].

14.1　PET Radiopharmaceuticals for Amyloid Detection

Radiopharmaceuticals able to bind amyloid deposits have been developed to detect brain amyloid deposits in patients with suspected Alzheimer's disease (AD). Some of these radiopharmaceuticals have shown a binding affinity also for other types of amyloid deposits, particularly in the heart.

The first PET radiopharmaceutical used to evaluate the presence of amyloid deposits was developed at the beginning of the 2000s and named Pittsburgh compound B (PiB); this molecule is a derivative of thioflavin T (a dye for histological specimens), and it is labeled with ^{11}C. The first study using this radiopharmaceutical in vivo dates to 2004 [7]. In 2013, the first prospective study evaluating the diagnostic utility of PiB for the diagnosis of CA was published [8]. The authors reported a significant early radiopharmaceutical uptake in the myocardium (around 15–25 min after the injection) in all the ten patients with amyloidosis and in no control subject ($n = 5$). This suggested a possible use of this radiopharmaceutical to diagnose cardiac involvement in the setting of systemic amyloidosis. Nonetheless, ^{11}C-labeled radiopharmaceuticals have a very short half-life (about 20 min); therefore, this kind of approach can be only used in centers equipped with a cyclotron. Since 2009, ^{18}F-labeled PET radiopharmaceuticals with high affinity for beta-amyloid have been developed. The first of these compounds was ^{18}F-florbetapir, a structural analogue of stilbene dyes used in histological studies [9–13]. In 2014, the first pilot study showed the affinity of ^{18}F-florbetapir for myocardial amyloid deposits [14]. The authors evaluated nine patients with CA and five controls with hypertrophic cardiomyopathy. The study involved the acquisition of dynamic images for a global duration of 60 min, to derive the retention index (RI) of the myocardium, and static reconstructions obtained by elaborating data acquired between 10 and 60 min. Patients with CA showed a significantly greater radiopharmaceutical accumulation in the myocardium compared to controls in terms of both SUV and target-to-background ratio. The analysis of static images did not allow a differential diagnosis between AL- and ATTR-CA, but RI assessment evidenced a greater retention of ^{18}F-florbetapir in AL- than ATTR-CA. Afterwards, autoradiographic studies demonstrated that ^{18}F-florbetapir specifically binds to amyloid deposits in CA [15].

The second ^{18}F-labeled PET radiopharmaceutical approved by the Food and Drug Administration to search for amyloid tissue deposits in vivo is ^{18}F-flutemetamol. This radiopharmaceutical has a molecular structure similar to PiB, as well as similar kinetics and binding affinity for brain amyloid. Compared to PiB, it is more easily used in a clinical setting because of its longer half-life (about 108 min) [16]. The first report of a myocardial uptake of ^{18}F-flutemetamol in CA was published in 2014 [17], followed by a pilot study including nine patients with CA and three control subjects that found a significantly greater radiopharmaceutical uptake in the myocardium in patients with CA compared to controls [18]. ^{18}F-flutemetamol has been evaluated also in patients with variant ATTRv-CA, with a study reporting the ability of this radiopharmaceutical to accumulate in the heart in patients with the V30M mutation [19]. The affinity of flutemetamol for ATTR amyloid deposits was further confirmed by *postmortem* histofluorescence analysis. In a recent study, the authors highlighted the ability of cyano-flutemetamol to specifically bind to amyloid deposits in case of both wild-type and variant ATTR-CA [20].

The latest radiopharmaceutical introduced has been ^{18}F-florbetaben [21]. Its molecular structure is similar to ^{18}F-florbetapir, and even its affinity for beta-amyloid is similar, and significantly lower than that of PiB or ^{18}F-flutemetamol (Table 14.1). Even this radiopharmaceutical has shown an affinity for amyloid deposits in the heart. In the first pilot study, the authors compared patients with CA (five with AL and five with ATTR) with a control group of patients with hypertensive heart disease. The authors reported a similar performance in differentiating CA from hypertensive heart disease [22]. More recently, Kircher et al. evaluated the performance of ^{18}F-florbetaben for the diagnosis of CA compared to echocardiography, cardiac magnetic resonance (CMR), and bone tracer scintigraphy. They also tried to use the quantitative data from PET-CT with ^{18}F-florbetaben to evaluate the amyloid burden and monitor the response to treatment. The authors analyzed 14 patients with CA (5 ATTR, 8 AL, 1 AA) and 8 patients with suspected CA and final diagnosis of non-infiltrative cardiomyopathy. PET-CT with ^{18}F-florbetaben allowed discriminating between CA and non-infiltrative cardiomyopathy and showed that RI was higher in AL- than ATTR-CA. In four patients, a follow-up PET-CT scan was available. Changes in the RI corresponded well to treatment response, as assessed by cardiac biomarkers and performance status, suggesting a possible role of this radiopharmaceutical to evaluate the response to treatment [23].

All these studies have considered PET-CT findings from very early phases of tissue distribution of the radiopharmaceutical. A study published in 2020 evaluated the cardiac uptake of ^{18}F-florbetaben in a group of 40 patients with CA (20 AL and 20 ATTR) compared with a control group of 20 patients with hypertrophic cardiomyopathy [24]. In this case, images were acquired dynamically for 60 min after the injection of the radiopharmaceutical, and then late static images of the thorax were acquired after 110 min from injection. The dynamic data were then retrospectively reconstructed to obtain three static acquisitions lasting 10 min each, after 5, 30, and 50 min after the injection. Patients with AL-CA displayed a high, persistent cardiac uptake in all the static scans, whereas patients with ATTR and those with non-CA

Table 14.1 Molecular characteristics of PET amyloid radiopharmaceuticals

Radiopharmaceutical	Ki for β-amyloid (nmol/L)	Molecular weight (kDa)	Molecular structure
[11]C-PiB	0.87 ± 0.18	25,532	$C_{13}{}^{11}CH_{12}N_2OS$
[18]F-flutemetamol	0.74 ± 0.38	27,331	$C_{14}H_{11}{}^{18}FN_2OS$
[18]F-florbetapir	2.87 ± 0.17	35,942	$C_{20}H_{25}{}^{18}FN_2O_3$
[18]F-florbetaben	2.22 ± 0.54	35,844	$C_{21}H_{26}{}^{18}FNO_3$

Ki is the binding affinity constant for beta-amyloid [28]

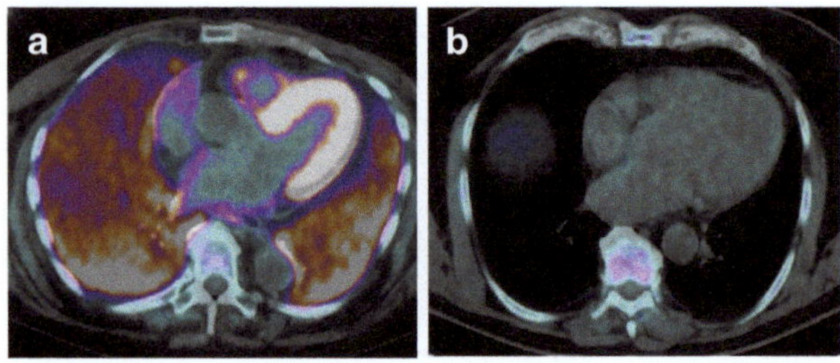

Fig. 14.1 Positron-emission tomography scans obtained 60 min after the injection of ^{18}F-florbetaben. (**a**) A 46-year-old woman with lambda IgG light-chain cardiac amyloidosis. (**b**) A 73-year-old man with transthyretin cardiac amyloidosis

showed an uptake decrease soon after the early scan. Semiquantitative assessment demonstrated higher mean standardized uptake value (SUV_{mean}) in patients with AL, sustained over the whole acquisition period (early SUVmean: 5.55, interquartile range [IQR]: 4.00–7.43, vs. delayed SUV_{mean}: 3.50, IQR: 2.32–6.10; p = NS), compared with patients with ATTR (early SUV_{mean}: 2.55, IQR: 1.80–2.97, vs. delayed SUV_{mean}: 1.25, IQR: 0.90–1.60; p < 0.001) and patients with non-CA (early SUV_{mean}: 3.50, IQR: 1.60–3.37, vs. delayed SUV_{mean}: 1.40, IQR: 1.20–1.60; p < 0.001). Similar results were found comparing heart-to-background ratio and molecular volume. These findings suggest a greater stability of the binding between ^{18}F-florbetaben and AL amyloid compared to ATTR amyloid, allowing to confirm or discard the presence of AL-CA by a single static acquisition after at least 30 min from radiopharmaceutical injection (Fig. 14.1).

[18]F-labeled sodium fluoride (^{18}F-Na) is a PET radiopharmaceutical used for the diagnosis of bone diseases [25]. ^{18}F-Na has been proposed as a novel tool to diagnose ATTR-CA, but its sensitivity for the detection of ATTR amyloid deposits seems modest [26, 27]. This may suggest that the affinity of the SPECT radiopharmaceuticals for ATTR-CA does not depend only on their link with the calcium deposits in the amyloid matrix, but also from other molecular mechanisms. The relatively low sensitivity and higher costs of ^{18}F-Na PET compared to SPECT will probably limit the use of this radiopharmaceutical in clinical practice.

14.2   Conclusions

Planar scintigraphy with bone tracers is currently recommended in patients with suspected CA; it cannot alone lead to a definite diagnosis of CA in all patients, as it cannot identify cases of AL-CA. PET-CT with specific radiopharmaceuticals for amyloid deposition could be the first diagnostic tool in patients with suspected AL-CA, possibly leading to an earlier diagnosis and avoiding the need for highly invasive procedures such as endomyocardial biopsy. There is also preliminary evidence that PET-CT with ^{18}F-flutemetamol may prove useful in patients with ATTRv-CA and that serial PET-CT scans may track the response to treatment.

References

1. Perugini E, Guidalotti PL, Salvi F, et al. Noninvasive etiologic diagnosis of cardiac amyloidosis using 99mTc-3,3-diphosphono-1,2-propanodicarboxylic acid scintigraphy. J Am Coll Cardiol. 2005;46:1076–84.
2. Gillmore JD, Maurer MS, Falk RH, et al. Nonbiopsy diagnosis of cardiac transthyretin amyloidosis. Circulation. 2016;133:2404–12.
3. Cappelli F, Gallini C, Di Mario C, et al. Accuracy of 99mTc-Hydroxymethylene diphosphonate scintigraphy for diagnosis of transthyretin cardiac amyloidosis. J Nucl Cardiol. 2019;26:497–504.
4. Garcia-Pavia P, Rapezzi C, Adler Y, et al. Diagnosis and treatment of cardiac amyloidosis: a position statement of the ESC working group on myocardial and pericardial diseases. Eur Heart J. 2021;42:1554–68.
5. Camici PG, Rosen SD, Terence J, et al. Positron emission tomography. In: Ell PJ, Gambhir SS, editors. . Nuclear medicine in clinical diagnosis and treatment: Elsevier; 2005. p. 1075–91.
6. Meikle SR, Dahlbom M. Positron emission tomography. In: Ell PJ, Gambhir SS, editors. . Nuclear medicine in clinical diagnosis and treatment: Elsevier; 2005. p. 1827–43.
7. Klunk WE, Engler H, Nordberg A, et al. Imaging brain amyloid in Alzheimer's disease with Pittsburgh compound-B. Ann Neurol. 2004;55:306–19.
8. Antoni G, Lubberink M, Estrada S, et al. In vivo visualization of amyloid deposits in the heart with 11C-PiB and PET. J Nucl Med. 2013;54:213–20.
9. Choi SR, Golding G, Zhuang Z, et al. Preclinical properties of 18F-AV-45: a PET agent for Abeta plaques in the brain. J Nucl Med. 2009;50:1887–94.
10. Wong DF, Rosenberg PB, Zhou Y, et al. In vivo imaging of amyloid deposition in Alzheimer disease using the radioligand 18F-AV-45 (florbetapir corrected. F 18). J Nucl Med. 2010;51:913–20.
11. Clark CM, Schneider JA, Bedell BJ, et al. Use of florbetapir-PET for imaging beta-amyloid pathology. JAMA. 2011;305:275–83.
12. Lister-James J, Pontecorvo MJ, Clark C, et al. Florbetapir f-18: a histopathologically validated Beta-amyloid positron emission tomography imaging agent. Semin Nucl Med. 2011;41:300–4.
13. Yang L, Rieves D, Ganley C. Brain amyloid imaging—FDA approval of florbetapir F18 injection. N Engl J Med 2012;367:885–887.
14. Dorbala S, Vangala D, Semer J, et al. Imaging cardiac amyloidosis: a pilot study using ^{18}F-florbetapir positron emission tomography. Eur J Nucl Med Mol Imaging. 2014;41:1652–62.
15. Park MA, Padera RF, Belanger A, et al. 18F-florbetapir binds specifically to myocardial light chain and transthyretin amyloid deposits: autoradiography study. Circ Cardiovasc Imaging. 2015;8:pii: e002954.
16. Vandenberghe R, Van Laere K, Ivanoiu A, et al. 18F-flutemetamol amyloid imaging in Alzheimer disease and mild cognitive impairment: a phase 2 trial. Ann Neurol. 2010;68:319–29.
17. Lhommel R, Sempoux C, Ivanoiu A, et al. Is 18F-flutemetamol PET/CT able to reveal cardiac amyloidosis? Clin Nucl Med. 2014;39:747–9.
18. Dietemann S, Nkoulou R. Amyloid PET imaging in cardiac amyloidosis: a pilot study using 18F-flutemetamol positron emission tomography. Ann Nucl Med. 2019;33:624–8.
19. Möckelind S, Axelsson J, Pilebro B, et al. Quantification of cardiac amyloid with [18F]Flutemetamol in patients with V30M hereditary transthyretin amyloidosis. Amyloid. 2020;27:191–9.
20. Abrahamson EE, Padera RF, Davies J, et al. The flutemetamol analogue cyano-flutemetamol detects myocardial AL and ATTR amyloid deposits: a post-mortem histofluorescence analysis. Amyloid. 2022;21:1–19.
21. Rowe CC, Ackerman U, Browne W, et al. Imaging of amyloid beta in Alzheimer's disease with 18F-BAY94-9172, a novel PET tracer: proof of mechanism. Lancet Neurol. 2008;7:129–35.
22. Law WP, Wang WY, Moore PT, Mollee PN, Ng AC. Cardiac amyloid imaging with 18F-florbetaben PET: a pilot study. J Nucl Med. 2016;57:1733–9.

23. Kircher M, Ihne S, Brumberg J, et al. Detection of cardiac amyloidosis with 18F-Florbetaben-PET/CT in comparison to echocardiography, cardiac MRI ad DPD-scintigraphy. Eur J Nucl Med Mol Imaging. 2019;46:1407–16.
24. Genovesi D, Vergaro G, Giorgetti A, et al. [18F]-florbetaben PET/CT for differential diagnosis among cardiac immunoglobulin light chain, transthyretin amyloidosis, and mimicking conditions. JACC Cardiovasc Imaging. 2021;14:246–55.
25. Park PSU, Raynor WY, Sun Y, et al. 18F-sodium fluoride PET as a diagnostic modality for metabolic, autoimmune, and osteogenic bone disorders: cellular mechanisms and clinical applications. Int J Mol Sci. 2021;22:6504.
26. Martineau P, Finnerty V, Giraldeau G, et al. Examining the sensitivity of 18F-NaF PET for the imaging of cardiac amyloidosis. J Nucl Cardiol. 2021;28:209–18.
27. Zhang LX, Martineau P, Finnerty V, et al. Comparison of 18F-sodium fluoride positron emission tomography imaging and 99mTc-pyrophosphate in cardiac amyloidosis. J Nucl Cardiol. 2022;29:1132–40.
28. Vallabhajosula S. Positron emission tomography radiopharmaceuticals for imaging brain beta-amyloid. Semin Nucl Med. 2011;41:283–99.

The Role of Tissue Biopsy: Identification of the Amyloid Precursor and Beyond

15

Angela Pucci, Veronica Musetti, Francesco Greco, Angela Dispenzieri, and Michele Emdin

15.1 Introduction

Amyloidosis is a heterogeneous disease including either systemic or localized disorders with different causes, various clinical presentations, and several patterns of tissue involvement [1]. It is characterized by the extracellular deposition of insoluble proteinaceous amorphous material forming rigid, insoluble, non-branching fibrils [2, 3]. On tissue biopsy, these fibrils may be shown by Congo red histochemical staining under a polarized light microscope as green, yellow, or orange deposits [4].

The amyloid deposition may cause organ failure; in the heart, the myocardial damage depends upon the amyloidogenic protein, the pattern, and the extent of amyloid deposition [2, 3, 5]. Recently, other mechanisms, first inflammation and fibrosis, have been shown to play a role in myocardial dysfunction [6, 7].

A. Pucci (✉)
Department of Histopathology, Pisa University Hospital, Pisa, Italy
e-mail: a.pucci@ao-pisa.toscana.it

V. Musetti · M. Emdin
Health Science Interdisciplinary Center, Scuola Superiore Sant'Anna, Pisa, Italy

Fondazione Toscana Gabriele Monasterio, Pisa, Italy
e-mail: v.musetti@santannapisa.it; emdin@ftgm.it

F. Greco
Fondazione Toscana Gabriele Monasterio, Pisa, Italy

Fondazione Pisana per la Scienza ONLUS, San Giuliano Terme (PI), Italy
e-mail: f.greco@fpscience.it

A. Dispenzieri
Division of Hematology, Mayo Clinic, Rochester, MN, USA
e-mail: dispenzieri.angela@mayo.edu

Table 15.1 Cardiac amyloidosis subtypes

Amyloidosis type	Protein	Frequency of heart involvement	Underlying pathologic conditions
AL	Immunoglobulin light chain	70%	Monoclonal protein-secreting disorders
ATTRwt	Transthyretin	100%	Aging-related
ATTRv	Transthyretin	30–100%, depending on mutation	Mutations of various gene proteins
AA	Serum amyloid A	5%	Inflammatory/autoimmune process, chronic infections, unknown etiology
AFib	Fibrinogen α	Rare	Mutations of various gene proteins
AApoAI	Apolipoprotein A-I	Rare, depending on mutation	Mutations of various gene proteins
AApoAII	Apolipoprotein A-II	Rare, depending on mutation	Mutations of various gene proteins
AApoAIV	Apolipoprotein A-IV	Unknown	Progressive renal dysfunction
Aβ2M	β2-microglobulin	80%	Iatrogenic, long-term dialysis
AGel	Gelsolin	5%	Mutations of various gene proteins

Modified with permission from Garcia-Pavia et al. [9]

So far, 42 amyloidogenic proteins have been identified, 9 of them causing cardiac amyloidosis (CA) [8, 9] (Table 15.1). The most common amyloidogenic precursors of CA are the immunoglobulin light chains and the transthyretin (TTR) protein, responsible for light chains (AL-CA) and TTR CA (ATTR-CA), respectively [9, 10]. CA may also be due to chronic inflammatory or infectious diseases [9].

In CA, the amyloid deposits can be detected in all the cardiac structures, first ventricular and atrial myocardium, the atrial deposits likely depending upon the hemodynamic effects of ventricular diastolic dysfunction [11]. Isolated forms of CA are also well known, first isolated atrial amyloidosis (IAA) that can be found in chronic heart failure with no association with systemic disease. IAA is related to the atrial stretch with local overproduction of atrial natriuretic peptide (ANP) that constitutes the amyloidogenic protein in the atria [12, 13]. In calcific cardiac valve stenosis, apolipoprotein-related amyloid deposits have been shown in many cases (up to 88% of aortic valves and 45% of mitral valves), adjacent to the calcified areas [14]. Isolated amyloid deposits may also be found in the aortic media of elderly (>50–60 years of age) patients, representing the most under-recognized isolated form of amyloidosis [15, 16]. The amyloidogenic protein of aortic media is named "medin," and it is an internal cleavage product of its precursor lactadherin (i.e., the milk fat globule epidermal growth factor 8) [17]. In the thoracic aortic media layer, medin may form aggregates and lead or contribute to the pathogenesis of thoracic aortic aneurysm and/or dissection [18].

Imaging techniques have dramatically improved the diagnosis of CA [19]. In ATTR-CA, non-biopsy diagnosis is possible in patients without monoclonal gammopathy by using 99mTc-hydroxymethylene diphosphonate (99mTc-HMDP) scintigraphy, associated with concordant results of echocardiography or cardiac magnetic resonance (CMR) [20–23]. In the remaining cases, such as in difficult or controversial cases and in localized (organ) amyloidosis, tissue biopsy represents not only the most reliable tool for investigating amyloidosis, but also the gold standard for diagnosis and typing of amyloidosis [24, 25]. Tissue analysis may also provide diagnosis of amyloidosis in unexpected or non-diagnosed cases, contribute to characterization of amyloidosis, and disclose pattern and extent of amyloid burden such as possible associated lesions [7].

Routinely, formalin-fixed and paraffin-embedded (FFPE) tissue samples represent suitable specimens for adequate analysis and full characterization of amyloid deposits by means of histology, histochemical (first, Congo red) staining, immunohistochemistry, and proteomics [26–28]. Such results may be achieved in experienced centers because reliable data require expertise and a rigorous methodology.

15.1.1 Tissue Analyses in Cardiac Amyloidosis

15.1.1.1 Histology

Histopathological analysis of CA is a multistep procedure requiring different types of investigations aimed at diagnosis and treatment of amyloidosis. It is also providing new insights into the pathogenetic mechanisms leading to CA and to cardiac dysfunction [26, 29]. Pathological investigations may include different analyses, i.e., gross examination and accurate sampling of explanted hearts (from cardiac transplantation recipients, cardiac valve donors, or *postmortem* procedures), appropriate processing of endomyocardial or surgical myocardial biopsy specimens, specific histochemical staining for amyloid (Congo red, thioflavin, etc.), and immunohistochemistry by using specific antisera raised against amyloidogenic proteins [25, 29]. Routinely performed hematoxylin and eosin (HE) staining on histological slides may be useful to evidence amorphous eosinophilic deposits in the myocardium, which may be consistent with a hypertrophic or restrictive phenotype of CA, but specific stainings are required for a definite diagnosis of CA (Fig. 15.1a, b).

15.1.1.2 Histochemistry

Congo red staining represents the most widely used and standardized histochemical staining to show amyloid deposits by light microscopy under polarized light [30, 31]. Although in a few cases the amyloid deposits can be suspected on light microscopy, at least in advanced cases showing large and amorphous aggregates on HE-stained histological sections, they have to be demonstrated by a specific histochemical staining for amyloid. Congo red staining shows amyloid deposits as a red or salmon-pink substance with a characteristic apple-green birefringence under polarized light (Figs. 15.1b and 15.2b). To improve its sensitivity, the Congo red staining has to be performed on 8–10 μm thick sections; it has to be examined under

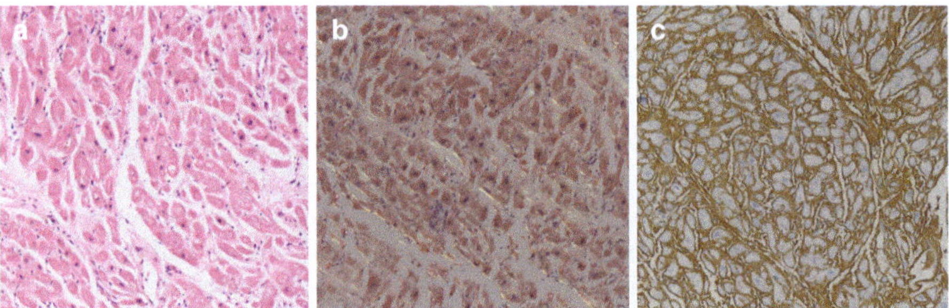

Fig. 15.1 Cardiac amyloidosis (CA): amyloid deposits are shown in a formalin-fixed and paraffin-embedded (FFPE) endomyocardial biopsy from the left ventricle of a patient with AL-CA, λ+. Amorphous and eosinophilic material is present in the interstitium between the myocytes (**a**). Congo red staining under polarized light shows apple-green birefringence corresponding to the amyloid deposits with an interstitial pattern (**b**). Immunohistochemistry shows intense and diffuse immunostaining for immunoglobulin λ light chain in the myocardial interstitium, by the immunoperoxidase technique (**c**). (**a**) Hematoxylin and eosin staining; (**b**) Congo red staining under polarized light; (**c**) Immunoperoxidase staining and hematoxylin counterstaining. Original magnification, 10×

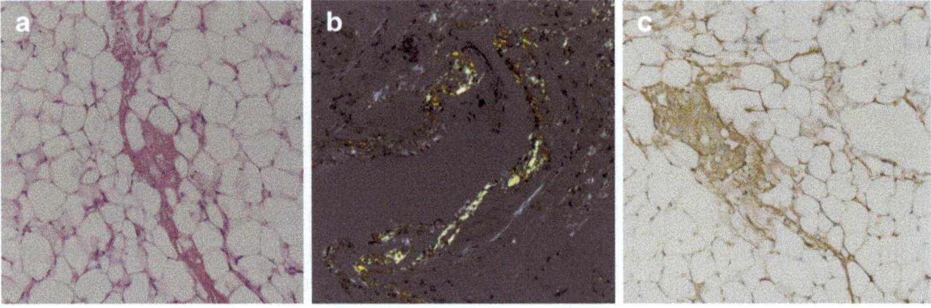

Fig. 15.2 Amyloid deposits in an abdominal fat biopsy form a patient with AL-CA, λ+. In the fibro-adipose tissue (**a**), limited deposits of amyloid are shown by Congo red staining under polarized light (**b**) and immunohistochemistry reveals the positivity for immunoglobulin λ light chain by using the immunoperoxidase technique (**c**). (**a**) Hematoxylin and eosin staining; (**b**) Congo red staining under polarized light; (**c**) Immunoperoxidase staining and hematoxylin counterstaining. Original magnification, 10×

polarized light to differentiate amyloid from collagen, fibrin, or red blood cells [26]. It is also advisable to get a positive control for amyloid on the same Congo red-stained histological slide, in order to exclude false-negative results. Other histochemical stainings (as thioflavin T or S) may also be applied for detecting amyloid, but Congo red represents the most diffusely used staining.

The distribution of Congo red positivity on cardiac tissue may be quite variable, depending on the extent of the amyloid deposits, which may be interstitial and/or nodular, focal or diffuse, perivascular, or into the vessel wall [26].

The Masson's trichrome staining highlights the connective fibrous tissue with intense blue staining, and it may be quite helpful to compare amyloid with fibrosis, as it gives a blue-violet appearance to amyloid deposits, but it is not specific for amyloid [7, 26].

15.1.1.3 Immunohistochemistry

Immunohistochemistry is widely used in histopathology laboratories for the diagnosis and the characterization of several diseases. For amyloid typing, it requires dedicated expertise, availability of specific antibodies, and standardized protocols, to avoid diagnostic failure or misdiagnosis, i.e., false-negative or -positive results. It can be used on FFPE section by immunoperoxidase technique, or on cryostat sections by indirect immunofluorescence, and even on ultrathin section of glutaraldehyde-fixed samples by immunoelectron transmission microscopy [26, 28, 32]. FFPE has been shown to be suitable for amyloid characterization in most cases, using rigorous protocols [7, 28, 29, 32]. The specific antisera must be appropriately tested; tissue processing, effective antigenic unmasking, as well as quality of the available antibodies are crucial (Figs. 15.1c and 15.2c). Over-fixation of tissue specimens may interfere with tissue antigenicity giving unreliable results. The use of an automated immunostainer with standardized and reproducible protocols may also help to sensibly improve the results and their reproducibility.

Transmission electron microscopy (TEM) and post-embedding immunogold techniques may be very useful for detection and typing of amyloid deposits [32, 33]. TEM is particularly useful in the early detection of amyloid because of its high resolution, although the focal and irregular distribution of amyloid deposits might limit its sensitivity. The tissue sample must be fixed by 2.5% glutaraldehyde or 2% Karnovsky (i.e., 2% paraformaldehyde and 2% glutaraldehyde) solution and embedded in Araldite resin, with or w/o previous osmium tetroxide postfixation. On ultrathin sections, the amyloid fibrils can be morphologically identified, whereas amyloid typing can be performed by using the post-embedding immunogold technique [32]. Briefly, ultrathin sections are incubated with specific primary antibodies, and the reaction is detected by the subsequent incubation with an appropriate secondary antibody bound to colloidal gold particles of 5–15 nm diameter.

15.1.2 Mass Spectrometry-Based Proteomics

In recent years, the capability of mass spectrometry-based bottom-up proteomics to identify and quantify proteins from complex tissue samples has been used to type amyloid [34–36]. Proteomics offers the advantage of an unbiased identification of the protein content, overcoming the need of multiple antibodies.

The typical sample used for proteomics typing of CA is endomyocardial biopsies (EMBs) or umbilical fat biopsies. EMBs are more suited for proteomics because the amyloid deposits often constitute a conspicuous component of the biopsy. Umbilical fat samples instead are mostly composed of adipocytes with limited amyloid deposits. Since proteomics can provide the relative amount of each protein in the sample, a simple analysis of the whole biopsy would be dominated by the proteins constituting the tissue bulk. Thus, sample enrichment in amyloid proteins or a background subtraction should be taken into consideration.

Formalin fixation preserves the tissue by reticulating the proteins. FFPE samples can be used for proteomics analysis, but a short fixation time is recommended to avoid excessive sample loss during protein extraction [37]. FFPE samples are usually mounted on glass slides, stained with Congo red, and only the positive areas (i.e., sample enrichment) are selected under a fluorescence microscope and excised by laser capture microdissection (LCM), and then transferred into a tube cap for in-liquid analysis [35, 36, 38]. Recently, a protocol was developed to characterize the amyloid protein without the need of prior LCM, starting from fresh frozen EMBs, more difficult to collect and store [39]. Umbilical fat samples are usually analyzed as fresh frozen homogenized [40, 41]. In this case, the proteomics profile of the homogenized sample is compared to the profile of control tissue to take into account the tissue background [40].

In the bottom-up proteomics workflow, extracted proteins are denatured, reduced to remove disulfide bounds, and alkylated. Proteins are then digested with trypsin, and the resulting peptides are purified. Peptides are separated by liquid chromatography and injected into the mass spectrometer, where mass spectra of peptides and their fragments are acquired. Mass spectra are compared to in silico-generated databases to provide peptide identification [42]. Peptides are then grouped and assigned to the corresponding proteins. Protein intensity is calculated based on the intensity of its peptides (Fig. 15.3).

There is no standard method to characterize the amyloid protein from the list of identified and quantified proteins in the sample. A commonly used method involves the ranking of the proteins based on the number of assigned fragmentation spectra [36]. The amyloidogenic protein with the highest position in the rank is marked as the depositing protein. This method is commonly used for LCM-enriched samples, since for these samples, the proteomics profile is dominated by the proteins in the deposit. For samples analyzed as a whole, such as umbilical fat biopsies, the proteomics profile is compared to the profile of healthy controls to remove the background contribution [40]. In this latter case, a score is computed for each protein by taking into account the ratio between the number of assigned fragmentation spectra in the diseased and the healthy tissue. Proteins co-precipitating in the deposit such as serum amyloid P-component, ApoE, and ApoA-IV are detected in the same analysis and constitute an "universal amyloid signature," which can be used as a high-confidence signal of amyloidosis presence [43].

The use of proteomics is still limited by the expensive equipment required and by the need of highly specialized personnel [44]. The use of proteomics for amyloid characterization can be improved by technique standardization and agreements on the best practices, including sample collection, data analysis, and diagnostic reporting [45].

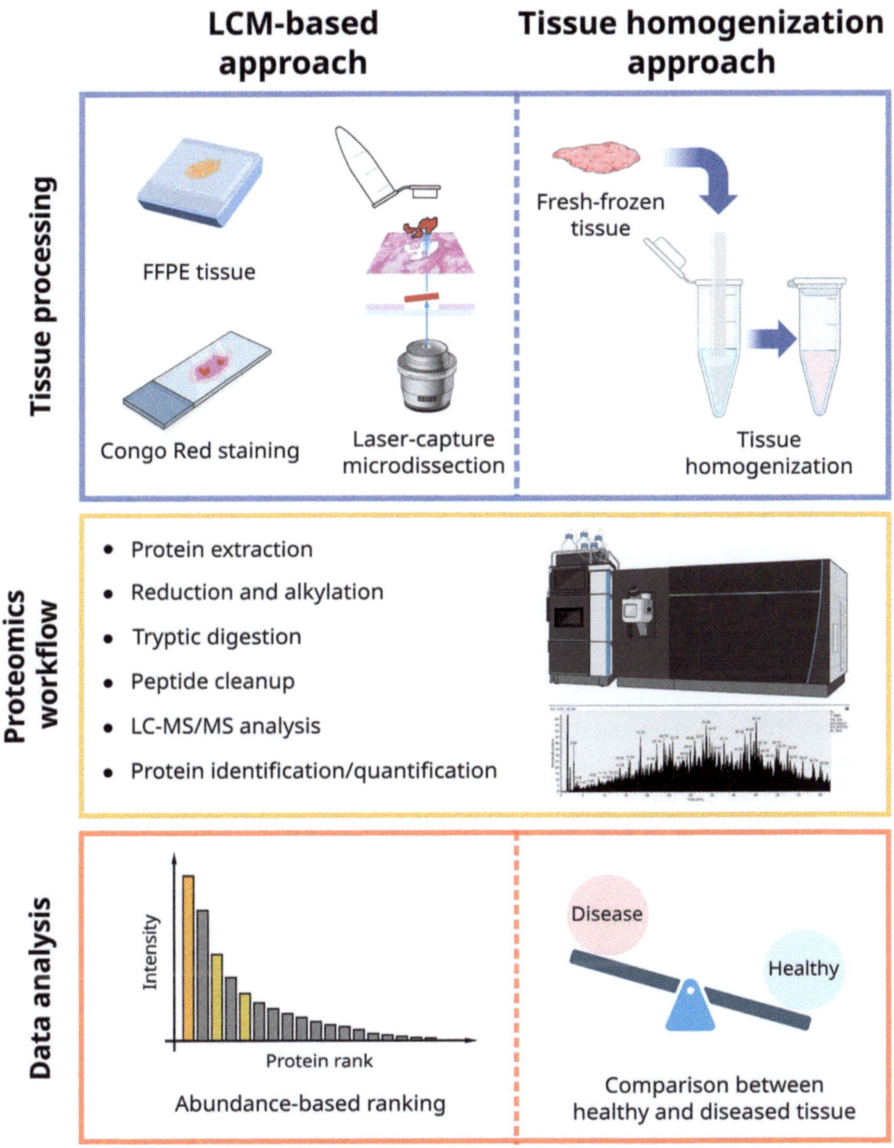

Fig. 15.3 Scheme of two possible approaches to proteomics-based amyloid typing. In the laser capture microdissection (LCM)-based approach, amyloid protein enrichment occurs during Congo red-positive region isolation. In the tissue homogenization approach, the sample is processed without prior enrichment. The proteomics workflow does not substantially differ between these two methods, but in the tissue homogenization approach, the contribution of the background is removed by comparing the protein profile of the sample with the protein profile of healthy tissue

15.2 Tissue Biopsy in Cardiac Amyloidosis

15.2.1 Endomyocardial Biopsy (EMB)

EMB may prove very useful for the diagnosis of CA, but it is an invasive procedure that must be performed in referral and experienced centers [7] (Fig. 15.1). It is performed in patients with suspected CA and inconclusive peripheral biopsy [25, 26]. EMB is mostly performed in the right ventricle (RV), but left ventricular (LV) EMB may be more sensitive, and in experienced centers, it shows a low risk of complications [7, 46, 47]. In the myocardium, the amyloid deposits may be interstitial, quite diffuse, and surrounding the individual myocytes, or patchy and nodular [10]. In AL-CA, they are mainly pericellular and reticular, often associated with inflammatory infiltrates, mainly T-lymphocytes and macrophages, which may contribute to tissue damage [5, 7, 48]. In ATTR-CA, amyloid deposits are usually irregular and patchy, displaying two main patterns, i.e., nodular and interstitial (*pattern A*), or thin interstitial and vascular (*pattern B*) [49].

15.2.2 Surrogate Biopsy Sites

In systemic forms of amyloidosis, different *surrogate* sites, first the abdominal periumbilical fat, may give positive results for diagnosis and typing of CA, depending upon the disease extent and the amyloidogenic protein [24].

Abdominal (periumbilical) fine needle biopsy and fat pad excisional biopsy (FPEB) are quite widely used for the diagnosis and characterization of CA [32, 50, 51] (Fig. 15.2). Fat biopsy was first introduced by Westermark and Stenkvist in 1973 [52]. This technique has a few advantages; it is a quite easy and low-cost procedure with high patient tolerance, lacking significant complications [24]. In qualified centers, the abdominal fat tissue aspirate/biopsy shows a high sensitivity in AL amyloidosis with 70–90% positive results and reaches 67% sensitivity in ATTRv, whereas it has a low (14%) sensitivity in wtTTR [50, 53–56].

15.2.3 Other Biopsy Sites

Bone marrow biopsy is usually part of clinical evaluation in AL amyloidosis, amyloid deposits being found in about 50–60% of patients [24].

Minor salivary gland biopsy (from the labial mucosa) shows variable sensitivity (up to 86%) in AL amyloidosis [57]. As to gastrointestinal biopsies, they may show amyloid deposits in elderly male patients with AL amyloidosis [58]. Biopsies of the upper gastrointestinal tract are apparently more often positive in AL κ + forms and in AA amyloidosis, whereas the large intestine and rectum biopsies are more frequently positive in AL λ + forms and in ATTR. Other sites, such as gingiva or skin, are less sensitive and are rarely biopsied [24].

15.3   Advantages and Limitations of Tissue Biopsy

The observation of the diseased tissue is the most straightforward method to assess the nature and entity of the amyloid deposition and to explore concomitant pathologies. Tissue-based techniques, especially proteomics, can also provide direct measurement of the co-precipitating proteins in the deposit, which constitutes a diagnostic fingerprint of amyloidosis [43].

In the presence of monoclonal gammopathy, tissue biopsy is recommended, especially in the case of positive/inconclusive cardiac magnetic resonance [59]. In such cases, tissue biopsy is the only way to characterize the amyloid type and to administer the correct treatment.

EMB is the recommended site for tissue biopsy in CA, but the biopsy procedure is invasive and requires highly specialized personnel [60]. Less invasive biopsy sites can be sampled, such as umbilical fat, skin, or lip, but a negative result from such specimens does not rule out the presence of the disease [61].

Tissue sampling can suffer from sampling biases; then it is crucial that more fragments, possibly from different organ's areas, are collected, especially in the early stages of the disease [62].

15.4   Tissue Biopsy: Beyond the Diagnostic Purpose and Future Directions

In CA, tissue sampling may be crucial for diagnostic purposes, but also to investigate the pathogenetic mechanisms, to evaluate the efficacy of treatments, and potentially to detect the disease in its early stages. Tissue analyses are fundamental to evaluate the effects of the amyloid deposition on the target organ, the properties of aggregated fibrils, and the in vivo interactions between fibrils and organ tissue. The tissue biopsy also allows for the recognition of less common or even new forms of amyloidosis [63].

The protein deposition in the tissue is a complex process. Tissue biopsies have been used to study the ratio between protein deposits and tissue fibrosis in AL- and ATTR-CA, correlating these data with the extracellular volume detected by CMR [7]. Moreover, the histopathological evaluation of EMB allowed to correlate the deposition pattern with the amyloid type [64]. EMBs were also investigated to detect microcalcification and macrophage infiltration in AL and ATTR patients in order to elucidate the role of scintigraphy trackers in CA [48].

Tissue biopsies have also been used to investigate the localization and the gene expression of the natriuretic peptides in the myocardium of CA [65], such as the protein profile of the myocardium from ATTR and AL patients as compared to healthy controls to elucidate the possible biological pathways involved in cardiac tissue response to amyloid [66, 67].

CA produces a mechanical disruption of heart fibers; the mechanical properties of the tissue and the possible correlations between the loss of cardiac function and the degree of amyloidosis can be investigated in ex vivo samples [68].

15.5 Conclusions

In CA, tissue biopsy is a crucial step in the diagnostic workflow and in some cases represents the only tool to reach the definite diagnosis. Despite its invasiveness, especially for EMB, direct tissue sampling provides high-value information through advanced techniques such as immunohistochemistry and proteomics, most potentials still being unexplored. Tissue biopsy not only gives a picture of the organ state at the sampling time, but it may also provide relevant data on the mechanisms of protein deposition, on the amyloidogenic protein-organ tissue interplays, and on the effects of treatments.

References

1. Benson M, Buxbaum J, Eisenberg D, Merlini G, Saraiva M, Sekijima Y, et al. Amyloid nomenclature 2020: update and recommendations by the international society of amyloidosis (ISA) nomenclature committee. Amyloid. 2020;27:217–22. https://doi.org/10.1080/13506129.2020.1835263.
2. Merlini G, Bellotti V. Molecular mechanisms of amyloidosis. N Engl J Med. 2003;349(6):583–96.
3. Flodrova P, Flodr P, Pika T, et al. Cardiac amyloidosis: from clinical suspicion to morphological diagnosis. Pathology. 2018;50(3):261–8. https://doi.org/10.1016/j.pathol.2017.10.012.
4. Yakupova EI, Bobyleva LG, Vikhlyantsev IM, et al. Congo red and amyloids: history and relationship. Biosci Rep. 2019;39(1):BSR20181415. https://doi.org/10.1042/BSR20181415.
5. Kristen AV, Brokbals E, Aus dem Siepen F, et al. Amyloid load: a prognostic and predictive biomarker in patients with light-chain amyloidosis. J Am Coll Cardiol. 2016;68(1):13–24. https://doi.org/10.1016/j.jacc.2016.04.035.
6. Siegismund CS, Escher F, Lassner D, et al. Intramyocardial inflammation predicts adverse outcome in patients with cardiac AL amyloidosis. Eur J Heart Fail. 2018;20(4):751–7. https://doi.org/10.1002/ejhf.1039.
7. Pucci A, Aimo A, Musetti V, Barison A, Vergaro G, Genovesi D, Giorgetti A, Masotti S, Arzilli C, Prontera C, Pastormerlo LE, Coceani MA, Ciardetti M, Martini N, Palmieri C, Passino C, Rapezzi C, Emdin M. Amyloid deposits and fibrosis on left ventricular endomyocardial biopsy correlate with extracellular volume in cardiac amyloidosis. J Am Heart Assoc. 2021;10(20):e020358. https://doi.org/10.1161/JAHA.120.020358.
8. Buxbaum JN, Dispenzieri A, Eisenberg DS, et al. Amyloid nomenclature 2022: update, novel proteins, and recommendations by the International Society of Amyloidosis (ISA) Nomenclature Committee. Amyloid. 2022;29(4):213–9. https://doi.org/10.1080/13506129.2022.2147636.
9. Garcia-Pavia P, Rapezzi C, Adler Y, et al. Diagnosis and treatment of cardiac amyloidosis: a position statement of the ESC Working Group on Myocardial and Pericardial Diseases. Eur Heart J. 2021;42(16):1554–68.
10. Maleszewski JJ. Cardiac amyloidosis: pathology, nomenclature, and typing. Cardiovasc Pathol. 2015;24(6):343–50. https://doi.org/10.1016/j.carpath.2015.07.008.
11. Vergaro G, Aimo A, Rapezzi C, et al. Atrial amyloidosis: mechanisms and clinical manifestations. Eur J Heart Fail. 2022;24(11):2019–28.
12. Looi LM. Isolated atrial amyloidosis: a clinicopathologic study indicating increased prevalence in chronic heart disease. Hum Pathol. 1993;24(6):602–7. https://doi.org/10.1016/0046-8177(93)90239-d.
13. Richter S, Jahnke C, Klingel K, Paetsch I. Isolated atrial amyloidosis. Eur Heart J. 2020;41(28):2695. https://doi.org/10.1093/eurheartj/ehaa370.

14. Sud K, Narula N, Aikawa E, Arbustini E, Pibarot P, Merlini G, Rosenson RS, Seshan SV, Argulian E, Ahmadi A, Zhou F, Moreira AL, Côté N, Tsimikas S, Fuster V, Gandy S, Bonow RO, Gursky O, Narula J. The contribution of amyloid deposition in the aortic valve to calcification and aortic stenosis. Nat Rev Cardiol. 2023;20(6):418–28. https://doi.org/10.1038/s41569-022-00818-2. Erratum in: Nat Rev Cardiol. (2023), Feb 17

15. Mucchiano G, Cornwell GG 3rd, Westermark P. Senile aortic amyloid. Evidence for two distinct forms of localized deposits. Am J Pathol. 1992;140(4):871–7.

16. Larsson A, Söderberg L, Westermark GT, et al. Unwinding fibril formation of medin, the peptide of the most common form of human amyloid. Biochem Biophys Res Commun. 2007;361(4):822–8. https://doi.org/10.1016/j.bbrc.2007.06.187.

17. Stubbs JD, Lekutis C, Singer KL, et al. cDNA cloning of a mouse mammary epithelial cell surface protein reveals the existence of epidermal growth factor-like domains linked to factor VIII-like sequences. Proc Natl Acad Sci U S A. 1990;87(21):8417–21. https://doi.org/10.1073/pnas.87.21.8417.

18. Westermark GT, Westermark P. Localized amyloids important in diseases outside the brain—lessons from the islets of Langerhans and the thoracic aorta. FEBS J. 2011;278(20):3918–29. https://doi.org/10.1111/j.1742-4658.2011.08298.x.

19. Jerome S, Farrell MB, Warren J, Embry-Dierson M, Schockling EJ. Cardiac amyloidosis imaging, part 3: interpretation, diagnosis, and treatment. J Nucl Med Technol. 2023;51(2):102–16. https://doi.org/10.2967/jnmt.123.265492.

20. Maurer MS, Bokhari S, Damy T, Dorbala S, Drachman BM, Fontana M, Grogan M, Kristen AV, Lousada I, Nativi-Nicolau J, Cristina Quarta C, Rapezzi C, Ruberg FL, Witteles R, Merlini G. Expert consensus recommendations for the suspicion and diagnosis of transthyretin cardiac amyloidosis. Circ Heart Fail. 2019;12(9):e006075. https://doi.org/10.1161/CIRCHEARTFAILURE.119.006075.

21. Brownrigg J, Lorenzini M, Lumley M, Elliott P. Diagnostic performance of imaging investigations in detecting and differentiating cardiac amyloidosis: a systematic review and meta-analysis. ESC Heart Fail. 2019;6(5):1041–51. https://doi.org/10.1002/ehf2.12511.

22. Chatzantonis G, Bietenbeck M, Elsanhoury A, Tschöpe C, Pieske B, Tauscher G, Vietheer J, Shomanova Z, Mahrholdt H, Rolf A, Kelle S, Yilmaz A. Diagnostic value of cardiovascular magnetic resonance in comparison to endomyocardial biopsy in cardiac amyloidosis: a multi-centre study. Clin Res Cardiol. 2021;110(4):555–68. https://doi.org/10.1007/s00392-020-01771-1.

23. Martinez-Naharro A, Baksi AJ, Hawkins PN, Fontana M. Diagnostic imaging of cardiac amyloidosis. Nat Rev Cardiol. 2020;17(7):413–26. https://doi.org/10.1038/s41569-020-0334-7.

24. Wisniowski B, Wechalekar A. Confirming the diagnosis of amyloidosis. Acta Haematol. 2020;143(4):312–21. https://doi.org/10.1159/000508022.

25. Leone O, Veinot JP, Angelini A, Baandrup UT, Basso C, Berry G, Bruneval P, Burke M, Butany J, Calabrese F, d'Amati G, Edwards WD, Fallon JT, Fishbein MC, Gallagher PJ, Halushka MK, McManus B, Pucci A, Rodriguez ER, Saffitz JE, Sheppard MN, Steenbergen C, Stone JR, Tan C, Thiene G, van der Wal AC, Winters GL. 2011 consensus statement on endomyocardial biopsy from the Association for European Cardiovascular Pathology and the Society for Cardiovascular Pathology. Cardiovasc Pathol. 2012;21(4):245–74. https://doi.org/10.1016/j.carpath.2011.10.001.

26. Musetti V, Greco F, Castiglione V, Aimo A, Palmieri C, Genovesi D, Giorgetti A, Emdin M, Vergaro G, McDonnell LA, Pucci A. Tissue characterization in cardiac amyloidosis. Biomedicines. 2022;10(12):3054. https://doi.org/10.3390/biomedicines10123054.

27. Dasari S, Theis JD, Vrana JA, Rech KL, Dao LN, Howard MT, Dispenzieri A, Gertz MA, Hasadri L, Highsmith WE, Kurtin PJ, McPhail ED. Amyloid typing by mass spectrometry in clinical practice: a comprehensive review of 16,175 samples. Mayo Clin Proc. 2020;95(9):1852–64. https://doi.org/10.1016/j.mayocp.2020.06.029.

28. Barreca A, Bottasso E, Veneziano F, Giarin M, Nocifora A, Martinetti N, Attanasio A, Biancone L, Benevolo G, Roccatello D, Cassoni P, Papotti MG. Amyloidosis Group of the "Rete Interregionale Piemonte e Valle d'Aosta per le Malattie Rare". Immunohistochemical

typing of amyloid in fixed paraffin-embedded samples by an automatic procedure: comparison with immunofluorescence data on fresh-frozen tissue. PLoS One. 2021;16(8):e0256306. https://doi.org/10.1371/journal.pone.0256306.

29. Riefolo M, Conti M, Longhi S, Fabbrizio B, Leone O. Amyloidosis: What does pathology offer? The evolving field of tissue biopsy. Front Cardiovasc Med. 2022;9:1081098. https://doi.org/10.3389/fcvm.2022.1081098.

30. Howie AJ. "green (or apple-green) birefringence" of Congo red-stained amyloid. Amyloid. 2015;22(3):205–6. https://doi.org/10.3109/13506129.2015.1054026.

31. Picken MM, Herrera GA. The burden of "sticky" amyloid: typing challenges. Arch Pathol Lab Med. 2007;131(6):850–1. https://doi.org/10.5858/2007-131-850-TBOSAT.

32. Arbustini E, Verga L, Concardi M, Palladini G, Obici L, Merlini G. Electron and immunoelectron microscopy of abdominal fat identifies and characterizes amyloid fibrils in suspected cardiac amyloidosis. Amyloid. 2002;9(2):108–14. PMID: 12440483

33. Abildgaard N, Rojek AM, Møller HE, Palstrøm NB, Nyvold CG, Rasmussen LM, Hansen CT, Beck HC, Marcussen N. Immunoelectron microscopy and mass spectrometry for classification of amyloid deposits. Amyloid. 2020;27(1):59–66. https://doi.org/10.1080/13506129.2019.1688289.

34. Hill MM, Dasari S, Mollee P, Merlini G, Costello CE, Hazenberg BPC, Grogan M, Dispenzieri A, Gertz MA, Kourelis T, McPhail ED. The clinical impact of proteomics in amyloid typing. Mayo Clin Proc. 2021;96(5):1122–7. https://doi.org/10.1016/j.mayocp.2020.12.002.

35. Lavatelli F, Vrana JA. Proteomic typing of amyloid deposits in systemic amyloidoses. Amyloid. 2011;18(4):177–82. https://doi.org/10.3109/13506129.2011.630762.

36. Vrana JA, Gamez JD, Madden BJ, Theis JD, Bergen HR, Dogan A. Classification of amyloidosis by laser microdissection and mass spectrometry-based proteomic analysis in clinical biopsy specimens. Blood. 2009;114(24):4957–9. https://doi.org/10.1182/blood-2009-07-230722.

37. Canetti D, Rendell NB, Di Vagno L, Gilbertson JA, Rowczenio D, Rezk T, Gillmore JD, Hawkins PN, Verona G, Mangione PP, Giorgetti S, Mauri P, Motta S, De Palma A, Bellotti V, Taylor GW. Misidentification of transthyretin and immunoglobulin variants by proteomics due to methyl lysine formation in formalin-fixed paraffin-embedded amyloid tissue. Amyloid. 2017;24(4):233–41. https://doi.org/10.1080/13506129.2017.1385452.

38. Mollee P, Boros S, Loo D, Ruelcke JE, Lakis VA, Cao KAL, Renaut P, Hill MM. Implementation and evaluation of amyloidosis subtyping by laser-capture microdissection and tandem mass spectrometry. Clin Proteomics. 2016;13(1):1–6. https://doi.org/10.1186/s12014-016-9133-x.

39. Noborn F, Thomsen C, Vorontsov E, Bobbio E, Sihlbom C, Nilsson J, Polte CL, Bollano E, Vukusic K, Sandstedt J, Dellgren G, Karason K, Oldfors A, Larson G. Subtyping of cardiac amyloidosis by mass spectrometry-based proteomics of endomyocardial biopsies. Amyloid. 2022;30:1–13. https://doi.org/10.1080/13506129.2022.2127088.

40. Brambilla F, Lavatelli F, Di Silvestre D, Valentini V, Rossi R, Palladini G, Obici L, Verga L, Mauri P, Merlini G. Reliable typing of systemic amyloidoses through proteomic analysis of subcutaneous adipose tissue. Blood. 2012;119(8):1844–7. https://doi.org/10.1182/blood-2011-07-365510.

41. Lavatelli F, Perlman DH, Spencer B, Prokaeva T, McComb ME, Théberge R, Connors LH, Bellotti V, Seldin DC, Merlini G, Skinner M, Costello CE. Amyloidogenic and associated proteins in systemic amyloidosis proteome of adipose tissue. Mol Cell Proteomics. 2008;7(8):1570–83. https://doi.org/10.1074/mcp.M700545-MCP200.

42. Steen H, Mann M. The ABC's (and XYZ's) of peptide sequencing. Nat Rev Mol Cell Biol. 2004;5(9):699–711. https://doi.org/10.1038/nrm1468.

43. Vrana JA, Theis JD, Dasari S, Mereuta OM, Dispenzieri A, Zeldenrust SR, Gertz MA, Kurtin PJ, Grogg KL, Dogan A. Clinical diagnosis and typing of systemic amyloidosis in subcutaneous fat aspirates by mass spectrometry-based proteomics. Haematologica. 2014;99(7):1239–47. https://doi.org/10.3324/haematol.2013.102764.

44. Benson MD, Berk JL, Dispenzieri A, Damy T, Gillmore JD, Hazenberg BP, Lavatelli F, Picken MM, Röcken C, Schönland S, Ueda M, Westermark P. Tissue biopsy for the diagnosis of

amyloidosis: experience from some centres. Amyloid. 2022;29(1):8–13. https://doi.org/10.108 0/13506129.2021.1994386.

45. Canetti D, Rendell NB, Gilbertson JA, Botcher N, Nocerino P, Blanco A, Di Vagno L, Rowczenio D, Verona G, Mangione PP, Bellotti V, Hawkins PN, Gillmore JD, Taylor GW. Diagnostic amyloid proteomics: experience of the UK National Amyloidosis Centre. Clin Chem Lab Med. 2020;58(6):948–57. https://doi.org/10.1515/cclm-2019-1007.

46. Yilmaz A, Kindermann I, Kindermann M, Mahfoud F, Ukena C, Athanasiadis A, Hill S, Mahrholdt H, Voehringer M, Schieber M, Klingel K, Kandolf R, Böhm M, Sechtem U. Comparative evaluation of left and right ventricular endomyocardial biopsy: differences in complication rate and diagnostic performance. Circulation. 2010;122(9):900–9. https://doi. org/10.1161/CIRCULATIONAHA.109.924167.

47. Rubiś P, Rudnicka-Sosin L, Jurczyszyn A, Janion M, Podolec P. The paramount importance of repeated left ventricular endomyocardial biopsy during the diagnosis of restrictive cardiomyopathy due to AL cardiac amyloidosis. Kardiol Pol. 2016;74(8):796. https://doi.org/10.5603/KP.2016.0114.

48. Stats MA, Stone JR. Varying levels of small microcalcifications and macrophages in ATTR and AL cardiac amyloidosis: implications for utilizing nuclear medicine studies to subtype amyloidosis. Cardiovasc Pathol. 2016;25(5):413–7. https://doi.org/10.1016/j.carpath.2016.07.001.

49. Bergström J, Gustavsson A, Hellman U, Sletten K, Murphy CL, Weiss DT, Solomon A, Olofsson BO, Westermark P. Amyloid deposits in transthyretin-derived amyloidosis: cleaved transthyretin is associated with distinct amyloid morphology. J Pathol. 2005;206(2):224–32. https://doi.org/10.1002/path.1759.

50. Garcia Y, Collins A, Stone J. Abdominal fat pad excisional biopsy for the diagnosis and typing of systemic amyloidosis. Hum Pathol. 2018;72:71–9. https://doi.org/10.1016/j.humpath.2017.11.001.

51. van Gameren II, Hazenberg BP, Bijzet J, van Rijswijk MH. Diagnostic accuracy of subcutaneous abdominal fat tissue aspiration for detecting systemic amyloidosis and its utility in clinical practice. Arthritis Rheum. 2006;54(6):2015–21. https://doi.org/10.1002/art.21902.

52. Westermark P, Stenkvist B. A new method for the diagnosis of systemic amyloidosis. Arch Intern Med. 1973;132(4):522–3.

53. Aimo A, Emdin M, Musetti V, Pucci A, Vergaro G. Abdominal fat biopsy for the diagnosis of cardiac amyloidosis. JACC Case Rep. 2020;2(8):1182–5. https://doi.org/10.1016/j.jaccas.2020.05.062.

54. Quarta C, Gonzalez-Lopez E, Gilbertson J, Botcher N, Rowczenio D, Petrie A, et al. Diagnostic sensitivity of abdominal fat aspiration in cardiac amyloidosis. Eur Heart J. 2017;38:1905–8. https://doi.org/10.1093/eurheartj/ehx047.

55. Fine N, Arruda-Olson A, Dispenzieri A, Zeldenrust S, Gertz M, Kyle R, et al. Yield of noncardiac biopsy for the diagnosis of transthyretin cardiac amyloidosis. Am J Cardiol. 2014;113:1723–7. https://doi.org/10.1016/j.amjcard.2014.02.030.

56. Gertz M, Li C, Shirahama T, Kyle R. Utility of subcutaneous fat aspiration for the diagnosis of systemic amyloidosis (immunoglobulin light chain). Arch Intern Med. 1988;148:929–33. https://doi.org/10.1001/archinte.148.4.929.

57. Suzuki T, Kusumoto S, Yamashita T, Masuda A, Kinoshita S, Yoshida T, Takami-Mori F, Takino H, Ito A, Ri M, Ishida T, Komatsu H, Ueda M, Ando Y, Inagaki H, Iida S. Labial salivary gland biopsy for diagnosing immunoglobulin light chain amyloidosis: a retrospective analysis. Ann Hematol. 2016;95(2):279–85. https://doi.org/10.1007/s00277-015-2549-y.

58. Freudenthaler S, Hegenbart U, Schönland S, Behrens HM, Krüger S, Röcken C. Amyloid in biopsies of the gastrointestinal tract-a retrospective observational study on 542 patients. Virchows Arch. 2016;468(5):569–77. https://doi.org/10.1007/s00428-016-1916-y. Epub 2016 Feb 25

59. Rapezzi C, Aimo A, Serenelli M, Barison A, Vergaro G, Passino C, Panichella G, Sinagra G, Merlo M, Fontana M, Gillmore J, Quarta CC, Maurer MS, Kittleson MM, Garcia-Pavia P, Emdin M. Critical comparison of documents from scientific societies on cardiac amyloi-

dosis: JACC state-of-the-art review. J Am Coll Cardiol. 2022;79(13):1288–303. https://doi.org/10.1016/j.jacc.2022.01.036.

60. Mollee P, Renaut P, Gottlieb D, Goodman H. How to diagnose amyloidosis. Intern Med J. 2014;44(1):7–17. https://doi.org/10.1111/imj.12288.

61. Gillmore JD, Wechalekar A, Bird J, Cavenagh J, Hawkins S, Kazmi M, Lachmann HJ, Hawkins PN, Pratt G. Guidelines on the diagnosis and investigation of AL amyloidosis. Br J Haematol. 2015;168(2):207–18. https://doi.org/10.1111/bjh.13156.

62. Crotty TB, Li CY, Edwards WD, Suman VJ. Amyloidosis and endomyocardial biopsy: correlation of extent and pattern of deposition with amyloid immunophenotype in 100 cases. Cardiovasc Pathol. 1995;4(1):39–42. https://doi.org/10.1016/1054-8807(94)00023-K.

63. Dogan A. Amyloidosis: insights from proteomics. Ann Rev Pathol. 2017;2017:277–304. https://doi.org/10.1146/annurev-pathol-052016-100200.

64. Larsen BT, Mereuta OM, Dasari S, Fayyaz AU, Theis JD, Vrana JA, Grogan M, Dogan A, Dispenzieri A, Edwards WD, Kurtin PJ, Maleszewski JJ. Correlation of histomorphological pattern of cardiac amyloid deposition with amyloid type: A histological and proteomic analysis of 108 cases. Histopathology. 2016;68(5):648–56. https://doi.org/10.1111/his.12793.

65. Takemura G, Takatsu Y, Doyama K, Itoh H, Saito Y, Koshiji M, Ando F, Fujiwara T, Nakao K, Fujiwara H. Expression of atrial and brain natriuretic peptides and their genes in hearts of patients with cardiac amyloidosis. J Am Coll Cardiol. 1998;31(4):754–65. https://doi.org/10.1016/s0735-1097(98)00045-x.

66. Kourelis T, Dasari S, Fayyaz AU, Grogan M, Ramirez-Alvarado M, Redfield M, Abou Ezzeddine OF, Dispenzieri A, McPhail ED. A proteomic atlas of cardiac amyloidosis. Blood. 2019;134(Supplement_1):1790–0. https://doi.org/10.1182/blood-2019-124802.

67. Di Silvestre D, Brambilla F, Lavatelli F, Chirivì M, Canetti D, Bearzi C, Rizzi R, Bijzet J, Hazenberg BPC, Bellotti V, Gillmore JD, Mauri P. The protein network in subcutaneous fat biopsies from patients with AL amyloidosis: more than diagnosis? Cell. 2023;12(5):699. https://doi.org/10.3390/cells12050699.

68. Petre RE, Quaile MP, Wendt K, Houser SR, Wald J, Goldman BI, Margulies KB. Regionally heterogeneous tissue mechanics in cardiac amyloidosis. Amyloid. 2005;12(4):246–50. https://doi.org/10.1080/13506120500386824.

Julian D. Gillmore, Alberto Aimo, and Pablo Garcia-Pavia

The diagnostic workup of cardiac amyloidosis (CA) includes two phases: suspicion and diagnosis [1]. The suspicion of CA should arise when "red flags" for this condition are present, particularly when increased left ventricular (LV) wall thickness has no clear explanation or is disproportionate to the possible cause. The diagnosis phase should follow a specific algorithm and includes amyloid typing, which is critical to guide specific treatment [1].

16.1　When Cardiac Amyloidosis Should Be Suspected

Some red flags are extracardiac signs and symptoms that are often associated with CA, such as carpal tunnel syndrome, proteinuria, macroglossia, and skin bruises. Cardiac red flags include a disproportionate increase in N-terminal pro-B-type

J. D. Gillmore
National Amyloidosis Centre, Division of Medicine, University College London, Royal Free Hospital, London, UK
e-mail: j.gillmore@ucl.ac.uk

A. Aimo (✉)
Interdisciplinary Center for Health Sciences, Scuola Superiore Sant'Anna, Pisa, Italy

Cardiology Division, Fondazione Toscana Gabriele Monasterio, Pisa, Italy
e-mail: aimoalb@ftgm.it

P. Garcia-Pavia
Heart Failure and Inherited Cardiac Diseases Unit, Department of Cardiology, Hospital Universitario Puerta de Hierro Majadahonda, CIBERCV, Madrid, Spain

Universidad Francisco de Vitoria (UFV), Pozuelo de Alarcon, Spain

European Reference Network for Rare, Low Prevalence and Complex Diseases of the Heart-ERN GUARD-Heart, Pavia, Italy
e-mail: pablo.garciap@uam.es

M. Emdin et al. (eds.), *Cardiac Amyloidosis*,
https://doi.org/10.1007/978-3-031-51757-0_16

natriuretic peptide (NT-proBNP) compared to the degree of cardiac dysfunction, disproportionally low QRS voltage compared to LV mass, persistent troponin elevation, unexplained right-heart failure (HF) or pericardial effusion, or conduction system disease. Table 16.1 lists the red flags that can be found in patients with amyloid light-chain (AL) or transthyretin (ATTR) amyloidosis, which in turn accounts for almost all cases of CA. Additionally, CA should be suspected in two settings: (1)

Table 16.1 Red flags of amyloidosis

Extracardiac/cardiac	Type	Red flag	Amyloidosis type where it is most frequently found
Extracardiac	Clinical	Polyneuropathy	ATTRv, AL
		Dysautonomia	ATTR, AL
		Skin bruising	AL
		Macroglossia	AL
		Deafness	ATTRwt
		Carpal tunnel syndrome	ATTRv, ATTRwt
		Ruptured biceps tendon	ATTRwt
		Lumbar spinal stenosis	ATTRwt
		Vitreous deposits	ATTRv
		Family history	ATTRv
	Laboratory	Kidney disease	AL
		Proteinuria	AL
Cardiac	Clinical	Hypotension or normotensive if previously hypertensive	ATTR, AL
	ECG	Pseudoinfarct pattern	All
		Low/decreased QRS voltage to degree of LV thickness	All
		AV conduction disease	All
	Laboratory	Disproportionally elevated NT-proBNP to degree of HF	All
		Persisting elevated troponin	All
	Echocardiogram	Granular sparkling of myocardium	All
		Increased RV wall thickness	All
		Increased valve thickness	All
		Pericardial effusion	All
		Apical sparing	All
	CMR	Subendocardial LGE	All
		Elevated native T1 values	All
		Increased ECV	All
		Abnormal gadolinium kinetics	All

AL amyloid light-chain amyloidosis, *ATTRv* variant transthyretin amyloidosis, *ATTRwt* wild-type transthyretin amyloidosis, *AV* atrioventricular, *CMR* cardiac magnetic resonance, *ECG* electrocardiogram, *ECV* extracellular volume, *HF* heart failure, *LGE* late gadolinium enhancement, *LV* left ventricular, *NT-proBNP* N-terminal pro-B-type natriuretic peptide, *RV* right ventricular
Modified with permission from Garcia-Pavia et al. [1]

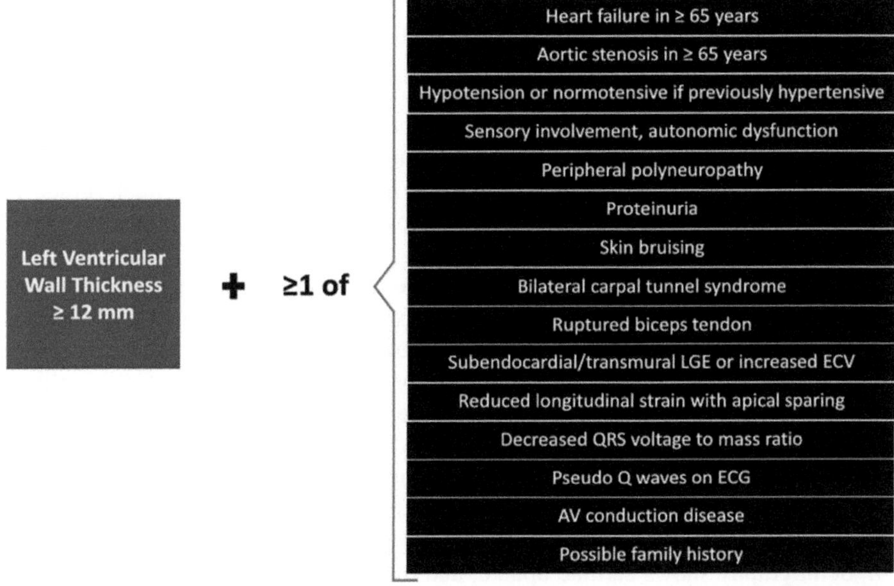

Fig. 16.1 Screening of cardiac amyloidosis. *AV* atrio-ventricular, *ECG* electrocardiogram, *ECV* extracellular volume, *LGE* late gadolinium enhancement. Reprinted with permission from: Garcia-Pavia et al. [1]

when cardiac involvement is accompanied by systemic conditions such as plasma cell dyscrasia, nephrotic syndrome, or peripheral neuropathy, and (2) when there is a combination of increased LV wall thickness, no LV dilation, HF, aortic stenosis, or some red flags, particularly in patients older than 65 years [1]. A position statement by the European Society of Cardiology (ESC) Working Group on Myocardial and Pericardial Diseases tried to enucleate a schematic algorithm to guide clinicians through the suspicion phase (Fig. 16.1).

16.2 Diagnostic Algorithm

Once CA is suspected, a timely diagnosis should be made as patient outcomes depend largely on early initiation of therapy, particularly in AL-CA. The ESC position statement has introduced a diagnostic algorithm focusing on identifying these subtypes by the initial use of scintigraphy with bone tracers coupled to assessment for monoclonal proteins by serum and urine protein electrophoresis and quantification of serum-free light chains [1]. The results of these tests could lead to four scenarios:

1. Scintigraphy does not show cardiac uptake, and no monoclonal protein is found. CA is unlikely, and alternative diagnoses should be considered. If the suspicion

of CA persists, consider CMR followed by cardiac or extracardiac biopsy, as bone scintigraphy could be negative in some ATTRv mutations (e.g., Phe84Leu ATTRv, Ser97Tyr) and in rare subtypes of CA.

2. Scintigraphy shows cardiac uptake, and no monoclonal protein is found. If cardiac uptake is intense (grade 2 or 3 on the Perugini scale), ATTR-CA may be diagnosed with no need for histology. Genetic testing is needed to differentiate variant (v) from wild-type (wt) disease. When cardiac uptake is weak (grade 1), histological confirmation of amyloid deposits is needed, possibly also in an extracardiac site.

3. Scintigraphy does not show cardiac uptake, and there is evidence of a monoclonal protein (i.e., at least one of the three exams searching for a monoclonal protein is positive). AL-CA must be ruled out promptly. Cardiovascular magnetic resonance (CMR) is an option to check for cardiac involvement: CA is unlikely when there are no signs of cardiac disease, while histological demonstration of amyloid deposits is required to diagnose AL-CA if CMR findings are supportive or inconclusive. Biopsy of the heart or another clinically affected organ is recommended. If CMR cannot be performed promptly, it is advisable to proceed directly to tissue biopsy.

4. Scintigraphy shows cardiac uptake, and there is evidence of a monoclonal protein. ATTR-CA with concomitant monoclonal gammopathy of unknown significance (or another plasma cell dyscrasia), AL-CA, or the coexistence of AL- and ATTR-CA is possible. Diagnosis of CA requires histology with amyloid typing, usually by an endomyocardial biopsy [1].

Figure 16.2 provides the diagnostic algorithm for CA according to the ESC.

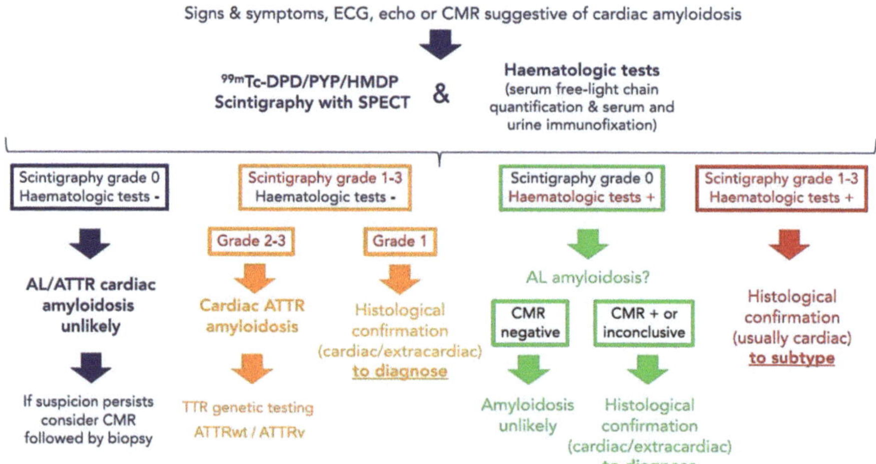

Fig. 16.2 Diagnostic algorithm for cardiac amyloidosis. *AL* amyloid light-chain amyloidosis, *ATTR* transthyretin amyloidosis (v, variant; wt, wild type), *CMR* cardiovascular magnetic resonance, *ECG* electrocardiogram, *SPECT* single-photon emission computed tomography, *TTR* transthyretin. Reprinted with permission from Garcia-Pavia et al. [1]

16.3 Different Approaches to the Suspicion and Diagnosis of CA

In 2021, five national or international scientific societies have issued guidelines or corresponding documents on CA: the ESC [1], the German Cardiac Society (*Deutsche Gesellschaft für Kardiologie*, DGK) [2], the Canadian Cardiovascular Society/Canadian Heart Failure Society (CCS/CHFS) [3, 4], the American Heart Association (AHA) [5, 6], and the Japanese Circulation Society (JCS) [7]. These documents proposed different approaches to the suspicion and diagnosis of CA, which we will recapitulate below.

16.3.1 Red Flags

The need for early diagnosis is stressed by all documents, which list several findings that may prompt a diagnostic workup for CA. Different red flags are listed in the five documents. Furthermore, the ESC [8] and DGK [2] documents recommend evaluation for CA in patients with LV wall thickness 12 mm or higher and at least one red flag is present, while the CCS/CHFS and AHA documents basically recommend to consider CA when red flags are present, regardless of LV wall thickness [3, 5]. Finally, the JCS guideline notes that some red flags are mandatory for diagnosis [7]. These differences highlight the current lack of knowledge on how the red flags should be utilized, prioritized, and combined when deciding on the timing of a diagnostic evaluation for CA in a population with a low prevalence of disease.

16.3.2 Diagnostic Algorithms

The two main decisional nodes in all proposed algorithms consist of the search of the monoclonal protein and bone scintigraphy with diphosphonate or pyrophosphate tracers, with the possible need for further histological exams [9]. The DGK statement diverges from the others because it contemplates multiple diagnostic pathways, one of them based on CMR; this last pathway mandatorily requires an endomyocardial biopsy to allow a definite diagnosis and to distinguish the CA subtype [2]. The diagnostic algorithms are summarized in Fig. 16.3.

The AHA and CCS/CHFS documents note that, while both bone scintigraphy and monoclonal light-chain screens may be performed simultaneously for convenience, the monoclonal light-chain screen takes priority, as bone scintigraphy findings must be interpreted on the light of the presence or absence of a monoclonal protein, and also because AL-CA should be promptly recognized and treated. When no monoclonal protein is found, the patient should undergo a bone scintigraphy or (when scintigraphy is not available) an endomyocardial biopsy [5]. The DGK statement also recommends that the search for a monoclonal protein precedes imaging in patients with suspected AL amyloidosis [2]. Conversely, the ESC document explicitly states that the search for a monoclonal protein and bone scintigraphy

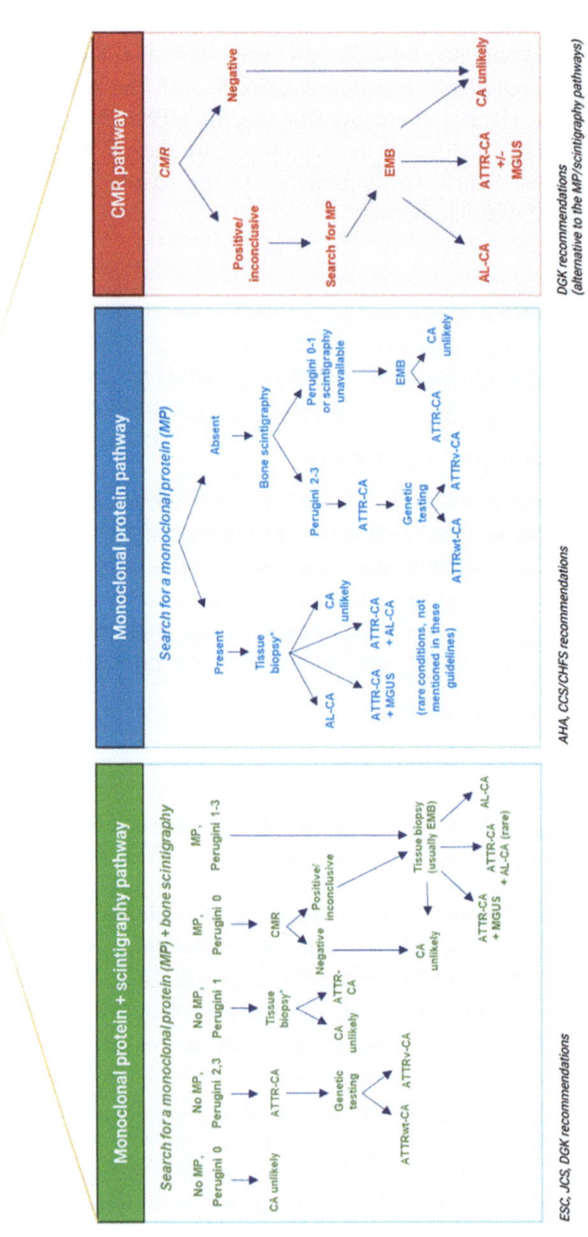

Fig. 16.3 Proposed diagnostic algorithms for cardiac amyloidosis. For details, see the original documents [2, 3, 5, 7, 8]. *AHA* American Heart Association, *CCS/CHFS* Canadian Cardiovascular Society/Canadian Heart Failure Society, *DGK* Deutsche Gesellschaft für Kardiologie (German Cardiac Society), *ESC* European Society of Cardiology, *JSC* Japanese Society of Cardiology, *MP* monoclonal protein, *NPs* cardiac natriuretic peptides (B-type natriuretic peptide, N-terminal B-type natriuretic peptide), *Tn* high-sensitivity troponins. Modified with permission from Rapezzi et al. [9]

should be performed together [8]. The notion of performing both exams in a single step emerges also from the JCS document, where four possible combinations of positive or negative results are considered [7]. When these exams are not performed in the same step, there is a risk of missing the coexistence of ATTR-CA and monoclonal gammopathy of unknown significance [9]. Indeed, this combination is not specifically mentioned in the AHA and CCS/CHFS algorithms [3, 5], while it is contemplated in the ESC statement: "[In patients with both a positive scintigraphy scan and a monoclonal protein], ATTR amyloidosis with concomitant [monoclonal gammopathy of unknown significance], AL amyloidosis, or coexistence of both AL and ATTR amyloidosis is possible" [8].

Overall, the divergence of the diagnostic pathways on the timing of bone scintigraphy and monoclonal light-chain screens in patients with suspected CA highlights another unresolved issue regarding the optimal diagnostic approach.

16.3.3 Echocardiography

Transthoracic echocardiography is the first-line imaging tool and may provide many red flags of CA. The AHA document stresses that echocardiography is useful to distinguish CA from cardiomyopathies with a hypertrophic phenotype, while it cannot differentiate AL- from ATTR-CA [5]. The CCS/CHFS statement [3], JCS guideline [7], and DGK statement [2] recommend the use of all available echocardiographic techniques, including speckle-tracking analysis, to diagnose CA. The ESC document is the only one to propose two echocardiographic scores to facilitate the diagnosis of cardiac involvement in patients with known AL amyloidosis, or in patients with unexplained hypertrophy and other red flags [8, 10] (Fig. 16.4). These scores may be seen as the first attempt to standardize the echocardiographic evaluation of patients with suspected CA.

16.3.4 Biomarkers

B-type natriuretic peptides and troponins within the normal range virtually exclude CA. Conversely, elevated biomarkers may indicate cardiac involvement in systemic amyloidosis, but are not specific for CA. Only the JCS guideline provides formal recommendations about biomarkers, stating that both NT-proBNP and hs-troponin might help diagnose CA (class IIa, level of evidence C) [7]. The JCS guideline also mentions the possible utility of retinol-binding protein 4, which binds to TTR and could stabilize the tetramer, for identifying subjects with ATTRv [7].

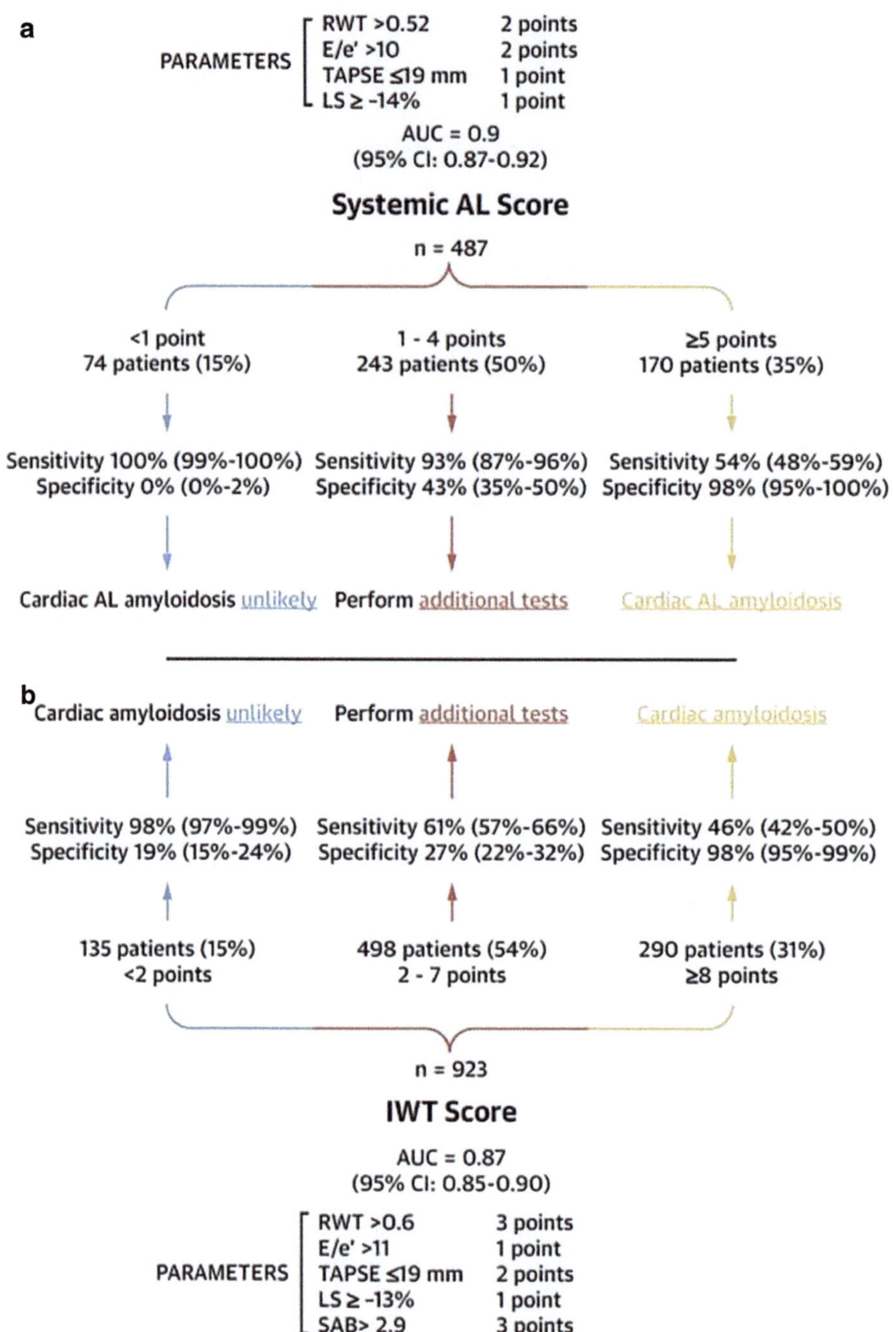

Fig. 16.4 Diagnostic algorithms with echocardiographic scores in two different clinical scenarios. Proposed diagnostic algorithms with highly sensitive and highly specific cutoffs to diagnose or exclude cardiac amyloidosis in patients with (**a**) systemic AL amyloidosis (AL score) and (**b**) increased wall thickness (IWT score). Reprinted with permission from Boldrini et al. [10]

16.3.5 Bone Scintigraphy

The ^{99m}Tc phosphates currently most often used in Europe are ^{99m}Tc-DPD (3,3-diphosphono-1,2-propanodicarboxylate) and ^{99m}Tc-HMDP (hydroxymethylene). By contrast, ^{99m}Tc-PYP (pyrophosphate) is the only tracer available in the United States, Canada, and Japan. The diagnostic criteria for positive planar scintigraphy are reported in Table 16.2. Single-photon emission computed tomography imaging enables a more accurate assessment of tracer uptake in the myocardium and blood pool and is recommended by all societies to avoid false-positive findings [9].

16.3.6 CMR

CMR is highly sensitive in detecting cardiac involvement in CA but cannot be used to distinguish amyloid subtypes [11]. In the AHA [5], CCS/CHFS [3], and JCS [7] documents, CMR is not an essential part of the diagnostic algorithm. The ESC statement identifies some specific instances where CMR can be important for diagnosis, as specified above [1]. Finally, the DGK statement is the only one to explicitly include a CMR-based diagnostic pathway that parallels the "scintigraphy-based" path and the "laboratory-based (monoclonal protein) path" [2].

16.3.7 Tissue Biopsy

All documents note that histologic diagnosis is required for AL amyloidosis (if a monoclonal protein is found) or there is a high clinical suspicion for CA despite negative or equivocal bone scintigraphy. The ESC document also emphasizes the role of histologic diagnosis if there are borderline findings on bone scintigraphy

Table 16.2 Criteria for positive scintigraphy with bone tracers

ESC [1]	DGK [2]	CCS/CHFS [3]	AHA [5]	JCS [6]
Perugini score $\geq$2 on a 99mTc-DPD or 99mTc-HMDP scan after 3 h	Perugini score $\geq$2 on a 99mTc-DPD or 99mTc-HMDP scan after 3 h	Perugini score $\geq$2 and/or a H/CL ratio $\geq$1.5 on a 99mTc-PYP scan after 1 or 3 h	Perugini score $\geq$2 and/or a H/CL ratio >1.5 on a 99mTc-PYP scan after 1 or 3 h	Perugini score $\geq$2 and/or a H/CL >1.5 on a 1-hour scan or >1.3 on a 3-h scan

AHA American Heart Association, *CCS/CHFS* Canadian Cardiovascular Society/Canadian Heart Failure Society, *DGK* Deutsche Gesellschaft für Kardiologie (German Cardiac Society), *DPD* 3,3-diphosphono-1,2-propanodicarboxylate, *ESC* European Society of Cardiology, *H/CL* heart/contralateral chest, *HMDP* hydroxymethylene, *PYP* pyrophosphate, *JCS* Japanese Circulation Society

A "positive bone scintigraphy" allows to diagnose amyloid transthyretin cardiac amyloidosis when no monoclonal protein is found

Reprinted with permission from Rapezzi et al. [9].

(Perugini score 1) [8]. Uniquely, the JCS guideline recommends a possible biopsy even if there is a positive bone scintigraphy scan and no monoclonal protein to make a definitive diagnosis of ATTR-CA [7]. As for the biopsy site, fat pad biopsy, renal biopsy (in patients with suspected renal amyloidosis) [3, 5], or bone marrow biopsy [3] are possible alternatives to endomyocardial biopsy. Importantly, a fat pad biopsy has low sensitivity, and a negative fat pad biopsy is not sufficient to exclude CA [5]. The JCS guideline proposes several additional sites for minimally invasive biopsy: abdominal wall liposuction biopsy, skin biopsy, lip biopsy, or digestive tract biopsy [7].

16.3.8 Genetic Testing

All documents agree that patients with a definite diagnosis of ATTR-CA should undergo a search for *TTR* gene mutations to distinguish wt from v disease [2, 3, 5, 7, 8]. Genetic testing should be performed regardless of age [5, 8]. The DGK document adds, "In selected cases, an extended genetic diagnosis of further amyloidosis genes (e.g., if AApoA1 is suspected) may also be considered" [2].

16.4   Conclusions

Diagnosing CA is challenging because of its phenotypic heterogeneity, multi-organ involvement often requiring the interaction among experts in different specialties and subspecialties, lack of a single noninvasive diagnostic tool, and still limited awareness in the medical community. Missing or delaying the diagnosis of CA may have a profound impact on patient outcome, as potentially lifesaving treatments (in particular, chemotherapy in the case of AL-CA) may be omitted or delayed. Several scientific societies have tried to provide algorithms able to guide clinicians through the phases of suspicion and diagnosis. Different approaches have been proposed, but the shared elements are the importance of red flags, the need to search for bone tracer uptake, and a monoclonal protein. A tissue biopsy is needed when a monoclonal protein is found and/or cardiac bone tracer uptake is weak. When CA is suspected and a monoclonal protein is found, further exams to confirm or rule out AL-CA are crucial. Finally, all patients diagnosed with ATTR-CA should undergo genetic testing to search for *TTR* gene mutations.

References

1. Garcia-Pavia P, Rapezzi C, Adler Y, Arad M, Basso C, Brucato A, Burazor I, Caforio ALP, Damy T, Eriksson U, Fontana M, Gillmore JD, Gonzalez-Lopez E, Grogan M, Heymans S, Imazio M, Kindermann I, Kristen AV, Maurer MS, Merlini G, Pantazis A, Pankuweit S, Rigopoulos AG, Linhart A. Diagnosis and treatment of cardiac amyloidosis. A position statement of the European Society of Cardiology Working Group on myocardial and pericardial diseases. Eur J Heart Fail. 2021;23:512–26.

2. Yilmaz A, Bauersachs J, Bengel F, Büchel R, Kindermann I, Klingel K, Knebel F, Meder B, Morbach C, Nagel E, Schulze-Bahr E, Aus dem Siepen F, Frey N. Diagnosis and treatment of cardiac amyloidosis: position statement of the German cardiac society (DGK). Clin Res Cardiol. 2021;110:479–506.

3. Fine NM, Davis MK, Anderson K, Delgado DH, Giraldeau G, Kitchlu A, Massie R, Narayan J, Swiggum E, Venner CP, Ducharme A, Galant NJ, Hahn C, Howlett JG, Mielniczuk L, Parent MC, Reece D, Royal V, Toma M, Virani SA, Zieroth S. Canadian Cardiovascular Society/Canadian Heart Failure Society joint position statement on the evaluation and management of patients with cardiac amyloidosis. Can J Cardiol. 2020;36:322–34.

4. O'Meara E, McDonald M, Chan M, Ducharme A, Ezekowitz JA, Giannetti N, Grzeslo A, Heckman GA, Howlett JG, Koshman SL, Lepage S, Mielniczuk LM, Moe GW, Swiggum E, Toma M, Virani SA, Zieroth S, De S, Matteau S, Parent MC, Asgar AW, Cohen G, Fine N, Davis M, Verma S, Cherney D, Abrams H, Al-Hesayen A, Cohen-Solal A, D'Astous M, Delgado DH, Desplantie O, Estrella-Holder E, Green L, Haddad H, Harkness K, Hernandez AF, Kouz S, LeBlanc MH, Lee D, Masoudi FA, McKelvie RS, Rajda M, Ross HJ, Sussex B. CCS/CHFS heart failure guidelines: clinical trial update on functional mitral regurgitation, SGLT2 inhibitors, ARNI in HFpEF, and tafamidis in amyloidosis. Can J Cardiol. 2020;36:159–69.

5. Kittleson MM, Maurer MS, Ambardekar AV, Bullock-Palmer RP, Chang PP, Eisen HJ, Nair AP, Nativi-Nicolau J, Ruberg FL. Cardiac amyloidosis: evolving diagnosis and management: a scientific statement from the American Heart Association. Circulation. 2020;142:e7–e22.

6. Addendum to: cardiac amyloidosis: evolving diagnosis and management: a scientific statement from the American Heart Association. Circulation. 2021;144:e10.

7. Kitaoka H, Izumi C, Izumiya Y, Inomata T, Ueda M, Kubo T, Koyama J, Sano M, Sekijima Y, Tahara N, Tsukada N, Tsujita K, Tsutsui H, Tomita T, Amano M, Endo J, Okada A, Oda S, Takashio S, Baba Y, Misumi Y, Yazaki M, Anzai T, Ando Y, Isobe M, Kimura T, Fukuda K. JCS 2020 guideline on diagnosis and treatment of cardiac amyloidosis. Circ J. 2020;84:1610–71.

8. Garcia-Pavia P, Rapezzi C, Adler Y, Arad M, Basso C, Brucato A, Burazor I, Caforio ALP, Damy T, Eriksson U, Fontana M, Gillmore JD, Gonzalez-Lopez E, Grogan M, Heymans S, Imazio M, Kindermann I, Kristen AV, Maurer MS, Merlini G, Pantazis A, Pankuweit S, Rigopoulos AG, Linhart A. Diagnosis and treatment of cardiac amyloidosis. A position statement of the European Society of Cardiology Working Group on Myocardial and Pericardial Diseases. Eur J Heart Fail. 2021;42:1554–68.

9. Rapezzi C, Aimo A, Serenelli M, Barison A, Vergaro G, Passino C, Panichella G, Sinagra G, Merlo M, Fontana M, Gillmore J, Quarta CC, Maurer MS, Kittleson MM, Garcia-Pavia P, Emdin M. Critical comparison of documents from scientific societies on cardiac amyloidosis: JACC state-of-the-art review. J Am Coll Cardiol. 2022;79:1288–303.

10. Boldrini M, Cappelli F, Chacko L, Restrepo-Cordoba MA, Lopez-Sainz A, Giannoni A, Aimo A, Baggiano A, Martinez-Naharro A, Whelan C, Quarta C, Passino C, Castiglione V, Chubuchnyi V, Spini V, Taddei C, Vergaro G, Petrie A, Ruiz-Guerrero L, Moñivas V, Mingo-Santos S, Mirelis JG, Dominguez F, Gonzalez-Lopez E, Perlini S, Pontone G, Gillmore J, Hawkins PN, Garcia-Pavia P, Emdin M, Fontana M. Multiparametric echocardiography scores for the diagnosis of cardiac amyloidosis. JACC Cardiovasc Imaging. 2020;13:909–20.

11. Dorbala S, Cuddy S, Falk RH. How to image cardiac amyloidosis: a practical approach. JACC Cardiovasc Imaging. 2020;13:1368–83.

Alberto Aimo, Giuseppe Vergaro, and Julian D. Gillmore

In this chapter, we will examine three topics: (1) the follow-up of subjects at risk of developing cardiac amyloidosis (CA), (2) the prediction of future disease evolution in patients diagnosed with CA, and (3) the assessment of treatment response in patients diagnosed with CA.

17.1 Follow-Up of Subjects at Risk of Developing CA

17.1.1 AL-CA

Patients with monoclonal gammopathy of unknown significance (MGUS) or other plasma cell dyscrasias are not routinely screened for cardiac disease, although they have a higher risk of AL-CA than the general population. A regular measurement of N-terminal pro-B-type natriuretic peptide (NT-proBNP) has been proposed in patients with MGUS to promptly detect the development of AL-CA [1], although the optimal timing of such measurement has not been defined.

Cardiac involvement must always be searched in patients with systemic AL amyloidosis, as it affects the treatment strategy and is a crucial determinant of outcome. Accordingly, the cardiac biomarkers (NT-proBNP and troponin T) are included in

A. Aimo (✉) · G. Vergaro
Interdisciplinary Center for Health Sciences, Scuola Superiore Sant'Anna, Pisa, Italy

Cardiology Division, Fondazione Toscana Gabriele Monasterio, Pisa, Italy
e-mail: a.aimo@santannapisa.it; vergaro@ftgm.it

J. D. Gillmore
National Amyloidosis Centre, Division of Medicine, University College London, Royal Free Hospital, London, UK
e-mail: j.gillmore@ucl.ac.uk

© The Author(s), under exclusive license to Springer Nature Switzerland AG 2024
M. Emdin et al. (eds.), *Cardiac Amyloidosis*,
https://doi.org/10.1007/978-3-031-51757-0_17

the laboratory exams for the initial diagnostic workup; symptoms of cardiac disease must be actively sought; echocardiogram with strain assessment and, in certain circumstances, cardiovascular magnetic resonance are suggested when there is some evidence of cardiac disease [2]. Cardiac involvement is defined as mean left ventricular (LV) wall thickness > 12 mm in the absence of other causes of LV hypertrophy or an NT-proBNP level > 332 ng/L in the absence of renal failure or atrial fibrillation [2].

17.1.2 ATTR-CA

Individuals harboring a pathogenic mutation in the *TTR* gene have an increased risk of developing a cardiac and/or neurological phenotype, according to the specific mutation. According to the guidelines and similar documents published in 2021, "first-degree relatives" [3] and possibly other biologically related relatives of patients with ATTRv-CA [3–7] should undergo a genetic screening to determine their mutation carrier status. Genetic testing should not be proposed to minors [4, 6], while it could be offered to young adults when results could guide lifestyle choices or reproductive planning [4].

There is little guidance regarding monitoring of *TTR* mutation carriers. The European Society of Cardiology (ESC) document advises to "search for disease manifestations [starting] around 10 years before the age of disease onset in affected family members or as soon as symptoms compatible with amyloidosis develop" [4]. The Japanese Cardiology Society (JCS) guideline states that "the carrier should be followed on a periodic basis [...] and psychological support and screening tests for the onset of amyloidosis should be provided" [6]. The American Heart Association document notes that "what methods (imaging or biomarkers) should be used to monitor disease progression, the timing of initiation of therapy in ATTRv carriers remains an area of uncertainty" [7].

17.2 Risk Prediction in Patients Diagnosed with CA

Only some documents provide some details about risk prediction in patients diagnosed with CA. Specifically, the ESC statement lists two scores for AL-CA, 1 for ATTRwt-CA and 2 for ATTRv- or ATTRwt-CA (Table 17.1) [4], and the JCS guideline reminds that NT-proBNP and hs-troponin can help refine risk stratification in patients with ATTRwt-CA [6]. The choice between different scores and the ways to tailor the therapeutic strategy are left to the discretion of treating physicians.

Table 17.1 Scoring systems in amyloid light-chain (AL) and transthyretin (ATTR) cardiac amyloidosis (CA)

Kumar et al. (Mayo) [8]		Grogan et al. [9]		NAC (Gillmore et al.) [10]		Cheng et al. [11]	
AL-CA		ATTRwt-CA		ATTRv- and ATTRwt-CA		ATTRv- and ATTRwt-CA	
Parameters: FLC difference $\geq$ 18 mg/dL Troponin T $\geq$ 0.025 ng/mL NT-proBNP $\geq$1800 ng/L		**Parameters:** Troponin T > 0.05 ng/mL NT-proBNP >3000 ng/L		**Parameters:** eGFR <45 mL/min/1.73 m^2 NT-proBNP >3000 ng/L		**Parameters:** Mayo/NAC score (0–2 points) Furosemide or equivalent daily dose: No diuretic therapy (0 points), $\leq$0.5 mg/kg (1 point), >0.5 and $\leq$1 mg/kg (2 points), >1 mg/kg (3 points) NYHA classes I–IV (1–4 points)	
Stage	**5-year survival**	**Stage**	**Median survival**	**Stage**	**Median survival**	**Stage**	**Median survival**
Stage I (0 parameters)	68%	Stage I (0 parameters)	66 months	Stage I (0 parameters)	69 months	Score 1–3	91 months
Stage II (1 parameter)	60%	Stage II (1 parameter)	40 months	Stage II (1 parameter)	47 months	Score 4–6	39 months (Mayo) 36 months (NAC)
Stage III (2 parameters)	28%	Stage III (2 parameters)	20 months	Stage III (2 parameters)	24 months	Score 7–9	20.3 months (Mayo/ NAC)
Stage IV (3 parameters)	14%						

The Mayo scoring system for amyloid light-chain (AL) amyloidosis is recommended by the NCCN Clinical Practice Guidelines on Systemic Light Chain Amyloidosis [2]. The score by Lillenes et al. is not reported [11]. *ATTR* amyloid transthyretin amyloidosis (*v* variant, *wt* wild type), *BNP* B-type natriuretic peptide, *eGFR* estimated glomerular filtration rate, *FLC-diff* difference between involved and uninvolved free light chain, *NAC* National Amyloidosis Centre, *NT-proBNP* N-terminal pro-B-type natriuretic peptide, *NYHA* New York Heart Association

17.3 Assessment of Treatment Response in Patients with CA

17.3.1 AL-CA

The notion of monitoring the response to treatment is well established in the hematologic field, including in the management of patients with AL-CA. Both hematologic and cardiac responses must be evaluated to define if the current treatment must be continued or replaced. Hematologic response is categorized as complete, very good partial, partial, no response, or progression. Cardiac response instead is categorized as response vs. progression [2] (Table 17.2). Other criteria have been introduced to assess organ response in patients with kidney or liver disease or with polyneuropathy [2].

Extracellular volume measurement by cardiovascular magnetic resonance provides an estimate of the amount of myocardial amyloid and has been recently proposed as an additional tool for the assessment of cardiac response in AL-CA [12]. In a cohort of 176 patients with AL-CA from the UK National Amyloidosis Centre (NAC), ECV was measured at the time of diagnosis and then at 6, 12, and 24 months after starting chemotherapy. CMR response was graded as progression ($\geq$0.05 increase in ECV), stability (<0.05 change), or regression ($\geq$0.05 decrease). At 6 months, CMR regression was observed in 3% of patients (all with hematological complete or very good partial response), and progression in 32% (61% in partial or

Table 17.2 Criteria for hematologic and cardiac response

Hematological response		Cardiac response	
Complete	Normalization of the FLC levels and ratio, negative serum, and urine immunofixation	Response	NT-proBNP response (>30% and >300 ng/L decrease in patients with baseline NT-proBNP $\geq$650 ng/L) or NYHA class response ($\geq$2 class decrease in subjects with baseline NYHA class III or IV)
Very good partial	Reduction in the dFLC to <40 mg/L		
Partial	A greater than 50% reduction in the dFLC		
No response	Less than a PR		
Progression	From CR, any detectable monoclonal protein or abnormal FLC ratio (light chain must double) From PR, 50% increase in serum M protein to >0.5 g/dL or 50% increase in urine M protein to >200 mg/d (a visible peak must be present) Serum FLC increase of 50% to >100 mg/L	Progression	NT-proBNP progression (>30% and >300 ng/L increase) or cTnT progression ($\geq$33% increase) or LVEF progression ($\geq$10% decrease)

CR complete response, *cTnT* cardiac troponin T, *dFLC* difference between involved and not involved free light chains, *FLC* free light chain, *LVEF* left ventricular ejection fraction, *NT-proBNP* N-terminal pro-B-type natriuretic peptide, *NYHA* New York Heart Association, *PR* partial response

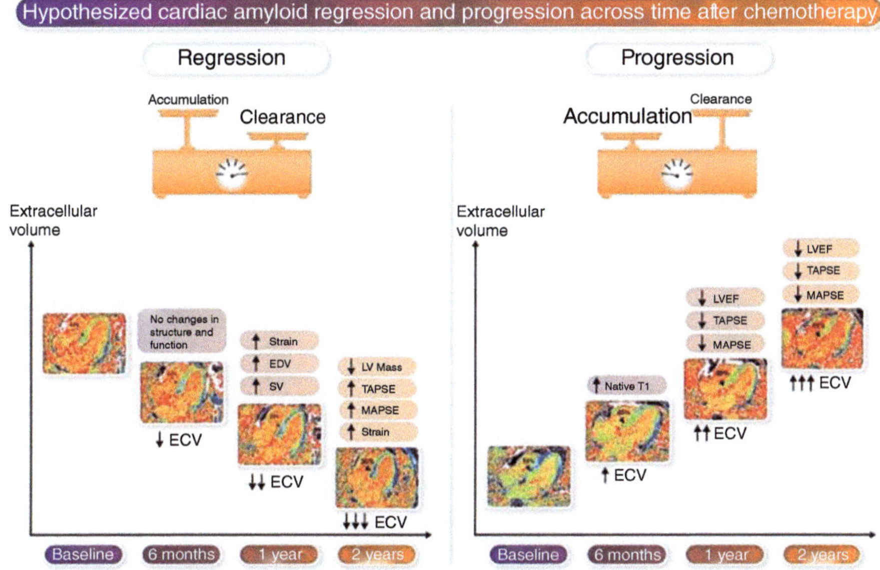

Fig. 17.1 Cardiovascular magnetic resonance-based assessment of the response to treatment in cardiac amyloid light-chain amyloidosis *ECV* extracellular volume, *EDV* end-diastolic volume, *LV* left ventricle, *LVEF* LV ejection fraction, *MAPSE* mitral annular plane systolic excursion, *TAPSE* tricuspid annular plane systolic excursion. Reprinted from Martinez-Naharro et al. [12]

no response). CMR regression at 1 year was observed in 22%, and in 38% at 2 years, with a good association with hematologic complete or very good partial response. Importantly, CMR response at 6 months predicted death (36 events over 40 ± 15 months), with a hazard ratio of 3.82 (95% confidence interval [CI] 1.95–7.49, $p < 0.001$) for CMR progression, and remained prognostic after adjusting for known predictors (hematologic response, NT-proBNP, and longitudinal strain). According to the proposed model, changes in ECV would be early signs of the trajectory of cardiac structure and function, and ultimately outcome (Fig. 17.1). The authors then envisage a future management of AL-CA informed by the hematologic, NT-proBNP, and CMR response, which would provide "a comprehensive clinical picture that could help clinicians to better tailor chemotherapy treatment in each individual patient" [12].

17.3.2 ATTR-CA

A 2021 document by the ESC Working Group on Myocardial and Pericardial Diseases introduced a system to detect the progression of cardiac involvement in patients with ATTR amyloidosis receiving disease-modifying therapies [13]. Several tools for patient monitoring were listed and categorized into three domains: clinical and functional, laboratory, and imaging and ECG markers (Table 17.3). The

Table 17.3 Proposed system to detect the progression of amyloid transthyretin cardiac amyloidosis in treated patients

Domain	Marker	Clinical feature	Threshold indicating disease progression	Recommended frequency of measurement
Clinical and functional markers	Clinical and medical history	Cardiovascular-related hospitalizations	Worsening indicated by any hospitalization (related to HF decompensation) in a 6-month period	6 months
	NYHA class	Stepwise class change (plus or minus) should indicate progression or amelioration/improvement, respectively	One class increase (must be measured during a 30-day period of stability)	6 months
	EQ-5D tool and KCCQ	Description of measurements	Five-point decrease in KCCQ represents deterioration; 10-point decrease in KCCQ represents moderate deterioration; 10% decline in EQ-5D score represents deterioration	6–12 months
	Functional capacity	6MWT	Decrease of 30–40 m every 6 months (in the absence of obvious non-cardiovascular cause)	6 months
Laboratory markers	Biomarkers and laboratory markers	30% increase in NT-proBNP with 300 ng/L cutoff	To be measured during a 30-day period of clinical stability and under same atrial rhythm	6 months
		Troponin (high-sensitivity) assay	30% increase	6 months
		Clinical staging system	Advance in NAC staging score	6 months

Table 17.3 (continued)

Domain	Marker	Clinical feature	Threshold indicating disease progression	Recommended frequency of measurement
Imaging and ECG markers	Echocardiography	LV measures wall thickness/mass	≥2 mm increase in LV wall thickness	6–12 months
		Systolic function measurements	≥5% decrease in LVEF decrease; ≥5 mL decrease in stroke volume and ≥1% increase in LV global longitudinal strain	12 months
		Diastolic dysfunction worsening, e.g., using diastolic functioning grade	Stepwise increase in diastolic functioning grade; consistent deterioration in diastolic function	12 months
	ECG/Holter	ECG	New onset of arrhythmic/conduction disturbances New-onset BBB New-onset AV block (of any degree) Sinus pauses, sinus node dysfunction, AF with a very slow ventricular response without pharmacologic treatment (<50 bpm)	6 months

AF atrial fibrillation, *AV* atrioventricular, *BBB* bundle branch block, *ECG* electrocardiogram, *EQ-5D* EuroQol five dimensions, *HF* heart failure, *KCCQ* Kansas City Cardiomyopathy Questionnaire, *LV* left ventricular, *NAC* National Amyloidosis Centre, *NT-proBNP* N-terminal pro-B-type natriuretic peptide, *NYHA* New York Heart Association, *QoL* quality of life, *6MWT* 6-minute walking test. Reprinted with permission from Garcia-Pavia et al. [13]. CMR-derived ECV has been proposed as a possible tool to track changes in cardiac amyloid following patisiran treatment. In 16 patients with ATTRv-CA receiving patisiran for 12 months, Fontana et al. found a small reduction in ECV compared to untreated patients (adjusted mean difference between groups: −6.2% [95% CI −9.5% to −3.0%]; $p = 0.001$), accompanied by a decrease in NT-proBNP and cardiac uptake of bone tracer and an increase in 6-minute walking distance (Fig. 17.2) [15]

presence of at least one marker from each domain denotes an appreciable progression of cardiac disease [13]. This system may be employed in patients with either wild-type (wt) or variant (v) ATTR-CA and was endorsed also by the International Society of Amyloidosis guidelines on ATTRv-CA [14]. The same guidelines proposed a minimum set of tools to monitor progression of polyneuropathy, which may accompany cardiac involvement in patients with ATTRv amyloidosis. Briefly, these tools are the Neuropathy Impairment Score (NIS; exploring sensory and motor

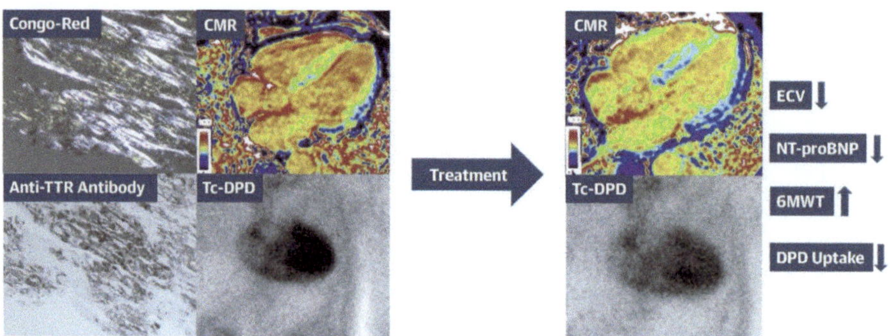

Fig. 17.2 Evidence of regression of cardiac amyloid in response to patisiran treatment*6MWT* 6-minute walking test, *CMR* cardiovascular magnetic resonance, *NT-proBNP* N-terminal pro-B-type natriuretic peptide, *Tc-DPD* 99mTc-dicarboxypropane *diphosphonate*, *TTR* transthyretin. Reprinted with permission from Fontana et al. [15]

function), *polyneuropathy* disability (*PND*; investigating motor function), 6- or 10-minute walking test (motor function), composite autonomic symptom score 31 (*COMPASS-31*), and Rasch-built Overall Disability *Scale* (*R-ODS*; autonomic disability). The frequency of assessment is 6–12 months for all tools except for COMPASS-31 (every 12 months) [14]. The evidence of disease progression demonstrates a limited efficacy of the disease-modifying treatment and may prompt a change in the therapeutic strategy.

We are not aware of other studies assessing ECV as a possible tool to track the response to therapies for ATTR-CA. Conversely, a few studies have tried to track the response to treatment through serial scintigraphy scans, as in the study by Fontana et al. In the phase 3 HELIOS-A trial, assessing the safety and efficacy of vutrisiran in patients with ATTRv amyloidosis, "^{99m}Tc scintigraphy assessment" was performed in 64 vutrisiran-treated patients at baseline, 35 (55%) of whom had Perugini grade ≥ 2 (moderate/intense) cardiac uptake of 99mTc; the tracer was not specified. Among the patients re-evaluated at 18 months, 28% (16/57) had a reduction from baseline in Perugini grade of cardiac uptake, 68% (39/57) had no change in grade, and 4% (2/57) worsened in grade. The regression of cardiac amyloid was confirmed when performing a quantitative assessment through the heart-to-contralateral lung (H/CL) ratio and normalized LV total uptake [16]. Another possible quantitative index is the heart-to-vertebral ratio, which avoids the intrinsic limitations of the H/CL ratio, including influences of blood pool and rib accumulations. In two patients from the ATTR-ACT trial, both visual assessment and heart-to-vertebral ratio were basically unchanged in a patient receiving placebo for 30 months, while both improved during 45 months of tafamidis treatment [17].

17.4 Conclusions

Cardiac involvement should always be searched in patients with AL amyloidosis. A grey zone of current recommendations is that the possible development of CA over time is not considered, and no indications are then provided as to whether cardiac biomarkers must be measured serially over time and which is the optimal timing of such measurement. As for ATTR-CA, the best way to follow asymptomatic gene carriers is currently unknown. Another important point, not touched by current guidelines, is whether mutation carriers with asymptomatic cardiac disease should start a disease-modifying treatment.

Risk stratification is important in both AL- and ATTR-CA to tailor the therapeutic strategy and follow-up based on the expected disease evolution. While risk stratification has been standardized through the development of specific score systems, the way this information should be translated into patient management remains to be defined.

Some CMR and scintigraphy studies suggest that blocking further amyloid deposition allows to reduce cardiac amyloid burden and also that tracking the response to disease-modifying therapies is feasible. Larger studies are needed to confirm these findings and define algorithms for patient management based on imaging findings. Single-photon emission computed tomography or positron-emission tomography allows to assess regional uptake and to quantify tracer uptake and might be considered as possible tools to assess treatment response.

References

1. Al Hamed R, Bazarbachi AH, Bazarbachi A, Malard F, Harousseau JL, Mohty M. Comprehensive review of AL amyloidosis: some practical recommendations. Blood Canc J. 2021;11:97.
2. https://www2.tri-kobe.org/nccn/guideline/hematologic/english/amyloidosis.pdf
3. Yilmaz A, Bauersachs J, Bengel F, Büchel R, Kindermann I, Klingel K, Knebel F, Meder B, Morbach C, Nagel E, Schulze-Bahr E, Aus dem Siepen F, Frey N. Diagnosis and treatment of cardiac amyloidosis: position statement of the German Cardiac Society (DGK). Clin Res Cardiol. 2021;110:479–506.
4. Garcia-Pavia P, Rapezzi C, Adler Y, Arad M, Basso C, Brucato A, Burazor I, Caforio ALP, Damy T, Eriksson U, Fontana M, Gillmore JD, Gonzalez-Lopez E, Grogan M, Heymans S, Imazio M, Kindermann I, Kristen AV, Maurer MS, Merlini G, Pantazis A, Pankuweit S, Rigopoulos AG, Linhart A. Diagnosis and treatment of cardiac amyloidosis. A position statement of the European Society of Cardiology Working Group on Myocardial and Pericardial Diseases. Eur J Heart Fail. 2021;42(16):1554–68.
5. Fine NM, Davis MK, Anderson K, Delgado DH, Giraldeau G, Kitchlu A, Massie R, Narayan J, Swiggum E, Venner CP, Ducharme A, Galant NJ, Hahn C, Howlett JG, Mielniczuk L, Parent MC, Reece D, Royal V, Toma M, Virani SA, Zieroth S. Canadian Cardiovascular Society/Canadian Heart Failure Society Joint Position Statement on the evaluation and management of patients with cardiac amyloidosis. Circ J. 2020;36:322–34.
6. Kitaoka H, Izumi C, Izumiya Y, Inomata T, Ueda M, Kubo T, Koyama J, Sano M, Sekijima Y, Tahara N, Tsukada N, Tsujita K, Tsutsui H, Tomita T, Amano M, Endo J, Okada A, Oda S,

Takashio S, Baba Y, Misumi Y, Yazaki M, Anzai T, Ando Y, Isobe M, Kimura T, Fukuda K. JCS 2020 Guideline on diagnosis and treatment of cardiac amyloidosis. Circ J. 2020;84:1610–71.

7. Kittleson MM, Maurer MS, Ambardekar AV, Bullock-Palmer RP, Chang PP, Eisen HJ, Nair AP, Nativi-Nicolau J, Ruberg FL. Cardiac amyloidosis: evolving diagnosis and management: a scientific statement from the American Heart Association. Circulation. 2020;142:e7–e22.

8. Kumar S, Dispenzieri A, Lacy MQ, Hayman SR, Buadi FK, Colby C, Laumann K, Zeldenrust SR, Leung N, Dingli D, Greipp PR, Lust JA, Russell SJ, Kyle RA, Rajkumar SV, Gertz MA. Revised prognostic staging system for light chain amyloidosis incorporating cardiac biomarkers and serum free light chain measurements. J Clin Oncol. 2012;30:989–95.

9. Grogan M, Scott CG, Kyle RA, Zeldenrust SR, Gertz MA, Lin G, Klarich KW, Miller WL, Maleszewski JJ, Dispenzieri A. Natural history of wild-type transthyretin cardiac amyloidosis and risk stratification using a novel staging system. J Am Coll Cardiol. 2016;68:1014–20.

10. Gillmore JD, Damy T, Fontana M, Hutchinson M, Lachmann HJ, Martinez-Naharro A, Quarta CC, Rezk T, Whelan CJ, Gonzalez-Lopez E, Lane T, Gilbertson JA, Rowczenio D, Petrie A, Hawkins PN. A new staging system for cardiac transthyretin amyloidosis. Eur Heart J. 2018;39:2799–806.

11. Cheng RK, Levy WC, Vasbinder A, Teruya S, De Los SJ, Leedy D, Maurer MS. Diuretic dose and NYHA functional class are independent predictors of mortality in patients with transthyretin cardiac amyloidosis. JACC CardioOncol. 2020;2:414–24.

12. Martinez-Naharro A, Patel R, Kotecha T, Karia N, Ioannou A, Petrie A, Chacko LA, Razvi Y, Ravichandran S, Brown J, Law S, Quarta C, Mahmood S, Wisniowski B, Pica S, Sachchithanantham S, Lachmann HJ, Moon JC, Knight DS, Whelan C, Venneri L, Xue H, Kellman P, Gillmore JD, Hawkins PN, Wechalekar AD, Fontana M. Cardiovascular magnetic resonance in light-chain amyloidosis to guide treatment. Eur Heart J. 2022;43:4722–35.

13. Garcia-Pavia P, Bengel F, Brito D, Damy T, Duca F, Dorbala S, Nativi-Nicolau J, Obici L, Rapezzi C, Sekijima Y, Elliott PM. Expert consensus on the monitoring of transthyretin amyloid cardiomyopathy. Eur J Heart Fail. 2021;23:895–905.

14. Ando Y, Adams D, Benson MD, Berk JL, Planté-Bordeneuve V, Coelho T, Conceição I, Ericzon BG, Obici L, Rapezzi C, Sekijima Y, Ueda M, Palladini G, Merlini G. Guidelines and new directions in the therapy and monitoring of ATTRv amyloidosis. Amyloid. 2022;29:143–55.

15. Fontana M, Martinez-Naharro A, Chacko L, Rowczenio D, Gilbertson JA, Whelan CJ, Strehina S, Lane T, Moon J, Hutt DF, Kellman P, Petrie A, Hawkins PN, Gillmore JD. Reduction in CMR derived extracellular volume with patisiran indicates cardiac amyloid regression. JACC Cardiovasc Imaging. 2021;14:189–99.

16. Mussinelli R, Garcia-Pavia P, Gillmore JD, Kale P, Berk JL, Maurer MS, Conceição I, Dicarli M, Solomon S, Chen C, Arum S, Vest J, Grogan M. 77 HELIOS-A: 18-month exploratory cardiac results from the phase 3 study of vutrisiran in patients with hereditary transthyretin-mediated amyloidosis. Eur Heart J Suppl. 2022;24:suac121–654.

17. Maeda-Ogata S, Tahara N, Tahara A, Bekki M, Honda A, Sugiyama Y, Igata S, Abe T, Sekijima Y, Ueda M, Ando Y, Fukumoto Y. Treatment response to Tafamidis quantitatively assessed by serial bone scintigraphy in transthyretin amyloid cardiomyopathy. J Nucl Cardiol. 2023;30(1):403–4.

Differential Diagnoses in Clinical Mimics

Annamaria Del Franco, Marco Merlo, Giulia Biagioni, Carlotta Mazzoni, Linda Pagura, Valentina Allegro, Francesco Cappelli, Maurizio Pieroni, and Iacopo Olivotto

Abbreviations

AFD	Anderson-Fabry disease
AL	Amyloid light-chain amyloidosis
AS	Aortic stenosis
ATTR	Amyloid transthyretin amyloidosis
CA	Cardiac amyloidosis

A. Del Franco · G. Biagioni · C. Mazzoni
Cardiomyopathy Unit, Careggi University Hospital, Florence, Italy
e-mail: delfrancoa@aou-careggi.toscana.it; biagionig@aou-careggi.toscana.it; carlotta.mazzoni@unifi.it

M. Merlo · L. Pagura · V. Allegro
Center for Diagnosis and Treatment of Cardiomyopathies, Cardiovascular Department, Azienda Sanitaria Universitaria Giuliano-Isontina (ASUGI), Trieste, Italy
e-mail: marco.merlo@units.it; linda.pagura@asugi.sanita.fvg.it; valentina.allegro@studenti.units.it

F. Cappelli
Cardiomyopathy Unit, Careggi University Hospital, Florence, Italy

Department of Experimental and Clinical Medicine, University of Florence, Florence, Italy
e-mail: cappellif@aou-careggi.toscana.it

M. Pieroni
Cardiovascular Department, San Donato Hospital, Arezzo, Italy
e-mail: maurizio.pieroni@unifi.it

I. Olivotto (✉)
Cardiomyopathy Unit, Careggi University Hospital, Florence, Italy

Department of Experimental and Clinical Medicine, University of Florence, Florence, Italy

Cardiology Unit, IRCCS Meyer Children's Hospital, Florence, Italy
e-mail: iacopo.olivotto@unifi.it

M. Emdin et al. (eds.), *Cardiac Amyloidosis*,
https://doi.org/10.1007/978-3-031-51757-0_18

CMR	Cardiac magnetic resonance
CS	Cardiac sarcoidosis
ECG	Electrocardiogram
EMB	Endomyocardial biopsy
FDG-PET	Fluorodeoxyglucose-positron-emission tomography
GLS	Global longitudinal strain
HCM	Hypertrophic cardiomyopathy
HF	Heart failure
LCDD	Light-chain deposition disease
LGE	Late gadolinium enhancement
LV	Left ventricular
LVEF	LV ejection fraction
PRKAG2	Protein kinase AMP-activated non-catalytic subunit gamma 2
SCD	Sudden cardiac death

Several conditions are characterized by left ventricular (LV) hypertrophy (most notably hypertrophic cardiomyopathy [HCM] and severe aortic stenosis [AS]), possibly associated with manifestations of systemic disease (as in Fabry disease) and plasma cell dyscrasia (as in light-chain deposition disease [LCDD]). An extensive evaluation including age, family history, extra-cardiac abnormalities, electrocardiographic pattern, and imaging findings is essential to determine the aetiology. Together with these, the prevalence of each cause should be taken into account once LV hypertrophy is identified. This chapter provides an overview of these conditions, listing them in order of prevalence and highlighting the characteristics that distinguish them from cardiac amyloidosis (CA) (central figure).

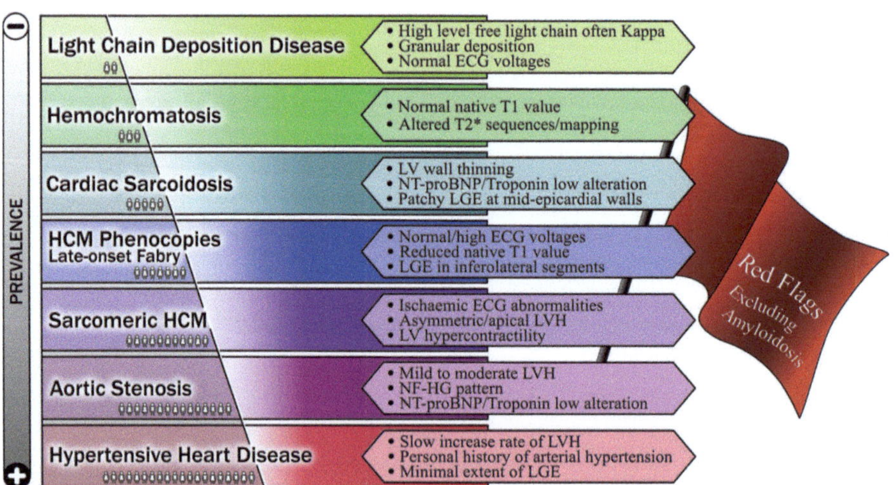

Clinical diagnoses resembling cardiac amyloidosis are listed in order of prevalence, with distinguishing aspects highlighted

ECG electrocardiogram, *HCM* hypertrophic cardiomyopathy, *LGE* late gadolinium enhancement, *LV* left ventricular, *LVH* left ventricular hypertrophy, *NF-HG* normal flow-high gradient, *NT-proBNP* N-terminal pro-brain natriuretic peptide

18.1 Hypertensive Heart Disease

Pressure overload is the most frequent cause of pathologic LV hypertrophy—as hypertensive artery disease is widely spread in the general population—with a global prevalence of 18.6 million cases (95% UI: 13.5–24.9 million) [1]. A picture of LV hypertrophy, which might be misinterpreted with CA, is unlikely to result from a mild or well-controlled hypertension with medical therapy. On the other hand, those with secondary forms of hypertension or people of Afro-American origin may have more severe and unpredictable hypertrophy patterns and may manifest phenotypes resembling cardiomyopathies [2, 3]. Due to the high frequency of hypertension and, consequently, the hypertrophic phenotype in the Afro-American community, the early identification of CA may be challenging. For secondary forms of hypertension, instead, extracardiac symptoms aid in reaching a proper diagnosis.

Some imaging features enhance the ability to discriminate between different cases. Unlike individuals with hypertensive heart disease, patients with CA show a faster rate of increasing septal and relative wall thickness, a decrease in LV myocardial strain, and a more impaired left atrial function [4]. Although up to 50% of patients with LV hypertrophy driven by arterial hypertension might have fibrosis identified as late gadolinium enhancement (LGE) by cardiac magnetic resonance (CMR), the LGE distribution in hypertensive patients is modest (few segments are affected) and presents a different pattern (patchy or linear in mid-wall) from CA [5]. It is also possible for such diseases to coexist, and while a history of hypertension could delay the other diagnosis, it does not appear to affect disease progression rate in CA patients [4].

18.2 Aortic Stenosis

Nearly 5% of 75 + -year-old individuals have at least a moderate AS [6, 7], of whom 8% have CA (typically wild-type amyloid transthyretin amyloidosis, ATTR) [8]. Myocyte hypertrophy and interstitial fibrosis are two histological abnormalities associated with AS, which result in the concentric thickening of the LV wall. Histology information after valve replacement might help in excluding CA, since in case of the sole AS (absence of another *noxa* such as amyloid fibrils), cellular hypertrophy and diffuse myocardial fibrosis—but not replacement fibrosis—might regress. Nevertheless, AS- and CA-related LV remodelling may coexist in some cases. Prevalence of CA is reported to be 5.6% [9] to 13% [10] for 65 + -year-old patients undergoing surgical or transcatheter valve replacement, respectively. Transthyretin-related CA is the most prevalent type, regardless of the complexity of screening for older adult patients with severe AS using bone scintigraphy, which could not be feasible in clinical routine practice. However, patients with CA have a distinctive phenotype, including older age, a history of carpal tunnel syndrome, higher LV wall thickness and a lower voltage/mass ratio, and higher high-sensitivity troponin T and N-terminal fragment of pro-B-type natriuretic peptide [10]. To rule out the coexistence of these two illnesses, the study of typical CA features should be considered while evaluating AS patients. In this scenario, a CMR examination has been suggested to support clinician suspicions of CA if LV hypertrophy is excessively high in both moderate AS patients and those without a previous history of hypertension. Additionally, a clinical score (RAISE) has been developed to predict the presence of CA; patients with AS and a score of 2 points should undergo bone scintigraphy and light-chain evaluation [11]. Specifically, this score considers left ventricular remodelling (hypertrophy/diastolic dysfunction), age, injury (high-sensitivity troponin T), systemic involvement, and electrical abnormalities (right bundle branch block/low voltages). AS and CA frequently harbour a low-flow, low-gradient pattern and thus require calcium scoring by computed tomography to confirm AS severity [12]. However, once diagnosed, CA should not modify treatment strategy, since patients with CA have comparable rates of complications and survival benefits from transcatheter valve replacement as those without [11]. Given the higher prevalence of CA in individuals with AS compared to the general population of the same age, a possible causal link between amyloid and AS has been proposed. It has been hypothesized that AS would increase LV afterload and predispose LV myocardium to the deposition of amyloid fibrils [13], whereas valve intervention could stabilize ATTR by lowering shear stress.

18.3 Hypertrophic Cardiomyopathy (Sarcomeric and Phenocopies)

Only 14% of individuals with unexplained LV hypertrophy are ultimately diagnosed with CA, while HCM is predominant in most cases (44%) [14]. Although clinically diagnosed HCM is believed to affect 1:3195 Americans in the United States [15], the actual prevalence of HCM increases to 1:500 or even 1:200 when healthy gene carriers are considered [16].

A careful interpretation of electrocardiogram (ECG) and echocardiogram offers many useful hints for a correct diagnosis, thus avoiding delaying or missing CA diagnosis. Main ECG differential features are the presence of repolarization abnormalities (more common in HCM) and the prolongation of QTc interval and low QRS values (prevalent in CA).

On echocardiogram, the distribution of hypertrophy (more often symmetric in CA and asymmetric in HCM), the function of the left ventricle (lower LV ejection fraction (LVEF) in CA), and the coexistence of pericardial effusion and increased atrioventricular valve thickness (common in CA) are the findings that are mostly used to differentiate CA from HCM.

Although asymmetric hypertrophy and LV outflow tract obstruction are echocardiographic hallmarks of HCM, their presence does not rule out the diagnosis of CA. In fact, CA patients could also display asymmetric septal hypertrophy in 15% of amyloid light chain (AL) cases [17] and 25% of ATTR, and potential LV outflow tract obstruction in fewer than 5% of cases [18]. Additionally, studies of surgical myectomy specimens have provided a thorough description of the occurrence of ATTR, by concluding that nearly 1 out of 5 individuals with a clinical diagnosis of

HCM could have had a different diagnosis, such as hypertensive heart disease, CA, or Anderson-Fabry disease (AFD) [19]. Similarly, the identification of a family history suggesting familial sarcomeric HCM, presence of hypertension, coronary artery disease, and advanced age may suggest a possible hypertensive or infiltrative origin of LV hypertrophy. Genetic test can further improve differential diagnosis: among patients submitted to extensive genetic testing for an HCM phenotype, 0.3% showed a pathogenic variant on the transthyretin gene [20].

In addition to the extent and distribution of LV hypertrophy, other echocardiographic signs and related score-based approaches have been suggested for the differential diagnosis between CA and HCM. Restrictive LV filling patterns can be observed in 5.9% of HCM patients at baseline and in up to 9.1% of them during follow-up (particularly in carriers of thin-filament variants) [21]. Therefore, diastolic dysfunction cannot represent per se a single discriminating parameter. On the other hand, a multiparametric assessment including concentric hypertrophy, global longitudinal strain (GLS), and E/e' ratio plays a critical role in the early detection of CA disease [22]. Moreover, the relative apical sparing (ratio between septal apical to base longitudinal strain) demonstrated good sensitivity and specificity and emerged as an independent predictor of CA [22]. Before LVEF deterioration begins, other parameters of systolic function, such as myocardial work [23], or of diastolic function, such as left atrial (LA) dimension/function [24], might help in distinguishing CA from HCM. Finally, LVEF-to-GLS ratio performed well in discriminating between the two disorders, even in the most difficult subgroup, i.e. maximum wall thickness 16 mm and LVEF >55%, regardless of CA type (AL vs. ATTR) [25].

In some cases, differential diagnosis remains challenging, mostly in subjects with milder phenotypes, as it is often the case in AL. In these settings, advanced imaging by CMR may provide a better morpho-functional characterization of cardiac chambers together with tissue characterization. In particular, CMR may reveal right ventricular involvement [26], detect the presence and extent of LGE, and evaluate the myocardial characteristics through newer techniques like T1 and T2 mapping and extracellular volume (ECV) assessment. While LGE typically has a diffuse subendocardial or transmural distribution, the mild amyloid deposition in the myocardium may be responsible for the atypical features of LGE in individuals with early-stage AL [27]. In this case, a modest GLS and global circumferential strain impairment, along with a larger extracellular volume and T1 value, both point to the diagnosis of CA [27].

Of note, individuals with systemic AA amyloidosis, often considered mainly a renal disease, may also have cardiac involvement in up to 10% of the cases [28].

The coexistence of HCM and CA should be considered whenever HCM has a clinical and morphological rapid progression compared to the slow disease progression occurring over a period of several years in 5–7% of patients with sarcomeric HCM [29].

Patients with unexplained LV hypertrophy should be evaluated for AFD, which accounts for 0.9% of cases [30]. Due to its X-linked nature, AFD primarily affects men, even though females may exhibit a range of clinical scenarios from healthy carriers to severe cardiomyopathy [31]. Classic AFD is characterized by the absence of alpha-galactosidase A activity and a paediatric onset with a wide range of clinical signs and symptoms, including neuropathic pain, angiokeratomas, gastrointestinal complaints, hearing loss, and corneal opacities. Proteinuria and initial cardiac involvement develop in the second–third decades of life and, if untreated, progress towards end-stage chronic renal disease and severe HCM. Late-onset AFD is characterized by residual alpha-galactosidase A activity leading to clinical manifestation occurring later in life and usually represented by a prevalent if not exclusive cardiac involvement. Cardiac damage is a dynamic process, initially sustained by intracellular glycolipid storage, then by myocardial hypertrophy and inflammation, and eventually by interstitial and replacement fibrosis [32]. This is consistent with the evolution of associated ECG changes (from short PR interval to bundle branch block and atrioventricular blocks), echocardiography findings (progressive wall thickening with worsening diastolic and then systolic dysfunction), and CMR findings (from reduced native T1 values to hypertrophy and increase of native T2 values with typical LGE in inferolateral segments). Some of these traits are common with CA, including concentric hypertrophic remodelling, primarily diastolic dysfunction [17], valvular thickening, and right ventricular hypertrophy, while others like LGE in the inferolateral wall can be rarely observed in CA [33]. On the contrary, other features are strikingly different and may help in differential diagnosis, like the high-voltage amplitude at the ECG, that in AFD reflects the increase in myocyte size (vs. myocyte atrophy in CA), or the native T1 reduction at CMR in the pre-fibrotic stages of AFD as the result of myocardial glycolipid storage that may pseudonormalize in later stages (vs. early native T1 increase in CA) [34].

First-level exams should guide differential diagnosis using distinct characteristics of CA vs. other disorders. In this context, an ECG-based algorithm proved to be highly sensitive and specific in the differentiation of AFD, CA, and HCM, by evaluating PQ interval minus P-wave duration in lead II, corrected QT duration, and Sokolow–Lyon index [35]. Likewise, speckle tracking imaging can suggest a diagnosis based on the location and distribution among the LV segments of the impaired longitudinal strain: CA displays a basal-apex gradient with apical sparing, whereas AFD exhibits an early involvement of inferolateral segments at the basal level [36].

An alternative diagnosis in the group of HCM phenocopies consists of the protein kinase AMP-activated non-catalytic subunit gamma 2 (PRKAG2) cardiomyopathy, which is usually characterized by a severe hypertrophic phenotype also involving the right ventricle, with LGE areas in the mostly hypertrophied segments including inferior and inferolateral walls (with patchy subendocardial or mid-wall distribution) [34]. A pathogenic mutation in PRKAG2 accounts for 0.15% of HCM patients. In PRKAG2 cardiomyopathy, a high prevalence of atrioventricular accessory pathways and atrioventricular blocks often requiring pacemaker implantation have been reported, even before the development of massive LV hypertrophy [20, 37].

Up to half of the individuals with sarcomeric HCM and its phenocopies may be diagnosed by genetic analysis. Endomyocardial biopsy (EMB) in heart failure (HF) with unexplained HCM has a class IIb indication according to ESC guidelines on the use of EMB [38] and a class IIA according to the most recent ESC and AHA/

ACC HF practice guidelines [39]. It remains indicated in a minority of cases when non-invasive means, including genetic studies, do not provide a definitive diagnosis (i.e. for the diagnosis of CA). Nowadays, the refinement of the diagnosis through gene analysis and in selected cases by endomyocardial biopsy appears even more crucial, given the availability of specific treatments, such as enzyme replacement therapy for AFD or steroid/alkylating therapy for AL.

18.4 Cardiac Sarcoidosis

In rare circumstances, cardiac sarcoidosis (CS) can simulate LV hypertrophy or resemble HCM with asymmetric LV hypertrophy and/or left ventricular outflow obstruction [40]. Sarcoidosis is a multisystem, granulomatous disease with an uncertain aetiology that is triggered by an immune response to an unknown antigen in genetically predisposed individuals [41]. Sarcoidosis is a worldwide condition affecting adults aged from 25 to 60 years old, with a prevalence of around 2–160 in 100,000, with the highest incidence in northern Europeans and African Americans, especially women [42]. Clinically evident cardiac involvement occurs in around 5% of sarcoidosis patients, with the rate increasing in silent individuals. However, according to autopsy investigations, the prevalence of cardiac involvement is estimated to be at least 25% of cases [43, 44].

The major clinical signs of CS include conduction abnormalities, ventricular arrhythmias including sudden cardiac death (SCD), and HF. Only a few characteristics are shared with CA, most notably pathological Q waves and atrioventricular or intraventricular conduction abnormalities [45], and—to a lesser extent—a myocardial wall thickness simulating LV hypertrophy [46]. In CS, echocardiographic features vary according to the disease phase, firstly showing a wall thickening due to inflammation of granulomatous lesions [47] and then followed by a wall thinning due to fibrous scar formation. At early stages or in silent cardiac damage, diagnosis of cardiac involvement is instead challenging—implying late or missed diagnosis—for several reasons: absence of a significant release of natriuretic peptides [48], isolated cardiac disease, and non-specificity of imaging findings [40]. With this regard, although CMR allows to identify small regions of myocardial damage as LGE, there is no specific pattern that is diagnostic for CS. LGE is most typically patchy and multifocal at mid-wall and epicardium—sparing the endocardial borders—and seen in basal segments. Still, LGE may become transmural and involve the right ventricle [49], like in CA; however, CS does not involve the atrium, a feature that helps distinguishing the two diseases [49].

When CMR demonstrates thinner walls, aneurysms, and segmental wall motion abnormalities in a noncoronary distribution, cardiac involvement is already at an advanced stage [50]. During the acute inflammatory stage, CMR may show regional wall motion abnormalities and increased wall thickness, whereas in chronic stage, myocardial wall thinning or aneurysm and increased signal are seen in LGE images. LGE has also a prognostic impact in identifying patients at a 30-fold increased risk of death, aborted SCD, or implantable cardioverter defibrillator shocks compared to patients without LGE [51]. Moreover, CMR, particularly with the new T2 mapping techniques, appears to be a promising tool for early detection and disease monitoring, although some limitations in differentiating active from chronic phase of the disease still remain.

In the context of an early and proper diagnosis, radionuclide imaging has a synergistic potential over CMR, by identifying at the same time the involvement of other tissues and monitoring the disease activity. In fact, hybrid imaging of fluorodeoxyglucose-positron-emission tomography (FDG-PET) and CMR has been proposed for an early detection of silent cardiac damage [52].

Even with an advanced multiparameter imaging acquisition, some cases may still require further investigation since CS and CA may exhibit the same degree of myocardial inflammation [53]. EMB may be helpful to correctly identify those cases falling in a grey diagnostic zone, despite a limited sensitivity due to the high sampling error associated with the focal nature of CS [54].

Finally, the coexistence of CS and CA, although extremely rare, should not be excluded *a priori*, particularly in subjects with AL and AA; for the latter, it seems that the activated inflammation-related pathways might favour the development of both disorders.

18.5 Haemochromatosis

Iron homeostasis dysfunction might result in its accumulation at cardiac level, with consequent oxidative damage due to the lack of a regulating mechanism for iron excretion and its high intake of cardiomyocytes. It is reported that 1 out of 500 people might develop symptoms of haemochromatosis, with 15% of these people exhibiting cardiac symptoms [55]. As a result of the interaction between hereditary and various patient or environmental variables, there is a wide range of cardiac patterns, spanning from dilated (the most frequent) to hypertrophic phenotype [55].

Iron overload can produce myocardial concentric or asymmetric hypertrophy, as well as progressive LV remodelling and dysfunction, if the underlying cause is not treated [56]. Similar to CA, bi-atrial enlargement and biventricular dilatation with systolic dysfunction are implied by disease progression, while impaired diastolic function and higher LV wall thickness parameters are evident since the beginning of the disease [57]. Speckle tracking imaging can early identify myocardial changes in terms of worse rotational and longitudinal deformation, starting from basal segments [58], even before the occurrence of LV hypertrophy. Echocardiography can highlight cardiac damage, but only CMR can guarantee a differential diagnosis, especially when T2* sequences/mapping are employed; the detection of high T2* values in the heart, resembling those found in the liver, identifies iron deposition with great specificity. Conversely, initial experience with T1 mapping techniques suggests that T1 may be more sensitive for the disease, by detecting missed myocardial iron deposition in 1 out of 3 subjects with normal T2*, and that T1 mapping is complementary to T2* [59]. Moreover, the predictive significance of CMR data has been recognized, with low T2 levels being associated with a higher risk of HF and arrhythmias [60].

18.6 Light-Chain Deposition Disease

The LCDD should be mentioned due to its pathophysiology similar to that of AL, although it is distinguished by the deposition of monoclonal immunoglobulin light-chain fragments that lack the properties required to form amyloid fibrils [61]. LCDD mainly targets the kidneys; however, other organs such as the heart, liver, and peripheral nervous system may also be affected. Cardiac involvement is rare and occurs in about one-third of LCDD cases [62].

Similar to AL, LCDD has been associated with multiple myeloma and other diseases such as lymphomas or Waldenström macroglobulinemia. Unlike AL, tissue deposits in LCDD are often composed by kappa light chains, are granular and not fibrillar, and are not stained by Congo red, thioflavin T, or serum amyloid P component. In individuals with plasma cell dyscrasias, it is unclear which clinical and biochemical variables can influence the type of light-chain deposition (amyloid fibrils or granular light chains).

LCDD is characterized by a nephrotic syndrome or a progressive chronic kidney disease, which frequently requires dialysis, and in some cases by HF [63]. In fact, cardiac LCDD should be evaluated as one of the possible differential diagnoses in HF patients with an unknown cause linked to a monoclonal protein in the blood or urine [64]. To make a clear diagnosis of LCDD, clinicians should verify urine and tissue deposits of light chains that are not organized in the form of amyloid fibrils; hence, a kidney biopsy with both electron microscopy analysis and immunofluorescence is needed to differentiate AL from LCDD [64].

Cardiac LCDD phenotypic presentation may vary, as evidenced by case reports/series, ranging from a dilated phenotype [64] with systolic dysfunction to those with clinical features similar to CA [62, 65], such as reduced LV global longitudinal strain with apical sparing, diastolic dysfunction, and increased T1 values in CMR imaging. It is interesting to note that the ECG does not show neither a low voltage nor a high voltage of the QRS complexes [65]. Patients with LCDD who have cardiac involvement show a considerably higher risk of treatment-related death following stem cell transplantation than LCDD patients without cardiac involvement. Lastly, cardiac involvement is associated with a shorter overall survival rate [62].

References

1. Roth GA, et al. Global burden of cardiovascular diseases and risk factors, 1990-2019: update from the GBD 2019 study. J Am Coll Cardiol. 2020;76(25):2982–3021. https://doi.org/10.1016/j.jacc.2020.11.010.
2. Elenkova A, Shabani R, Kinova E, Vasilev V, Goudev A, Zacharieva S. Global longitudinal strain as a marker for systolic function in patients with pheochromocytomas. Endocr Relat Cancer. 2020;27(10):561–70. https://doi.org/10.1530/ERC-20-0137.
3. Kokkinos PF, et al. Effects of regular exercise on blood pressure and left ventricular hypertrophy in African-American men with severe hypertension. N Engl J Med. 1995;333(22):1462–7. https://doi.org/10.1056/NEJM199511303332204.

4. Henein MY, Pilebro B, Lindqvist P. Disease progression in cardiac morphology and function in heart failure: ATTR cardiac amyloidosis versus hypertensive left ventricular hypertrophy. Heart Vessel. 2022;37(9):1562–9. https://doi.org/10.1007/s00380-022-02048-5.

5. Takeda M, Amano Y, Tachi M, Tani H, Mizuno K, Kumita S. MRI differentiation of cardiomyopathy showing left ventricular hypertrophy and heart failure: differentiation between cardiac amyloidosis, hypertrophic cardiomyopathy, and hypertensive heart disease. Jpn J Radiol. 2013;31(10):693–700. https://doi.org/10.1007/s11604-013-0238-0.

6. Lindroos M, Kupari M, Heikkilä J, Tilvis R. Prevalence of aortic valve abnormalities in the elderly: an echocardiographic study of a random population sample. J Am Coll Cardiol. 1993;21(5):1220–5. https://doi.org/10.1016/0735-1097(93)90249-z.

7. Thaden JJ, Nkomo VT, Enriquez-Sarano M. The global burden of aortic stenosis. Prog Cardiovasc Dis. 2014;56(6):565–71. https://doi.org/10.1016/j.pcad.2014.02.006.

8. Aimo A, et al. Redefining the epidemiology of cardiac amyloidosis. A systematic review and meta-analysis of screening studies. Eur J Heart Fail. 2022;24(12):2342–51. https://doi.org/10.1002/ejhf.2532.

9. Treibel TA, et al. Occult transthyretin cardiac amyloid in severe calcific aortic stenosis: prevalence and prognosis in patients undergoing surgical aortic valve replacement. Circ Cardiovasc Imaging. 2016;9(8):e005066. https://doi.org/10.1161/CIRCIMAGING.116.005066.

10. Scully PR, et al. Prevalence and outcome of dual aortic stenosis and cardiac amyloid pathology in patients referred for transcatheter aortic valve implantation. Eur Heart J. 2020;41(29):2759–67. https://doi.org/10.1093/eurheartj/ehaa170.

11. Nitsche C, et al. Prevalence and outcomes of concomitant aortic stenosis and cardiac amyloidosis. J Am Coll Cardiol. 2021;77(2):128–39. https://doi.org/10.1016/j.jacc.2020.11.006.

12. Ternacle J, et al. Aortic stenosis and cardiac amyloidosis: JACC review topic of the week. J Am Coll Cardiol. 2019;74(21):2638–51. https://doi.org/10.1016/j.jacc.2019.09.056.

13. Marcoux J, et al. A novel mechano-enzymatic cleavage mechanism underlies transthyretin amyloidogenesis. EMBO Mol Med. 2015;7(10):1337–49. https://doi.org/10.15252/emmm.201505357.

14. Aquaro GD, et al. Magnetic resonance for differential diagnosis of left ventricular hypertrophy: diagnostic and prognostic implications. J Clin Med. 2022;11(3):651. https://doi.org/10.3390/jcm11030651.

15. Maron MS, Hellawell JL, Lucove JC, Farzaneh-Far R, Olivotto I. Occurrence of clinically diagnosed hypertrophic cardiomyopathy in the United States. Am J Cardiol. 2016;117(10):1651–4. https://doi.org/10.1016/j.amjcard.2016.02.044.

16. Maron BJ, et al. Diagnosis and evaluation of hypertrophic cardiomyopathy. J Am Coll Cardiol. 2022;79(4):372–89. https://doi.org/10.1016/j.jacc.2021.12.002.

17. Marek J, et al. Comparison of echocardiographic parameters in Fabry cardiomyopathy and light-chain cardiac amyloidosis. Echocardiogr Mt Kisco N. 2018;35(11):1755–63. https://doi.org/10.1111/echo.14144.

18. Falk RH, Quarta CC. Echocardiography in cardiac amyloidosis. Heart Fail Rev. 2015;20(2):125–31. https://doi.org/10.1007/s10741-014-9466-3.

19. Alashi A, et al. Different histopathologic diagnoses in patients with clinically diagnosed hypertrophic cardiomyopathy after surgical myectomy. Circulation. 2019;140(4):344–6. https://doi.org/10.1161/CIRCULATIONAHA.119.040129.

20. Hoss S, et al. Genetic testing for diagnosis of hypertrophic cardiomyopathy mimics: yield and clinical significance. Circ Genomic Precis Med. 2020;13(2):e002748. https://doi.org/10.1161/CIRCGEN.119.002748.

21. Biagini E, et al. Prognostic implications of the Doppler restrictive filling pattern in hypertrophic cardiomyopathy. Am J Cardiol. 2009;104(12):1727–31. https://doi.org/10.1016/j.amjcard.2009.07.057.

22. Boldrini M, et al. Multiparametric echocardiography scores for the diagnosis of cardiac amyloidosis. JACC Cardiovasc Imaging. 2020;13(4):909–20. https://doi.org/10.1016/j.jcmg.2019.10.011.

23. Stassen J, et al. Left ventricular myocardial work to differentiate cardiac amyloidosis from hypertrophic cardiomyopathy. J Am Soc Echocardiogr Off Publ Am Soc Echocardiogr. 2023;36(2):252–4. https://doi.org/10.1016/j.echo.2022.08.015.
24. Higashi H, et al. Restricted left atrial dilatation can visually differentiate cardiac amyloidosis from hypertrophic cardiomyopathy. ESC Heart Fail. 2021;8(4):3198–205. https://doi.org/10.1002/ehf2.13442.
25. Pagourelias ED, et al. Echo parameters for differential diagnosis in cardiac amyloidosis: a head-to-head comparison of deformation and nondeformation parameters. Circ Cardiovasc Imaging. 2017;10(3):e005588. https://doi.org/10.1161/CIRCIMAGING.116.005588.
26. Liu H, et al. Distinguishing cardiac amyloidosis and hypertrophic cardiomyopathy by thickness and myocardial deformation of the right ventricle. Cardiol Res Pract. 2022;2022:4364279. https://doi.org/10.1155/2022/4364279.
27. Yue X, et al. The diagnostic value of multiparameter cardiovascular magnetic resonance for early detection of light-chain amyloidosis from hypertrophic cardiomyopathy patients. Front Cardiovasc Med. 2022;9:1017097. https://doi.org/10.3389/fcvm.2022.1017097.
28. Li B, et al. Cardiac AA amyloidosis in a patient with obstructive hypertrophic cardiomyopathy. Cardiovasc Pathol Off J Soc Cardiovasc Pathol. 2020;48:107218. https://doi.org/10.1016/j.carpath.2020.107218.
29. Tomberli B, Cappelli F, Perfetto F, Olivotto I. Abrupt onset of refractory heart failure associated with light-chain amyloidosis in hypertrophic cardiomyopathy. JAMA Cardiol. 2017;2(1):94–7. https://doi.org/10.1001/jamacardio.2016.3894.
30. Doheny D, Srinivasan R, Pagant S, Chen B, Yasuda M, Desnick RJ. Fabry disease: prevalence of affected males and heterozygotes with pathogenic GLA mutations identified by screening renal, cardiac and stroke clinics, 1995–2017. J Med Genet. 2018;55(4):261–8. https://doi.org/10.1136/jmedgenet-2017-105080.
31. Niemann M, et al. Differences in Fabry cardiomyopathy between female and male patients: consequences for diagnostic assessment. JACC Cardiovasc Imaging. 2011;4(6):592–601. https://doi.org/10.1016/j.jcmg.2011.01.020.
32. Pieroni M, et al. Cardiac involvement in Fabry disease: JACC review topic of the week. J Am Coll Cardiol. 2021;77(7):922–36. https://doi.org/10.1016/j.jacc.2020.12.024.
33. Kirschbaum SW, Baks T, Kofflard MJM, van Geuns R-JM. Case report. Cardiac amyloidosis mimicking Fabry's disease in cardiac magnetic resonance imaging. Clin Radiol. 2008;63(11):1274–6. https://doi.org/10.1016/j.crad.2008.03.010.
34. Ranganath PG, Tower-Rader A. Utility of cardiac magnetic resonance imaging in the diagnosis, prognosis, and treatment of infiltrative cardiomyopathies. Curr Cardiol Rep. 2021;23(7):87. https://doi.org/10.1007/s11886-021-01518-y.
35. Namdar M, et al. Value of electrocardiogram in the differentiation of hypertensive heart disease, hypertrophic cardiomyopathy, aortic stenosis, amyloidosis, and Fabry disease. Am J Cardiol. 2012;109(4):587–93. https://doi.org/10.1016/j.amjcard.2011.09.052.
36. Tanaka H. Efficacy of echocardiography for differential diagnosis of left ventricular hypertrophy: special focus on speckle-tracking longitudinal strain. J Echocardiogr. 2021;19(2):71–9. https://doi.org/10.1007/s12574-020-00508-3.
37. Pieroni M, et al. Beyond sarcomeric hypertrophic cardiomyopathy: how to diagnose and manage phenocopies. Curr Cardiol Rep. 2022;24(11):1567–85. https://doi.org/10.1007/s11886-022-01778-2.
38. Cooper LT, et al. The role of endomyocardial biopsy in the management of cardiovascular disease: a scientific statement from the American Heart Association, the American College of Cardiology, and the European Society of Cardiology. Circulation. 2007;116(19):2216–33. https://doi.org/10.1161/CIRCULATIONAHA.107.186093.
39. Heidenreich PA, et al. 2022 AHA/ACC/HFSA Guideline for the Management of Heart Failure: executive summary: a report of the American College of Cardiology/American Heart Association Joint Committee on Clinical Practice Guidelines. J Am Coll Cardiol. 2022;79(17):1757–80. https://doi.org/10.1016/j.jacc.2021.12.011.

40. Birnie DH, Nery PB, Ha AC, Beanlands RSB. Cardiac sarcoidosis. J Am Coll Cardiol. 2016;68(4):411–21. https://doi.org/10.1016/j.jacc.2016.03.605.

41. Baughman RP, Lower EE, du Bois RM. Sarcoidosis. Lancet Lond Engl. 2003;361(9363):1111–8. https://doi.org/10.1016/S0140-6736(03)12888-7.

42. Arkema EV, Cozier YC. Sarcoidosis epidemiology: recent estimates of incidence, prevalence and risk factors. Curr Opin Pulm Med. 2020;26(5):527–34. https://doi.org/10.1097/MCP.0000000000000715.

43. Iwai K, Tachibana T, Takemura T, Matsui Y, Kitaichi M, Kawabata Y. Pathological studies on sarcoidosis autopsy. I. Epidemiological features of 320 cases in Japan. Acta Pathol Jpn. 1993;43(7–8):372–6. https://doi.org/10.1111/j.1440-1827.1993.tb01148.x.

44. Patel MR, et al. Detection of myocardial damage in patients with sarcoidosis. Circulation. 2009;120(20):1969–77. https://doi.org/10.1161/CIRCULATIONAHA.109.851352.

45. Nery PB, Keren A, Healey J, Leug E, Beanlands RS, Birnie DH. Isolated cardiac sarcoidosis: establishing the diagnosis with electroanatomic mapping-guided endomyocardial biopsy. Can J Cardiol. 2013;29(8):1015.e1–3. https://doi.org/10.1016/j.cjca.2012.09.009.

46. Tahara N, et al. Cardiac sarcoidosis with thickening myocardium. J Nucl Cardiol Off Publ Am Soc Nucl Cardiol. 2022;29(6):3619–22. https://doi.org/10.1007/s12350-021-02719-2.

47. Takemura K, et al. A case of cardiac sarcoidosis mimicking cardiac amyloidosis on cardiovascular magnetic resonance. ESC Heart Fail. 2018;5(2):306–10. https://doi.org/10.1002/ehf2.12263.

48. Kiko T, et al. A multiple biomarker approach in patients with cardiac sarcoidosis. Int Heart J. 2018;59(5):996–1001. https://doi.org/10.1536/ihj.17-695.

49. Moraes GL, Higgins CB, Ordovas KG. Delayed enhancement magnetic resonance imaging in nonischemic myocardial disease. J Thorac Imaging. 2013;28(2):84–92. https://doi.org/10.1097/RTI.0b013e3182828f89. quiz 93–95, 2013

50. Muchtar E, Blauwet LA, Gertz MA. restrictive cardiomyopathy: genetics, pathogenesis, clinical manifestations, diagnosis, and therapy. Circ Res. 2017;121(7):819–37. https://doi.org/10.1161/CIRCRESAHA.117.310982.

51. Coleman GC, et al. Prognostic value of myocardial scarring on CMR in patients with cardiac sarcoidosis. JACC Cardiovasc Imaging. 2017;10(4):411–20. https://doi.org/10.1016/j.jcmg.2016.05.009.

52. Vita T, et al. Complementary value of cardiac magnetic resonance imaging and positron emission tomography/computed tomography in the assessment of cardiac sarcoidosis. Circ Cardiovasc Imaging. 2018;11(1):e007030. https://doi.org/10.1161/CIRCIMAGING.117.007030.

53. Young KA, et al. 18F-FDG/13N-ammonia cardiac PET findings in ATTR cardiac amyloidosis. J Nucl Cardiol Off Publ Am Soc Nucl Cardiol. 2023;30(2):726–35. https://doi.org/10.1007/s12350-021-02886-2.

54. Bennett MK, et al. Evaluation of the role of endomyocardial biopsy in 851 patients with unexplained heart failure from 2000–2009. Circ Heart Fail. 2013;6(4):676–84. https://doi.org/10.1161/CIRCHEARTFAILURE.112.000087.

55. Gulati V, Harikrishnan P, Palaniswamy C, Aronow WS, Jain D, Frishman WH. Cardiac involvement in hemochromatosis. Cardiol Rev. 2014;22(2):56–68. https://doi.org/10.1097/CRD.0b013e3182a67805.

56. Díez-López C, Comín-Colet J, González-Costello J. Iron overload cardiomyopathy: from diagnosis to management. Curr Opin Cardiol. 2018;33(3):334–40. https://doi.org/10.1097/HCO.0000000000000511.

57. Rozwadowska K, Raczak G, Sikorska K, Fijałkowski M, Kozłowski D, Daniłowicz-Szymanowicz L. Influence of hereditary haemochromatosis on left ventricular wall thickness: does iron overload exacerbate cardiac hypertrophy? Folia Morphol (Warsz). 2019;78(4):746–53. https://doi.org/10.5603/FM.a2019.0025.

58. Rozwadowska K, et al. Can two-dimensional speckle tracking echocardiography be useful for left ventricular assessment in the early stages of hereditary haemochromatosis? Echocardiogr Mt Kisco N. 2018;35(11):1772–81. https://doi.org/10.1111/echo.14141.

59. Torlasco C, et al. Role of T1 mapping as a complementary tool to T2* for non-invasive cardiac iron overload assessment. PLoS One. 2018;13(2):e0192890. https://doi.org/10.1371/journal.pone.0192890.
60. Habib G, et al. Multimodality Imaging in Restrictive Cardiomyopathies: An EACVI expert consensus document in collaboration with the "Working Group on myocardial and pericardial diseases" of the European Society of Cardiology Endorsed by The Indian Academy of Echocardiography. Eur Heart J Cardiovasc Imaging. 2017;18(10):1090–121. https://doi.org/10.1093/ehjci/jex034.
61. Gertz MA. Immunoglobulin light chain amyloidosis: 2020 update on diagnosis, prognosis, and treatment. Am J Hematol. 2020;95(7):848–60. https://doi.org/10.1002/ajh.25819.
62. Mohan M, et al. Clinical characteristics and prognostic factors in multiple myeloma patients with light chain deposition disease. Am J Hematol. 2017;92(8):739–45. https://doi.org/10.1002/ajh.24756.
63. Sayed RH, et al. Natural history and outcome of light chain deposition disease. Blood. 2015;126(26):2805–10. https://doi.org/10.1182/blood-2015-07-658872.
64. Aimo A, et al. Cardiac light-chain deposition disease relapsing in the transplanted heart. Amyloid Int J Exp Clin Investig Off J Int Soc Amyloidosis. 2017;24(2):135–7. https://doi.org/10.1080/13506129.2017.1334196.
65. Osanami A, et al. Cardiac light chain deposition disease mimicking immunoglobulin light chain amyloidosis: two branches of the same tree. Circ Cardiovasc Imaging. 2020;13(9):e010478. https://doi.org/10.1161/CIRCIMAGING.120.010478.

Applications of Artificial Intelligence in Amyloidosis

19

Andrea Barison, Daniela Tomasoni, Alessandro Filippeschi, Maria Giulia Bellicini, Carlo Alberto Avizzano, Marco Metra, and Martha Grogan

19.1 Artificial Intelligence and Machine Learning: Introduction and Use in Medicine

Driven by an increase in computational power and memory, computers are being more and more used to perform a wide range of complex tasks in many fields, including medicine [1]. The potential of artificial intelligence (AI) is almost unlimited, being theoretically able to improve early diagnosis, patients' management, treatments, and adherence to therapy.

Machine learning (ML), a subfield of AI, is designed to teach computers to make an inference from data (i.e., identify patterns and relationships and provide interpretation of data) using statistical algorithms and to make predictions based on this

A. Barison (✉)
Cardiology and Cardiovascular Medicine, Fondazione Toscana Gabriele Monasterio, Pisa, Italy

Institute of Life Sciences, Scuola Superiore Sant'Anna, Pisa, Italy
e-mail: abarison@ftgm.it

D. Tomasoni · M. G. Bellicini · M. Metra
Institute of Cardiology, ASST Spedali Civili di Brescia, Department of Medical and Surgical Specialties, Radiological Sciences, and Public Health, University of Brescia, Brescia, Italy
e-mail: m.bellicini003@unibs.it; marco.metra@unibs.it

A. Filippeschi · C. A. Avizzano
Institute of Mechanical Intelligence, Scuola Superiore Sant'Anna, Pisa, Italy

Department of Excellence in Robotics and AI, Scuola Superiore Sant'Anna, Pisa, Italy
e-mail: alessandro.filippeschi@santannapisa.it; carloalberto.avizzano@santannapisa.it

M. Grogan
Department of Cardiovascular Diseases, Mayo Clinic, Rochester, MN, USA
e-mail: grogan.martha@mayo.edu

© The Author(s), under exclusive license to Springer Nature Switzerland AG 2024
M. Emdin et al. (eds.), *Cardiac Amyloidosis*,
https://doi.org/10.1007/978-3-031-51757-0_19

inference. In the ML process, the machine is trained on a range of inputs associated with a known outcome so it can make an inference; based on this inference, the machine can process new unseen inputs and provide an outcome on its own. The more the new inputs are similar to those used in the machine training, the more accurate the outcome provided will be, so large amount of data should be input to ensure that the computer provides reliable outcomes. Deep learning (DL) is AI advanced from artificial neural networks that enables a computer to learn data using input and output variables similar to neurons. Machine learning and deep learning can be used to improve the diagnostic accuracy, outcome prediction, and precision medicine in treatment, but the full potential is yet to be reached [2–4]. Many DL network architectures are nowadays at the state of the art for detection, classification, segmentation, and localization that are fundamental tasks to achieve diagnosis support systems (DSS) powered by AI [5]. Moreover, diverse input such as images, biosignal time series, and patient clinical history can now be processed both in separate DL modules and together at once [6] to provide a classification of a disease. Rich datasets that include patients' data gathered at different screening complexity levels, that is, from simple measurement of the body mass to complex examinations such as PET or CT, are the key to develop DSS capable of detecting and classifying early-stage diseases even before the most informative data, i.e., those obtainable from complex examinations, are available. This is especially true for cardiac amyloidosis (CA).

Cardiac amyloidosis has traditionally been considered a rare disease, even if recent studies suggested that it has been underdiagnosed for many years [7]. Thus, AI represents a potential breakthrough to facilitate the diagnosis of CA. To date, the use of ML and DL in patients with CA has been almost limited to imaging or other quantifiable instrumental tests (Fig. 19.1). In the case of rare diseases, especially CA, the most common analytical problem is that of insufficient data and limited knowledge to provide a reliable input to the machine [8–10]. In this chapter, we will summarize evidence regarding the application of AI in patients with CA and the most challenging aspects in this field.

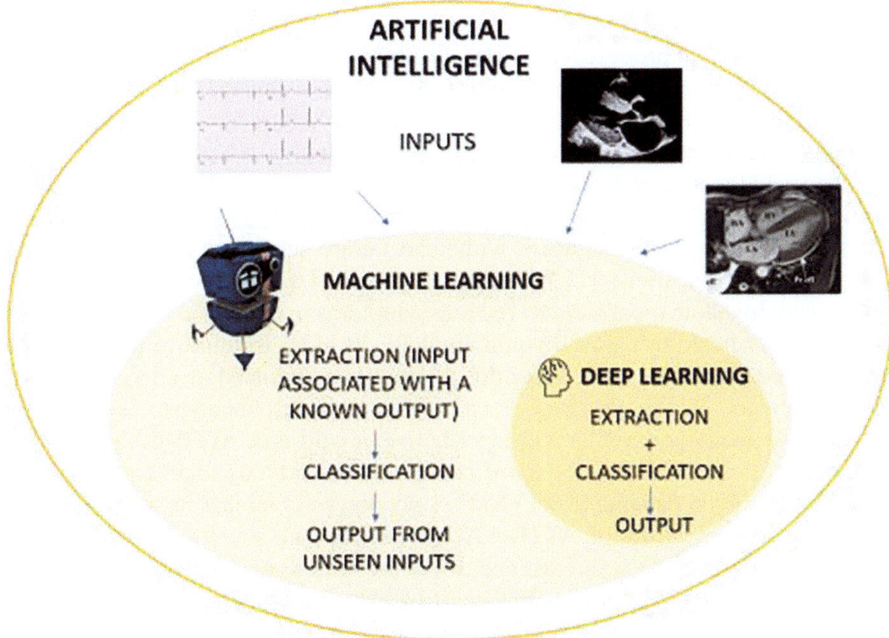

Fig. 19.1 Artificial intelligence in cardiac amyloidosis

19.2 Artificial Intelligence and Cardiac Amyloidosis: Diagnosis

For a long time, CA remained underdiagnosed both in subclinical and in clinical stages. However, it is now clear that its prevalence is higher than previously thought, and in the last years, the number of diagnoses has increased due to a greater awareness of the disease and the development of noninvasive diagnosis. Given the development of several new therapies that significantly improve the prognosis of patients with CA when initiated at an early stage of the disease, the issue of underdiagnosis/misdiagnosis of CA is becoming more urgent. In such a scenario, artificial intelligence (AI) represents a useful tool to improve the diagnostic accuracy of CA and to anticipate the diagnosis to an early stage.

To date, there are few studies regarding AI application in CA, and the sample size is generally small. However, these studies consistently showed that AI-based diagnosis of CA using clinical data, ECG, or cardiac imaging modalities (e.g., echocardiography, cardiac magnetic resonance, and PET) has better sensitivity and specificity than a diagnosis done by an experienced physician.

19.2.1 Clinical Variables and Biomarkers

García-García et al. proposed a statistical learning algorithm based on clinical variables in order to help the diagnosis of CA. Information generated by the patients in each admission and discharge episode was used as data vectors to facilitate their aggregation. The large volume of clinical histories implied a high dimensionality of the data, and the lack of diagnosis led to a severe class imbalance caused by the low prevalence of the disease. In the validation phase, the algorithm was applied to a large sample of patients diagnosed with heart failure presenting an excellent specificity and high sensitivity [11]. Hens et al. provided a validation of an AI-driven framework to automatically detect red flag symptoms in electronic health records in screening for hereditary transthyretin amyloidosis [12]. To improve the identification of patients at risk for CA, a pilot program was initiated at a large academic medical center. In this program, 9 cardiac/noncardiac phenotypes and 20 high-performing phenotype combinations predictive of wild-type ATTR-CA were operationalized in electronic health record configurations. Among 45,051 patients with heart failure, 4006 patients (8.9%) had ≥ 1 phenotype combination associated with increased risk of wild-type ATTR-CA. Across all data sources, two phenotypes (cardiomegaly and osteoarthrosis) and two combinations (carpal tunnel syndrome + heart failure and atrial fibrillation + heart block + cardiomegaly + osteoarthrosis) generated the highest proportions of patients for wild-type ATTR-CA screening [13].

Heart failure patients with CA display distinct biomarker patterns as compared to non-CA heart failure patients that are detectable by intelligent statistical approaches. Expert-independent ML prediction models for CA relying on routinely determined laboratory parameters were developed [14]. The first model included 12 routine laboratory parameters, via a simple and interpretable linear prediction model (logistic regression) that was backed by a complex machine learning algorithm (ensemble of decision trees) for variable selection. This model reached a diagnostic prediction accuracy in an unrelated prospective cohort consisting of heart failure patients with and without CA. Even more convincing was the prediction model proposed by a black-box algorithm (nonlinear complex machine learning model) that could be confirmed by the results obtained from the unrelated validation cohort [14].

19.2.2 Electrocardiogram

ECG data, unlike clinical data, are objective and standardized, easily obtained, stored, and analyzed for the development of AI models. AI-enhanced ECG can detect or raise the suspicion of hypertrophic cardiomyopathy (HCM), dilated cardiomyopathy, or cardiac contractile dysfunction using ECG patterns unrecognizable to the human eye [15–17]. ECG is usually abnormal in patients with clinically manifest CA. Abnormalities include various degrees of conduction block or disproportionally low QRS voltage. Also, pathological Q wave (the "pseudoinfarct pattern") is considered a red flag that could evoke the diagnosis of CA [18–20]. Thus, there is a strong rationale for the use of ECG data as inputs for the ML process in the diagnosis of CA [21]. Grogan et al. collected 12-lead ECG data from 2541 patients with AL- or ATTR-CA seen at Mayo Clinic between 2000 and 2019. Cases were matched for age and sex, with 2454 controls. A subset of 2997 (60%) cases and controls were used to train a deep neural network to predict the presence of CA with an internal validation set ($n = 999$; 20%) and a randomly selected holdout testing set ($n = 999$; 20%). The area under the receiver operating characteristic curve (AUC) was 0.91 (95% CI, 0.90–0.93), with a positive predictive value for detecting either type of CA of 0.86. A cutoff probability of 0.485 was determined by the Youden index. Using this cutoff, 426 (84%) of the holdout patients with CA were detected by the model. Among patients with CA with available pre-diagnosis ECG studies, the AI model successfully predicted the presence of CA more than 6 months before the clinical diagnosis in 59%. The best single-lead model was V5 with an AUC of 0.86 and a precision of 0.78, with other single leads performing similarly. The authors also performed experiments using single-lead and 6-lead ECG subsets. The 6-lead (bipolar leads) model had an AUC of 0.90 and a precision of 0.85 [22].

19.2.3 Echocardiography

As far as echocardiography is concerned, several ML-based studies have been published on automated chamber quantification, ejection fraction calculation, diastolic function assessment, and strain measurement, as, once again, they represent standardized and objective measurements that fit well in the setting of ML [15, 23]. In a case–control study including 138 subjects (74 patients with verified AL-CA and 64 patients with verified HCM), machine learning models utilizing traditional and advanced algorithms were established. Machine learning combined with speckle tracking echocardiography had a great performance in the differential diagnosis of CA and HCM and could automatically integrate plentiful variables to identify the most discriminative predictors without presumption [24]. Using 14,035 echocardiograms spanning a 10-year period, Zhang et al. trained and evaluated convolutional neural network models for multiple tasks, including automated identification of 23 viewpoints and segmentation of cardiac chambers across five common views. Results were evaluated through comparison to manual segmentation and measurements from 8666 echocardiograms obtained during the routine clinical workflow. Zhang et al. demonstrated the ability of ML to accurately identify the various echocardiographic views and automate cardiac structure measurements, which were comparable or superior to manual measurements. The authors also developed models to detect HCM and CA with C statistics of 0.93 and 0.87, respectively [13]. In a further study, including a total of 289 participants ($n = 50$ with CA; $n = 70$ with HCM; $n = 92$ with uremic cardiomyopathy; $n = 77$ with hypertensive heart disease), ML-based myocardial texture analysis using conventional two-dimensional transthoracic echocardiography effectively distinguished CA from non-CA left ventricular hypertrophy [25]. This discrimination usually poses an issue to cardiologists and represents a useful tool in order to reduce the number of misdiagnoses. Such results were further confirmed in a Chinese study, highlighting the potential of AI in the definition of the etiology behind left ventricular (LV) hypertrophy [26].

19.2.4 Advanced Imaging Techniques (Cardiovascular Magnetic Resonance and PET)

Several studies highlighted the usefulness of AI when applied to other imaging techniques [27–30]. Davies et al. presented a fully automated algorithm for the measurement of LV structure and function using cardiovascular magnetic resonance (CMR), which offers better outcomes compared to human performance in terms of precision and speed [29]. Myocardial texture mapping can also be studied throughout ML-based CMR. Antonopoulos et al. investigated whether radiomic features from T1 maps by CMR could enhance the diagnostic value of T1 mapping in distinguishing health from disease and classifying cardiac disease phenotypes. A total of 149 patients ($n = 30$ without cardiac disease; $n = 30$ with LV hypertrophy; $n = 61$ with HCM; and $n = 28$ with CA) undergoing a CMR scan were included in the study. The authors applied principal component analysis and unsupervised clustering in exploratory analysis, and then machine learning for feature selection of the best radiomic features that maximized the diagnostic value for cardiac disease classification. The first three principal components of the T1 radiomics were distinctively associated with different cardiac phenotypes. Unsupervised hierarchical clustering of the population by myocardial T1 radiomics was significantly associated with myocardial disease type (chi^2 = 55.98, $p < 0.0001$). After feature selection, internal validation, and external testing, a model of T1 radiomics had good diagnostic performance (AUC 0.753) for multinomial classification of disease phenotype (normal vs. LVH vs. HCM vs. CA). A subset of six radiomic features outperformed mean native T1 values for classification of cardiac disease (AUC of T1 vs. radiomics model for cardiac amyloid 0.769 vs. 0.840) [30]. Another study demonstrated that texture analysis based on T2-weighted images could feasibly differentiate CA from hypertrophic cardiomyopathy, even in patients with similar hypertrophy [31]. Martini et al. applied deep learning to automatically analyze CMR findings and establish the likelihood of CA among 206 subjects who underwent CMR due to unexplained LV hypertrophy or blood dyscrasia and suspected AL amyloidosis (Fig. 19.2) [28]. A DL approach evaluating late gadolinium enhancement acquisitions displayed a similar diagnostic performance for CA to an ML-based approach, which simulates CMR reading by experienced operators [28].

The potential of DL tools for characterizing the presence of CA from early acquired PET images, i.e., 15 min after [18F]-florbetaben tracer injection, has also been assessed by several groups [27, 32]. Sensitivity, specificity, and accuracy evaluated on the test dataset were high.

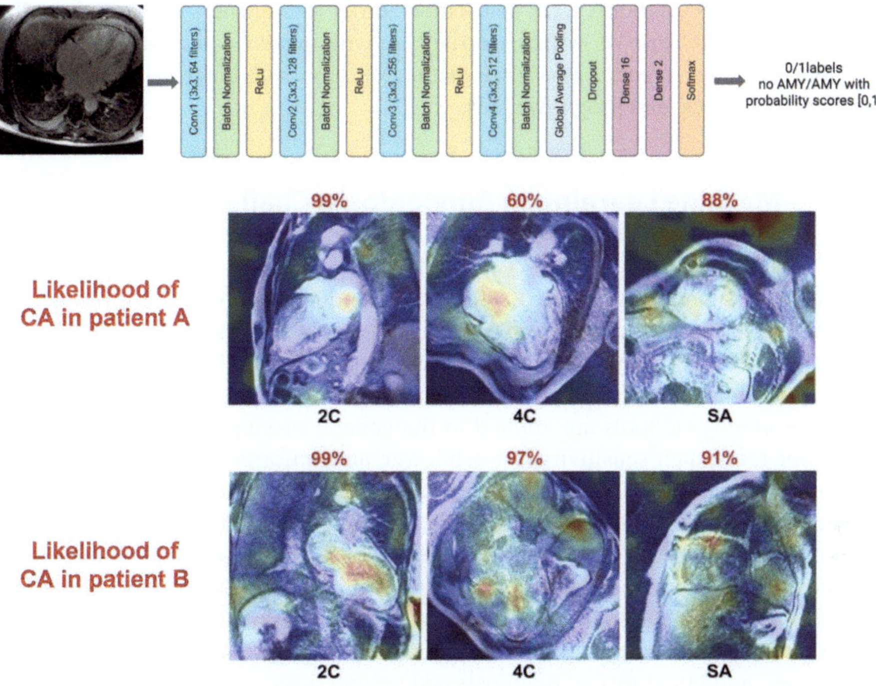

Fig. 19.2 Exemplar convolutional neural network (CNN) to detect cardiac amyloidosis (CA) from cardiovascular magnetic resonance imaging. Top: CNN architecture, whereby LGE images in different orientations were input into three base CNNs (2C, 4C, SAx) and the global CNN established the likelihood of CA based on the average prediction scores from the three individual CNNs. Bottom: Activation maps from two patients showing the most informative image elements from cardiovascular magnetic resonance. 2C two-chamber, 4C four-chamber, CA cardiac amyloidosis, SA short axis. Reproduced with permission from Martini et al. [28]

19.3 Artificial Intelligence in Amyloidosis: Outcome

Both ML and DL tools have been applied for risk prediction in cardiomyopathies. The models used multiple clinical parameters as input and were trained to predict ventricular tachycardia, heart failure, and/or appropriate implantable cardioverter defibrillator shocks [15]. Given limited knowledge as regards the natural history of CA, it might be more difficult to develop risk prediction models in patients with CA.

Bonnefous et al. used clustering analysis to identify typical clinical profiles in a large population of 1394 patients with suspected CA from the French Referral Center for Cardiac Amyloidosis database. Overall, 345 (25%) had a diagnosis of AL, 263 (19%) ATTRv, 402 (29%) ATTRwt, and 384 (28%) no amyloidosis. Seven clusters of patients with contrasting profiles and prognosis were identified. AL patients were distinctively located within a typical cluster and displayed the worst prognosis; ATTRv patients were distributed across four clusters with varying clinical presentations, one of which overlapped with patients without amyloidosis; ATTRwt patients spread across three distinct clusters with contrasting risk factors, biological profiles, and prognosis [33].

19.4 Machine Learning in Amyloidosis: Challenges and Future Perspectives

Of note, all the abovementioned studies are conduced training the machine with clinical, laboratory, electrocardiographic, and/or echocardiographic characteristics of patients that currently receive a diagnosis of CA (i.e., including mainly patients with symptoms and who often have an advanced disease). Therefore, when the resulting diagnostic tools are applied to the general (asymptomatic) population as screening tools, their sensitivity is much lower, and, unfortunately, the identification of similar but milder alterations than those of clinical patients could lead to the generation of incorrect outcomes. The advances in the field of AI (e.g., the introduction of a new method for high-dimensional pattern regression that estimates continuous instead of categorical variables) might allow to overcome these limitations. Soon as the diagnostic tools will be refined and the percentage and variety of diagnosed patients will be greater, AI-based models will improve our understanding of the disease and our ability of diagnosis and predict disease outcomes.

Several risks are also associated with relying on AI for selecting patients for the prescription of treatment. These risks include usability aspects of the DSS and AI system development issues. The former aspects are related to explicability trustworthiness of the DSS, its interoperability, and the possible loss of user's skills related to excessive reliance on the DSS tools [34]. The latter includes dataset creation issues, guarantees of input uniformity, and proper selection of both DL methods and DSS architecture.

Randomized trials must be conducted to demonstrate that an algorithm operates without bias in each population to which it will be applied [15].

The rarity of this kind of cardiopathy poses an issue in the determination of the size of the dataset to be used for training and validation of AI tools as well as the design of proper balancing of classes (i.e., disease levels) in the dataset. Dataset class balancing methods (e.g., data augmentation) are necessary steps in the creation of datasets when a large part of the dataset sample belongs to only one class [35].

The potential complexity of the information to be used as input for the components of DSS poses the design question of a balance between the size of the parameter space (i.e., the complexity of the networks) and the size of the dataset. In parallel, the same information complexity may lead to overly complex DL solutions that require larger datasets to avoid overfitting [36]. Finally, uniformity in the execution of examinations and in the labeling process, i.e., uniformity in the diagnosis, is another risk factor to take into account when adopting AI solutions for preliminary screenings. Uniform protocols and standardized equipment are a must both in the creation of the dataset and when using the developed tools for preliminary screening and diagnosis support.

19.5 Conclusions

Cardiac amyloidosis (CA) is a rare condition burdened by an extremely poor prognosis, namely when diagnosed at an advanced stage. CA remains often underdiagnosed due to a limited awareness among physicians. The use of artificial intelligence has been associated with improved diagnostic accuracy and should be largely applied in our clinical practice in order to anticipate the diagnosis and improve the outcome.

References

1. Sidey-Gibbons JAM, Sidey-Gibbons CJ. Machine learning in medicine: a practical introduction. BMC Med Res Methodol. 2019;19(1):64.
2. He B, Kwan AC, Cho JH, Yuan N, Pollick C, Shiota T, et al. Blinded, randomized trial of sonographer versus AI cardiac function assessment. Nature. 2023;616(7957):520–4.
3. Adler ED, Voors AA, Klein L, Macheret F, Braun OO, Urey MA, et al. Improving risk prediction in heart failure using machine learning. Eur J Heart Fail. 2020;22(1):139–47.
4. Johnson KW, Torres Soto J, Glicksberg BS, Shameer K, Miotto R, Ali M, et al. Artificial intelligence in cardiology. J Am Coll Cardiol. 2018;71(23):2668–79.
5. Ahsan MM, Siddique Z. Machine learning-based heart disease diagnosis: a systematic literature review. Artif Intell Med. 2022;128:102289.
6. Ayala Solares JR, Diletta Raimondi FE, Zhu Y, Rahimian F, Canoy D, Tran J, et al. Deep learning for electronic health records: a comparative review of multiple deep neural architectures. J Biomed Inform. 2020;101:103337.
7. Aimo A, Merlo M, Porcari A, Georgiopoulos G, Pagura L, Vergaro G, et al. Redefining the epidemiology of cardiac amyloidosis. A systematic review and meta-analysis of screening studies. Eur J Heart Fail. 2022;24(12):2342–51.
8. Lee J, Liu C, Kim J, Chen Z, Sun Y, Rogers JR, et al. Deep learning for rare disease: A scoping review. J Biomed Inform. 2022;135:104227.
9. Shehab M, Abualigah L, Shambour Q, Abu-Hashem MA, Shambour MKY, Alsalibi AI, et al. Machine learning in medical applications: a review of state-of-the-art methods. Comput Biol Med. 2022;145:105458.
10. Decherchi S, Pedrini E, Mordenti M, Cavalli A, Sangiorgi L. Opportunities and challenges for machine learning in rare diseases. Front Med (Lausanne). 2021;8:747612.
11. Garcia-Garcia E, Gonzalez-Romero GM, Martin-Perez EM, Zapata Cornejo ED, Escobar-Aguilar G, Cardenas Bonnet MF. Real-world data and machine learning to predict cardiac amyloidosis. Int J Environ Res Public Health. 2021;18(3):908.
12. Hens D, Wyers L, Claeys KG. Validation of an artificial intelligence driven framework to automatically detect red flag symptoms in screening for rare diseases in electronic health records: hereditary transthyretin amyloidosis polyneuropathy as a key example. J Peripher Nerv Syst. 2023;28(1):79–85.
13. Zhang J, Gajjala S, Agrawal P, Tison GH, Hallock LA, Beussink-Nelson L, et al. Fully automated echocardiogram interpretation in clinical practice. Circulation. 2018;138(16):1623–35.

14. Agibetov A, Seirer B, Dachs TM, Koschutnik M, Dalos D, Rettl R, et al. Machine learning enables prediction of cardiac amyloidosis by routine laboratory parameters: a proof-of-concept study. J Clin Med. 2020;9(5):1334.
15. Kim KH, Kwon JM, Pereira T, Attia ZI, Pereira NL. Artificial intelligence applied to cardiomyopathies: is it time for clinical application? Curr Cardiol Rep. 2022;24(11):1547–55.
16. Attia ZI, Kapa S, Lopez-Jimenez F, McKie PM, Ladewig DJ, Satam G, et al. Screening for cardiac contractile dysfunction using an artificial intelligence-enabled electrocardiogram. Nat Med. 2019;25(1):70–4.
17. Siontis KC, Noseworthy PA, Attia ZI, Friedman PA. Artificial intelligence-enhanced electrocardiography in cardiovascular disease management. Nat Rev Cardiol. 2021;18(7):465–78.
18. Ruberg FL, Grogan M, Hanna M, Kelly JW, Maurer MS. Transthyretin amyloid cardiomyopathy: JACC state-of-the-art review. J Am Coll Cardiol. 2019;73(22):2872–91.
19. Garcia-Pavia P, Rapezzi C, Adler Y, Arad M, Basso C, Brucato A, et al. Diagnosis and treatment of cardiac amyloidosis. A position statement of the European Society of Cardiology Working Group on myocardial and pericardial diseases. Eur J Heart Fail. 2021;23(4):512–26.
20. Merlo M, Pagura L, Porcari A, Cameli M, Vergaro G, Musumeci B, et al. Unmasking the prevalence of amyloid cardiomyopathy in the real world: results from Phase 2 of the AC-TIVE study, an Italian nationwide survey. Eur J Heart Fail. 2022;24(8):1377–86.
21. Goto S, Mahara K, Beussink-Nelson L, Ikura H, Katsumata Y, Endo J, et al. Artificial intelligence-enabled fully automated detection of cardiac amyloidosis using electrocardiograms and echocardiograms. Nat Commun. 2021;12(1):2726.
22. Grogan M, Lopez-Jimenez F, Cohen-Shelly M, Dispenzieri A, Attia ZI, Abou Ezzedine OF, et al. Artificial intelligence-enhanced electrocardiogram for the early detection of cardiac amyloidosis. Mayo Clin Proc. 2021;96(11):2768–78.
23. Alsharqi M, Woodward WJ, Mumith JA, Markham DC, Upton R, Leeson P. Artificial intelligence and echocardiography. Echo Res Pract. 2018;5(4):R115–R25.
24. Wu ZW, Zheng JL, Kuang L, Yan H. Machine learning algorithms to automate differentiating cardiac amyloidosis from hypertrophic cardiomyopathy. Int J Cardiovasc Imaging. 2023;39(2):339–48.
25. Zhang X, Liang T, Su C, Qin S, Li J, Zeng D, et al. Deep learn-based computer-assisted transthoracic echocardiography: approach to the diagnosis of cardiac amyloidosis. Int J Cardiovasc Imaging. 2023;39(5):955–65. https://doi.org/10.1007/s10554-023-02806-0.
26. Yu F, Huang H, Yu Q, Ma Y, Zhang Q, Zhang B. Artificial intelligence-based myocardial texture analysis in etiological differentiation of left ventricular hypertrophy. Ann Transl Med. 2021;9(2):108.
27. Santarelli MF, Genovesi D, Positano V, Scipioni M, Vergaro G, Favilli B, et al. Deep-learning-based cardiac amyloidosis classification from early acquired pet images. Int J Cardiovasc Imaging. 2021;37(7):2327–35.
28. Martini N, Aimo A, Barison A, Della Latta D, Vergaro G, Aquaro GD, et al. Deep learning to diagnose cardiac amyloidosis from cardiovascular magnetic resonance. J Cardiovasc Magn Reson. 2020;22(1):84.
29. Davies RH, Augusto JB, Bhuva A, Xue H, Treibel TA, Ye Y, et al. Precision measurement of cardiac structure and function in cardiovascular magnetic resonance using machine learning. J Cardiovasc Magn Reson. 2022;24(1):16.
30. Antonopoulos AS, Boutsikou M, Simantiris S, Angelopoulos A, Lazaros G, Panagiotopoulos I, et al. Machine learning of native T1 mapping radiomics for classification of hypertrophic cardiomyopathy phenotypes. Sci Rep. 2021;11(1):23596.
31. Huang S, Shi K, Zhang Y, Yan WF, Guo YK, Li Y, et al. Texture analysis of T2-weighted cardiovascular magnetic resonance imaging to discriminate between cardiac amyloidosis and hypertrophic cardiomyopathy. BMC Cardiovasc Disord. 2022;22(1):235.
32. Komori S, Cross DJ, Mills M, Ouchi Y, Nishizawa S, Okada H, et al. Deep-learning prediction of amyloid deposition from early-phase amyloid positron emission tomography imaging. Ann Nucl Med. 2022;36(10):913–21.

33. Bonnefous L, Kharoubi M, Bezard M, Oghina S, Le Bras F, Poullot E, et al. Assessing cardiac amyloidosis subtypes by unsupervised phenotype clustering analysis. J Am Coll Cardiol. 2021;78(22):2177–92.
34. Sutton RT, Pincock D, Baumgart DC, Sadowski DC, Fedorak RN, Kroeker KI. An overview of clinical decision support systems: benefits, risks, and strategies for success. NPJ Digit Med. 2020;3:17.
35. Chan HP, Hadjiiski LM, Samala RK. Computer-aided diagnosis in the era of deep learning. Med Phys. 2020;47(5):e218–e27.
36. Chen PC, Liu Y, Peng L. How to develop machine learning models for healthcare. Nat Mater. 2019;18(5):410–4.

Treatment of Amyloid Light-Chain Amyloidosis

Gabriele Buda, Paolo Morfino, Alberto Aimo, and Ashutosh D. Wechalekar

Abbreviations

AL	Amyloid light-chain amyloidosis
ASCT	Autologous stem cell transplantation
BMDex	Bortezomib-melphalan-dexamethasone
CR	Complete response
CyBorD	Cyclophosphamide-bortezomib-dexamethasone
dFLC	Difference between involved and uninvolved FLC
eGFR	Estimated glomerular filtration rate
FLCs	Free light chains
HDM/ASCT	Melphalan followed by ASCT
Ig	Immunoglobulin
IMiD	Immunomodulatory drug
mAb	Monoclonal antibody

G. Buda (✉)
Hematology Division, University Hospital of Pisa, Pisa, Italy
e-mail: g.buda@ao-pisa.toscana.it

P. Morfino
Interdisciplinary Center for Health Sciences, Scuola Superiore Sant'Anna, Pisa, Italy
e-mail: paolo.morfino@santannapisa.it

A. Aimo
Interdisciplinary Center for Health Sciences, Scuola Superiore Sant'Anna, Pisa, Italy

Cardiology Division, Fondazione Toscana Gabriele Monasterio, Pisa, Italy
e-mail: aimoalb@ftgm.it

A. D. Wechalekar
University College London and the Royal Free London NHS Foundation Trust, London, UK
e-mail: a.wechalekar@ucl.ac.uk

M. Emdin et al. (eds.), *Cardiac Amyloidosis*,
https://doi.org/10.1007/978-3-031-51757-0_20

MDex	Melphalan-dexamethasone
MM	Multiple myeloma
NT-proBNP	N-terminal pro-B-type natriuretic peptide
NYHA	New York Heart Association
PI	Proteasome inhibitor
PR	Partial response
VCD	Bortezomib-cyclophosphamide-dexamethasone
VGPR	Very good partial response

Amyloid light-chain (AL) amyloidosis is caused by abnormal production of immunoglobulin (Ig) κ or λ free light chains (FLC) by clonal plasma cells. FLCs transform into amyloid fibrils and progressively accumulate in organs and tissues, most often the heart, kidneys, and bone marrow, but also the liver, soft tissues, gastrointestinal tract, and peripheral nervous system [1]. AL amyloidosis is a rare condition, with an incidence of about 10 cases per million per year [2]. AL treatment has many similarities with multiple myeloma (MM), which is approximately five times more frequent and that must be necessarily excluded as a differential diagnosis [1, 3].

Patients newly diagnosed with AL amyloidosis should be addressed to a tertiary center with experience in multidisciplinary management of this condition, and they are possibly enrolled in clinical trials [4, 5]. The lack of reliable and affordable preclinical models has hampered translational research and pharmacological testing in AL amyloidosis. The treatment of AL amyloidosis consisted of melphalan and steroids (mainly prednisone) until the introduction of autologous hematopoietic stem cell transplantation (ASCT) in the 1990s, following the success of ASCT in MM [6]. Drug agents targeting molecular mechanisms of the disease were introduced in the late 2000s and include immunomodulatory drugs (IMiDs) and proteasome inhibitors (PIs). Daratumumab combined with cyclophosphamide-bortezomib-dexamethasone (CyBorD or VCD) is the only approved therapy for AL amyloidosis [3]. Further therapies for AL amyloidosis are emerging, including monoclonal antibodies (mAb) targeting AL amyloid (Fig. 20.1).

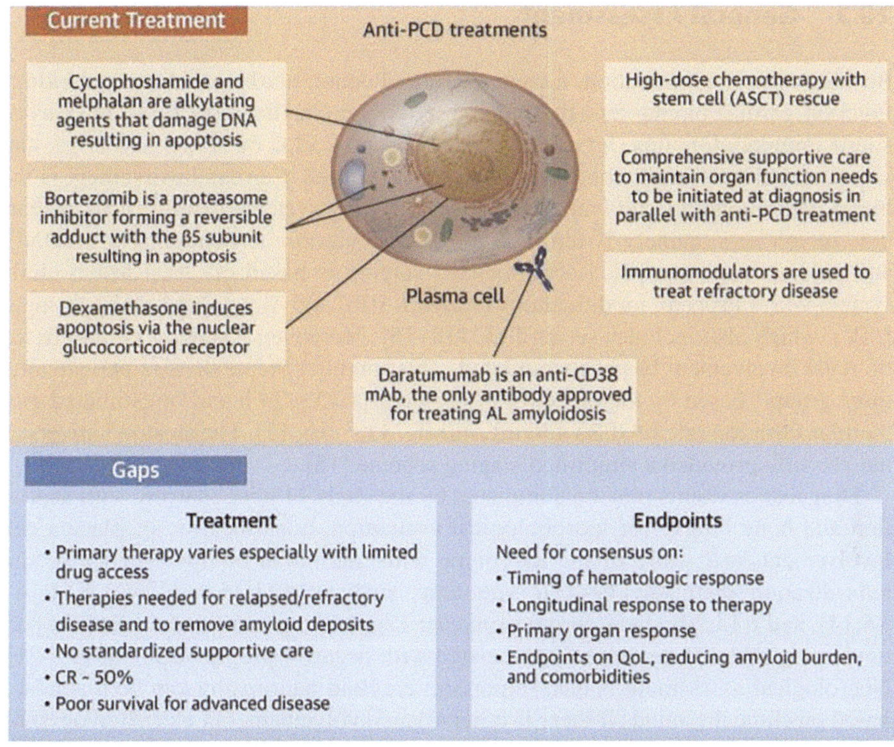

Fig. 20.1 Therapeutic targets in ALThis figure summarizes the current therapeutic targets in AL amyloidosis, as well as the gaps that still exist in treatment and in relevant endpoints. *AL* amyloid light chain, *ASCT* autologous stem cell transplantation, *CR* complete response, *PCD* plasma cell dyscrasia, *QoL* quality of life. Reprinted from Wechalekar et al. [1]

20.1 General Principles of Treatment

Early diagnosis and treatment have improved the outcomes of patients with AL amyloidosis, achieving sometimes stable remissions, although recurrences remain common [7–9]. Remission is achieved by reducing amyloid deposits and the production of amyloidogenic precursors by therapies targeting the clonal plasma cells [4]. Patients treated with current therapeutic regimens usually achieve an improvement in organ function after several months (median 10.4 months), and only 25–50% of all treated patients reach an organ response [10]. The major prognostic determinant in AL amyloidosis is cardiac involvement. The presence of myocardial damage requires a specific supportive therapy and is crucially important to plan the hematological therapeutic strategy [11, 12].

20.2 General Assessment

Besides clinical examination, a complete blood count, markers of liver and kidney function, cardiac biomarkers, thyroid and serum protein electrophoresis, an assay of single immunoglobulins (IgG, IgA, or IgM), κ and λ FLC on serum and urine, and serum and urinary immunofixation should be obtained. Cardiac involvement is the major determinant of survival. Thus, patient staging systems mainly focus on cardiac biomarkers, namely N-terminal pro-B-type natriuretic peptide (NT-proBNP) and cardiac troponins [4]. Recommended staging is based on 2004 Mayo clinic system with European modifications (stages I–IIIb) and Mayo 2012 update (stages I–IV), which also includes serum FLC [13–15]. Moreover, a staging system based on renal involvement has been validated. This staging scheme divides patients into three groups, based on the presence of proteinuria >5 g/24 h and/or estimated glomerular filtration rate (eGFR) <50 mL/min/1.73 m^2 [16, 17]. The Boston University has recently provided a simplified staging scheme [18].

Diagnostics exams may be completed by the study of bone marrow with aspiration and bone biopsy for morphological evaluation, quantification of plasma cell involvement, and study of the karyotype with traditional or fluorescence in situ hybridization methods [19–21]. Mutations such as t(11;14), t(4;14), t(14;16), t(6;14), and t(14;20); 1q + chromosome; or 17p deletion can be identified. In particular, the t(11;14) mutation is associated with negative prognosis in AL [19–21]. Neurological assessment is also important: amyloid neuropathy can be diagnosed based on clinical grounds if there is other organ involvement, but electromyography and nerve conduction studies are recommended [22]. Ultrasound and computed tomography imaging may help assess organ involvement, in particular kidney and liver, but also lungs, gastrointestinal tract, abdominal fat, and heart [23, 24].

As a final remark, advice on fertility preservation options is appropriate if patients wish to have children after therapy, as therapy can have negative effects on fecundity.

20.3 Assessment of Response

Response to therapy in AL amyloidosis reflects the direct effect of chemotherapy on the plasma cell clone and the impact on major organs' function. A good hematologic response is usually associated with better organ responses, but sometimes, there may be discrepancies [25]. Clinical response evaluation is based on hematological and organ criteria established by the International Society of Amyloidosis and is crucial in both the prognostic stratification and clinical management of patients [25, 26].

The hematological response can be assessed by calculating the difference between FLC (dFLC) involved and not involved in the amyloidogenic process. For example, in IgG λ amyloidosis, λ FLCs are the involved FLCs, and κ the noninvolved FLCs. A complete response (CR) is defined as the normalization of dFLC plus negative serum and urinary immunofixation. Very good partial response

(VGPR) is defined as dFLC <40 mg/L, partial response (PR) as dFLC reduction >50%, and absence of response as the other instances [25, 26]. The achievement of CR (grade B, level IIb) with involved FLC <20 mg/L or dFLC <10 mg/L (grade B, level III) represents the goal of treatment in AL amyloidosis, because it is associated with better outcomes [25, 27]. Current guidelines recommend an evaluation of hematological response at least monthly and reconsidering therapy if the patient does not achieve significant response, defined as the response <PR following two cycles or < VGPR following three cycles (grade C, level IV) [25]. Furthermore, an early good response (at least VGPR after 1 month) results in improved survival in all Mayo disease stages, and the prolonged treatment is associated with increased response (34.1%, 57.1%, and 65% ≥ VGPR at 1, 3, and 6 months, respectively) [28].

Cardiac response is defined as a reduction of NT-proBNP >30% and > 300 ng/L (if baseline levels are >650 ng/L) or New York Heart Association (NYHA) class response ≥2 (if baseline NYHA class 3 or 4). As for the other organs, renal response is defined as ≥30% decrease in proteinuria or drop below 0.5 g/24 h, in the absence of kidney progression, defined as >25% decrease in eGFR, while liver response as a ≥ 50% decrease in abnormal alkaline phosphatase value or decrease in radiographic liver size ≥2 cm [25, 26].

20.4 Autologous Bone Marrow Transplantation

Around 20–25% of patients with newly diagnosed AL amyloidosis are eligible for ASCT [29]. Current guidelines propose several criteria for the eligibility to ASCT (Table 20.1) [30]. In eligible subjects, guidelines recommend high-dose (200 mg/m^2) melphalan followed by transplant (HDM/ASCT) [26, 29–31]. There is some evidence that splitting the dose over 2 days results in decreased toxicity [32]. Dose reduction of melphalan to 140 based on the extent of renal involvement (eGFR ≤30) has resulted in improved outcome for patients at high risk and is then recommended [30].

In experienced centers, VGPR is achieved in approximately 70% of patients, and patients with a CR have a median survival of more than 15 years [33]. In a large series, 84% of patients undergoing ASCT achieved hematologic response, with VGPR rate of 33% and CR of 39%, which increased to 60% if associated with bortezomib treatment after transplant [33]. Young age, minimal cardiac involvement, κ light-chain disease, and full-dose melphalan conditioning have been associated with longer survival [34].

Induction therapy is usually not necessary, and patients can directly proceed to ASCT after stem cell mobilization [35]. When a delay in transplantation is expected, if the patient also has MM or the plasma cell burden exceeds 10% of bone marrow cells, 2–4 cycles of induction therapy are advisable [30, 32, 36]. Traditionally, CyBorD and bortezomib-melphalan-dexamethasone (BMDex) were the two most common strategies. However, daratumumab, which is an anti-CD38 human IgG-κ mAb previously administered for relapsed or refractory AL amyloidosis, has recently been included in the standard therapy [30]. In particular, the ANDROMEDA

Table 20.1 Eligibility criteria for ASCT in AL amyloidosis

Eligibility criteria	Exclusion criteria
• AL amyloidosis with end-organ damage confirmed with tissue biopsy • Clear evidence of a clonal PCD • Age 18–70 years • LVEF ≥40% • Oxygen saturation on room air >95% • eGFR >30 mL/min/1.73 m^2 • Cardiac TnI <0.1 ng/mL; TnT levels <60 ng/L, hs-TnT <75 ng/mL • Supine systolic blood pressure ≥ 90 mmHg • ECOG Performance Score ≤ 2 • NYHA class <3 • NT-proBNP <5000 pg/mL • Direct bilirubin <2 mg/dL • DLCO >50% • At least one major organ involvement (soft tissues or bone marrow alone is not considered) • Patients on chronic and stable schedule of dialysis if other eligibility criteria are met	• Symptomatic and/or refractory pleural effusions • Uncompensated heart failure • Symptomatic and/or refractory ventricular and atrial arrhythmias • Orthostatic hypotension refractory to therapy • Acquired factor X deficiency with a factor X level < 25% and/or active bleeding • Gastrointestinal involvement with bleeding or risk of bleeding

The table summarizes all broad eligibility and exclusion criteria for ASCT in patients with AL amyloidosis according to the 2021 EHA-ISA guidelines [30]. *AL* light-chain amyloidosis, *ASCT* autologous stem cell transplantation, *DLCO* diffusing capacity of the lungs for carbon monoxide, *ECOG* Eastern Cooperative Oncology Group, *eGFR* estimated glomerular filtration rate, *hs-* high sensitivity, *LVEF* left ventricular ejection fraction, *NYHA* New York Heart Association, *NT-proBNP* N-terminal pro-B-type natriuretic peptide, *PCD* plasma cell dyscrasia, *Tn* troponin

(A Study to Evaluate the Efficacy and Safety of Daratumumab in Combination With Cyclophosphamide, Bortezomib and Dexamethasone [CyBorD] Compared to CyBorD Alone in Newly Diagnosed Systemic Amyloid Light-Chain [AL] Amyloidosis) phase 3 trial demonstrated that daratumumab combined with CyBorD compared with CyBorD alone had a surprisingly high rate of at least VGPR (78.5% vs. 49.2%), as well as a decreased risk of major organ deterioration or hematologic progression or death (hazard ratio 0.58; 95% confidence interval 0.36–0.93) in patients with newly diagnosed AL [37]. Therefore, the preferred induction therapy before HDM/ASCT now includes daratumumab plus CyBorD [26, 37].

The guidelines do not recommend the routine use of maintenance or consolidation therapy following ASCT, which usually consists of the same regimen administered as induction treatment, because of limited clinical evidence [30]. On the other hand, consolidation therapy may be effective in patients who do not achieve at least VGPR and who were not treated with induction therapy [30, 38].

No clear demonstration has been provided of the better outcome of ASCT vs. conventional chemotherapy [3, 32]. For example, in a phase 3 trial in patients with new diagnosis of AL amyloidosis, melphalan combined with dexamethasone was associated with a longer overall survival compared with HDM/ASCT [39].

Nevertheless, ASCT is strongly recommended in patients with AL amyloidosis and symptomatic myeloma, and those with IgM-AL amyloidosis [25]. The prognosis of transplanted patients improves in high-volume centers and where candidates have been carefully selected. The advance in transplant techniques also resulted in a reduction of mortality during the acute phase, which is now around 3% in specialized centers [40]. However, patients with AL amyloidosis are at risk of transplant-related death due to sepsis, arrhythmias, intractable hypotension, gastrointestinal bleeding, or multiorgan failure, even more than those with MM, and then need to be managed in specialist centers with multidisciplinary teams [41].

20.5 Therapy in Patients Not Candidates to Transplantation

The standard of care for patients with a new diagnosis of AL amyloidosis and not eligible for ASCT consists of anti-plasma cell dyscrasia chemotherapy. For patients with cardiac stages I–IIIa, daratumumab-CyBorD is recommended, and CyBorD is a second option (Table 20.2). For patients with cardiac stage IIIb, dose-modified daratumumab-CyBorD or single-agent daratumumab should be considered, and dose-modified CyBorD alternatively [26]. In patients with advanced cardiac disease, collaboration with the cardiologist is crucial for the management of heart failure (HF). In relatively young patients and without severe extracardiac disease, heart transplantation should be discussed [25, 26]. For patients with neuropathy, single-agent daratumumab or lenalidomide-dexamethasone or oral MDex or carfilzomib-dexamethasone or venetoclax may be considered, but single-agent daratumumab is preferred [25].

Treatment with <u>alkylating agents</u> (melphalan and cyclophosphamide) combined with corticosteroids is a safe and tolerable option but is considered suboptimal. Alkylating agents impair cell proliferation and transcription by inducing guanine-based inter-strand cross-links and DNA damage [3]. The melphalan-dexamethasone (MDex) regimen leads to a hematological response in up to 76% of cases, but it is more effective when combined with bortezomib (BMDex) (hematological response of 57% vs. 81% at 3 months) [25, 42]. The use of MDex without bortezomib can be particularly effective in elderly or frail patients and/or those with cardiac dysfunction [43]. As alkylating agents are nonspecific therapies, adverse effects as cytopenia and gastrointestinal toxicities are commonly reported [3]. Usually, the MDex regimen is administered orally for four consecutive days at 28-day intervals at the following doses [44]: melphalan 0.22 mg/kg and dexamethasone 40 mg/kg.

The use of <u>PIs</u> (bortezomib, carfilzomib, ixazomib) has revolutionized the treatment of AL amyloidosis, because clonal plasma cells' vitality strongly relies on proteasome integrity, which mitigates the proteotoxicity induced by misfolded light chains [3]. The three approved PIs target the catalytic function of the proteasome [3]. The CyBorD regime, which was introduced in 2009, represents the first-choice therapy and provides a hematological response of 60–65% and a CR of 18–25% [15, 25, 45]. Bortezomib as a single agent or with dexamethasone is effective and well tolerated but should be used cautiously in patients with pulmonary disease

Table 20.2 Recommendations for non-transplant treatment of light-chain amyloidosis

Status	Patient		Risk assessment	Recommended treatments	
				First choice	Alternative
Newly diagnosed	Patients without significant neuropathy		Cardiac stage I–IIIa	Dara-CyBorD[a] (Grade A; Level Ia)	CyBorD[b] (Grade B; Level IIa) VMDex[a] (Grade A; Level Ia)
			Cardiac stages IIIb	Dose-modified Dara-CyBorD[c] (grade C; level IV) Single agent daratumumab[c] (grade B; level III)	Dose modified CyBorD[b] Or VMDex[b] (Grade C; Level IV)
	Patients with significant neuropathy		All stages*	Single-agent daratumumab[c] (grade C; level IV) Lenalidomide-dexamethasone[b] (grade C; level IV)	MelDex[b] or carfilzomib-Dex[c] or venetoclax[c] (grade C; level IV)
Relapsed	PI-naïve or prolonged response to first-line PI		All stages*	CyBorD/VMDex[b] (level B; grade III) Ixazomib-Dex[a] (grade A; level Ib)	Dara-V(C)D[c] (level C; grade IV)
	PI-exposed	Daratumumab-naïve	All stages*	Single agent daratumumab[b] (level B; grade IIb) Dara-V(C)D[c] (level C; grade IV)	Dara-RD[b] (level B; grade III) Isatuximab[c] (level C; grade IV)
		IMiD-naïve	All stages*	Lenalidomide-dexamethasone (±cyclophosphamide)[b] (level B; grade IIa)	IRD[b] (grade B; level IIb)
		Lenalidomide refractory	All stages*	Pomalidomide-dexamethasone[b] (level B; grade IIa)	Bendamustine[b] (level B; grade IIa)
		t(11;14)	All stages*	Venetoclax[c] (grade B; level III)	Venetoclax-bortezomib-dexamethasone[c] (grade C; level III) MelDex[c] (grade C; level IV)

Table 20.2 (continued)

				Recommended treatments	
Status	Patient		Risk assessment	First choice	Alternative
IgM-AL[**]			All stages[*]	Rituximab-bendamustine[c] (grade B; level IIb) ASCT[c] (grade B, level IIb)	Rituximab-bort-Dex[c] or rituximab-Cyclo-Dex[c] or CyBorD[c] or ibrutinib (±Ritux)[c] (level C; grade IV)

Therapeutic options for patients with AL amyloidosis not undergoing autologous stem cell transplant according to the 2021 EHA-ISA guidelines, *ACST* autologous stem cell transplantation, *CyBorD* cyclophosphamide-bortezomib-dexamethasone, *Dara* daratumumab, *Dex* dexamethasone, *IRD* ixazomib-lenalidomide-dexamethasone, *MelDex* oral melphalan-dexamethasone, *Ritux* rituximab, *VCD* bortezomib-cyclophosphamide-dexamethasone, *VD* bortezomib-dexamethasone, *VMDex* bortezomib-melphalan-dexamethasone. Stages: defined as per the European update of Mayo 2004 staging system

Modified from Wechalekar et al. [25]

[*]Dose modification and adjustments mandatory in patients with advanced end-organ damage (cardiac or other)

[**]IgM-related AL with lymphoid component in the bone marrow

[a,b,c]Levels of available evidence for the recommendation

because of the possible lung toxicity [25]. Bortezomib is used in most protocols together with steroids or with the addition of cyclophosphamide (according to the CyBorD scheme) for induction therapy. The CyBorD regimen is usually administered once a week in 28-day cycles at the following doses [46]:

- Cyclophosphamide: 500 mg orally.
- Bortezomib: 1.3–1.5 mg/m^2 subcutaneously.
- Dexamethasone: 20–40 mg orally.

Dose adjustments for renal disease progression are not required [15]. CyBorD may be less effective in patients with t(11;14) mutation, while cytogenetics related to high risk in MM, including t(4;14), t(14;16), del(17p), and gain of 1q21, have no effect on clinical outcomes [21, 25]. Combined therapy consisting of bortezomib-melphalan-dexamethasone and bortezomib-lenalidomide-dexamethasone was associated with significant hematologic remission, but adverse effects were more frequent compared with traditional CyBorD [47, 48].

Ixazomib is a second-generation PI given orally and is less neurotoxic than bortezomib [3]. Ixazomib appeared beneficial in relapsed or refractory AL amyloidosis both as a single agent and in combination with lenalidomide and dexamethasone [25, 49]. Carfilzomib is an irreversible second-generation PI with high efficacy compared to bortezomib in relapsed/refractory MM [3]. Cardiovascular and renal toxicity contraindicate its use in AL amyloidosis [25].

IMiD agents (thalidomide, lenalidomide, pomalidomide) impair cancer microenvironment by inhibiting angiogenesis and stimulating immune response. Thalidomide is rarely prescribed because of the high risk for neurological and gastrointestinal toxicity [25]. Lenalidomide is generally effective, especially in combined therapies, but is poorly tolerated at the full 25 mg daily dose [25]. Frequent adverse events include skin rashes, thrombotic complications, infections, fatigue, and impaired renal function. Pomalidomide is more tolerated and more effective [50]. IMiDs generally cause an elevation of serum NT-proBNP, which is often transient [25].

IMiD therapies based on lenalidomide and dexamethasone are administered in 28-day cycles in the following doses [51]:

- Lenalidomide: 15 mg orally for 21 consecutive days.
- Dexamethasone: 40 mg orally once a week.

Pomalidomide is usually associated with dexamethasone in 28-day cycles (2 mg per day of pomalidomide, with possible adjustments based on toxicity and response). Adverse events include neuropathy and fatigue [52].

As discussed above, the mAb daratumumab has proven dramatically effective as up-front treatment of patients with AL amyloidosis CIT. Intravenous daratumumab may be given in divided doses to reduce fluid volume, but the subcutaneous formulation is preferred.

Given the limited data, maintenance therapy in AL amyloidosis is not recommended. However, patients with AL and background of myeloma may benefit from maintenance treatment, as recommended by guidelines for MM [25]. Additionally, the role of consolidation therapy in AL amyloidosis has been poorly explored. Daily consolidation therapy is not recommended, but it may be considered in patients with VGPR or CR with persistent minimal residual disease and no organ response [25]. In this setting, the availability and low toxicity related to daratumumab provides novel perspectives.

To summarize, a combination of daratumumab-CyBorD is the gold standard in patients ineligible for ASCT. If daratumumab administration is not pursuable, then a bortezomib-based triplet combination, either CyBord (preferred by expert consensus) or BMDex, is recommended. Expert consensus recommends a therapeutic duration of at least two cycles after the optimal response. In patients with at least VGPR after three cycles, based on tolerance, treatment can be prolonged to a total of 6–8 cycles (Fig. 20.2) [25].

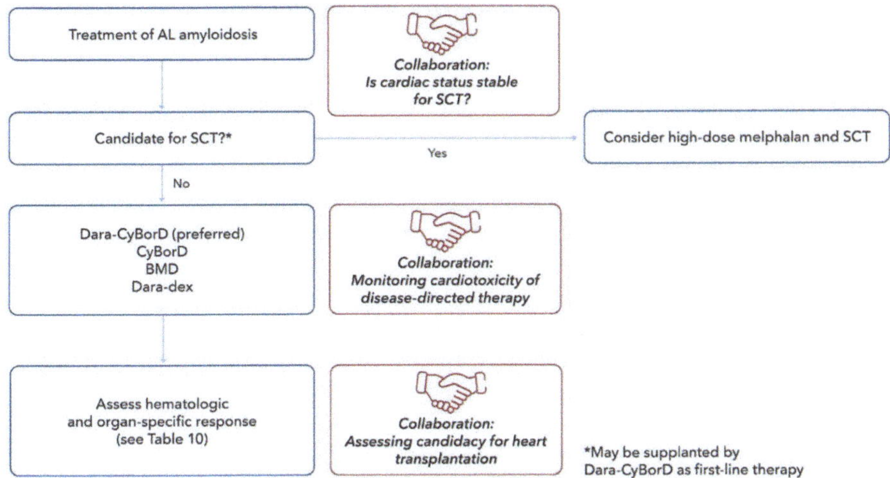

Fig. 20.2 Treatment options for patients with AL amyloidosisThe figure schematically summarizes the management options for patients with AL amyloidosis according to the 2023 American College of Cardiology guidelines. AL, light-chain amyloidosis, *BMD* bortezomib-melphalan-dexamethasone, *CyBorD* cyclophosphamide, bortezomib, and dexamethasone, *Dara* daratumumab, *dex* dexamethasone, *SCT* stem cell transplantation. Reprinted with permission from Kittleson et al. [62]

20.6 Therapy of Relapsing or Non-responding Patients

Patients who relapse or do not respond to therapy following either ASCT or standard chemotherapy may be treated with first- or second-generation PIs (carfilzomib or ixazomib) or IMiDs at lower doses than those used for MM, such as lenalidomide, thalidomide, or pomalidomide, or mAb, but also with bendamustine, and HDM/ASCT [25].

Ixazomib may prove effective in relapsed AL, as suggested by a phase 3 trial in patients with no previous exposure to PIs [53]. Serious concerns about carfilzomib toxicity exist [25]. Several observational studies and a phase 2 trial demonstrated that daratumumab results in high hematological response rate in AL-relapsed patients [54]. IMiD administration in relapsed AL needs further investigation because of the associated cardiotoxicity, which may be symptomatic. Thalidomide is generally associated with dexamethasone and sometimes with cyclophosphamide. However, its cardiac toxicity and the risk of neuropathy and thrombosis requiring antithrombotic prophylaxis make this therapeutic scheme much less used than lenalidomide- or pomalidomide-based regimens, which appear more tolerable [49]. Patients who had a durable response after an up-front transplant may still meet ASCT eligibility criteria and can then be considered for a second transplant [4].

Guideline-guided therapy for relapsed AL amyloidosis is summarized in Table 20.2 [25]:

- Patients PI-naïve or with prolonged response to first-line PI: CyBorD or bortezomib-melphalan-dexamethasone; ixazomib-dexamethasone; daratumumab; and bortezomib-(cyclophosphamide)-dexamethasone (V(C)D).
- Patients PI-exposed daratumumab-naïve: single-agent daratumumab, daratumumab-V(C)D, daratumumab and rituximab-dexamethasone, isatuximab.
- Patients PI-exposed and IMiDs-naïve: lenalidomide-dexamethasone-(cyclophosphamide), ixazomib-lenalidomide-dexamethasone.
- Patients refractory to lenalidomide: pomalidomide-dexamethasone, bendamustine.

20.7 Selective Anti-fibril Therapy

In the setting of AL amyloidosis, mAbs may be used to target amyloid fibrils, thus triggering their removal through immunological recruitment of phagocytic cells [55]. Although anti-fibril therapies are still not recommended outside of clinical trials, promising results encourage their utilization [25].

Birtamimab (NEOD001) is a humanized IgG1 mAb binding to a critical epitope exposed by misfolded AL amyloid fibrils [56]. Birtamimab was proven to be safe and well tolerated in patients with previously treated AL amyloidosis, but the phase 3 VITAL trial (NCT02312206) including newly diagnosed AL-CA patients was not likely to meet its primary endpoint (composite of all-cause mortality and cardiac hospitalizations) and was then halted after an interim futility analysis [57, 58]. However, post hoc analyses reported a significant improvement in survival and quality of life among patients with advanced disease (Mayo stage IV) receiving birtamimab plus standard therapy [59]. Based on these results, the phase 3 AFFIRM-AL trial (NCT04973137) enrolling patients with Mayo stage IV AL amyloidosis is ongoing.

The IgG1 mAb anselamimab (CAEL-101), which targets a neo-epitope of misfolded AL fibrils, represents another potential anti-fibril agent. CAEL-101 was safe and well tolerated in patients with AL amyloidosis, with some patients manifesting beneficial cardiac response (improved global longitudinal strain) [60, 61]. Two phase 3 trials enrolling patients with AL amyloidosis are ongoing (NCT04512235 and NCT04504825).

20.8 Conclusions

Recent therapeutic advances have revolutionized the management of patients with AL amyloidosis, but the management of this disease remains complex and requires specialized centers. The results of recent trials and the ongoing research activity let us hope for further progress in the near future.

References

1. Wechalekar AD, Fontana M, Quarta CC, et al. AL amyloidosis for cardiologists: awareness, diagnosis, and future prospects: JACC: cardiooncology state-of-the-art review. JACC CardioOncol. 2022;4(4):427–41.
2. Kumar N, Zhang NJ, Cherepanov D, et al. Global epidemiology of amyloid light-chain amyloidosis. Orphanet J Rare Dis. 2022;17(1):278.
3. Bianchi G, Zhang Y, Comenzo RL. AL amyloidosis: current chemotherapy and immune therapy treatment strategies: JACC: CardioOncology state-of-the-art review. JACC CardioOncol. 2021;3(4):467–87.
4. Cook J, Muchtar E, Warsame R. Updates in the diagnosis and management of AL amyloidosis. Curr Hematol Malig Rep. 2020;15(3):155–67.
5. Dispenzieri A, Buadi F, Kumar SK, et al. Treatment of immunoglobulin light chain amyloidosis: mayo stratification of myeloma and risk-adapted therapy (mSMART) consensus statement. Mayo Clin Proc. 2015;90(8):1054–81.
6. Sanchorawala V. High-dose Melphalan and autologous peripheral blood stem cell transplantation in AL amyloidosis. Acta Haematol. 2020;143(4):381–7.
7. Kyle RA, Larson DR, Therneau TM, et al. Long-term follow-up of monoclonal gammopathy of undetermined significance. N Engl J Med. 2018;378(3):241–9.
8. Muchtar E, Gertz MA, Kumar SK, et al. Improved outcomes for newly diagnosed AL amyloidosis between 2000 and 2014: cracking the glass ceiling of early death. Blood. 2017;129(15):2111–9.
9. Rajkumar SV, Gertz MA, Kyle RA. Primary systemic amyloidosis with delayed progression to multiple myeloma. Cancer. 1998;82(8):1501–5.
10. Kaufman GP, Dispenzieri A, Gertz MA, et al. Kinetics of organ response and survival following normalization of the serum free light chain ratio in AL amyloidosis. Am J Hematol. 2015;90(3):181–6.
11. Palladini G, Merlini G. How I treat AL amyloidosis. Blood. 2022;139(19):2918–30.
12. Palladini G, Merlini G. What is new in diagnosis and management of light chain amyloidosis? Blood. 2016;128(2):159–68.
13. Dispenzieri A, Gertz MA, Kyle RA, et al. Serum cardiac troponins and N-terminal pro-brain natriuretic peptide: a staging system for primary systemic amyloidosis. J Clin Oncol. 2004;22(18):3751–7.
14. Kumar S, Dispenzieri A, Lacy MQ, et al. Revised prognostic staging system for light chain amyloidosis incorporating cardiac biomarkers and serum free light chain measurements. J Clin Oncol. 2012;30(9):989–95.
15. Palladini G, Sachchithanantham S, Milani P, et al. A European collaborative study of cyclophosphamide, bortezomib, and dexamethasone in upfront treatment of systemic AL amyloidosis. Blood. 2015;126(5):612–5.
16. Palladini G, Hegenbart U, Milani P, et al. A staging system for renal outcome and early markers of renal response to chemotherapy in AL amyloidosis. Blood. 2014;124(15):2325–32.
17. Havasi A, Stern L, Lo S, et al. Validation of new renal staging system in AL amyloidosis treated with high dose melphalan and stem cell transplantation. Am J Hematol. 2016;91(10):E458–60.
18. Lilleness B, Ruberg FL, Mussinelli R, et al. Development and validation of a survival staging system incorporating BNP in patients with light chain amyloidosis. Blood. 2019;133(3):215–23.
19. Bochtler T, Hegenbart U, Kunz C, et al. Prognostic impact of cytogenetic aberrations in AL amyloidosis patients after high-dose melphalan: a long-term follow-up study. Blood. 2016;128(4):594–602.
20. Bryce AH, Ketterling RP, Gertz MA, et al. Translocation t(11;14) and survival of patients with light chain (AL) amyloidosis. Haematologica. 2009;94(3):380–6.
21. Bochtler T, Hegenbart U, Kunz C, et al. Translocation t(11;14) is associated with adverse outcome in patients with newly diagnosed AL amyloidosis when treated with bortezomib-based regimens. J Clin Oncol. 2015;33(12):1371–8.

22. Weber N, Mollee P, Augustson B, et al. Management of systemic AL amyloidosis: recommendations of the Myeloma Foundation of Australia Medical and Scientific Advisory Group. Intern Med J. 2015;45(4):371–82.
23. Merlini G, Seldin DC, Gertz MA. Amyloidosis: pathogenesis and new therapeutic options. J Clin Oncol. 2011;29(14):1924–33.
24. Gertz MA, Comenzo R, Falk RH, et al. Definition of organ involvement and treatment response in immunoglobulin light chain amyloidosis (AL): a consensus opinion from the 10th International Symposium on Amyloid and Amyloidosis, Tours, France, 18–22 April 2004. Am J Hematol. 2005;79(4):319–28.
25. Wechalekar AD, Cibeira MT, Gibbs SD, et al. Guidelines for non-transplant chemotherapy for treatment of systemic AL amyloidosis: EHA-ISA working group. Amyloid. 2023;30(1):3–17.
26. Writing C, Kittleson MM, Ruberg FL, et al. 2023 ACC expert consensus decision pathway on comprehensive multidisciplinary care for the patient with cardiac amyloidosis: a report of the American College of Cardiology solution set oversight committee. J Am Coll Cardiol. 2023;81(11):1076–126.
27. Sidana S, Dispenzieri A, Murray DL, et al. Revisiting complete response in light chain amyloidosis. Leukemia. 2020;34(5):1472–5.
28. Ravichandran S, Cohen OC, Law S, et al. Impact of early response on outcomes in AL amyloidosis following treatment with frontline Bortezomib. Blood Cancer J. 2021;11(6):118.
29. Palladini G, Milani P, Merlini G. Management of AL amyloidosis in 2020. Blood. 2020;136(23):2620–7.
30. Sanchorawala V, Boccadoro M, Gertz M, et al. Guidelines for high dose chemotherapy and stem cell transplantation for systemic AL amyloidosis: EHA-ISA working group guidelines. Amyloid. 2022;29(1):1–7.
31. Garcia-Pavia P, Rapezzi C, Adler Y, et al. Diagnosis and treatment of cardiac amyloidosis: a position statement of the ESC Working Group on Myocardial and Pericardial Diseases. Eur Heart J. 2021;42(16):1554–68.
32. Bomsztyk J, Khwaja J, Wechalekar AD. Recent guidelines for high-dose chemotherapy and autologous stem cell transplant for systemic AL amyloidosis: a practitioner's perspective. Expert Rev Hematol. 2022;15(9):781–8.
33. Sanchorawala V, Sun F, Quillen K, et al. Long-term outcome of patients with AL amyloidosis treated with high-dose melphalan and stem cell transplantation: 20-year experience. Blood. 2015;126(20):2345–7.
34. Sidana S, Sidiqi MH, Dispenzieri A, et al. Fifteen year overall survival rates after autologous stem cell transplantation for AL amyloidosis. Am J Hematol. 2019;94(9):1020–6.
35. Schonland SO, Lokhorst H, Buzyn A, et al. Allogeneic and syngeneic hematopoietic cell transplantation in patients with amyloid light-chain amyloidosis: a report from the European Group for Blood and Marrow Transplantation. Blood. 2006;107(6):2578–84.
36. Kourelis TV, Kumar SK, Gertz MA, et al. Coexistent multiple myeloma or increased bone marrow plasma cells define equally high-risk populations in patients with immunoglobulin light chain amyloidosis. J Clin Oncol. 2013;31(34):4319–24.
37. Kastritis E, Palladini G, Minnema MC, et al. Daratumumab-based treatment for immunoglobulin light-chain amyloidosis. N Engl J Med. 2021;385(1):46–58.
38. Al Saleh AS, Sidiqi MH, Sidana S, et al. Impact of consolidation therapy post autologous stem cell transplant in patients with light chain amyloidosis. Am J Hematol. 2019;94(10):1066–71.
39. Jaccard A, Moreau P, Leblond V, et al. High-dose melphalan versus melphalan plus dexamethasone for AL amyloidosis. N Engl J Med. 2007;357(11):1083–93.
40. D'Souza A, Dispenzieri A, Wirk B, et al. Improved outcomes after autologous hematopoietic cell transplantation for light chain amyloidosis: a Center for International Blood and Marrow Transplant Research Study. J Clin Oncol. 2015;33(32):3741–9.
41. Wechalekar AD, Goodman HJ, Lachmann HJ, et al. Safety and efficacy of risk-adapted cyclophosphamide, thalidomide, and dexamethasone in systemic AL amyloidosis. Blood. 2007;109(2):457–64.

42. Palladini G, Milani P, Foli A, et al. Oral melphalan and dexamethasone grants extended survival with minimal toxicity in AL amyloidosis: long-term results of a risk-adapted approach. Haematologica. 2014;99(4):743–50.
43. Campo C, da Silva Filho MI, Weinhold N, et al. Bortezomib-induced peripheral neuropathy: a genome-wide association study on multiple myeloma patients. Hematol Oncol. 2018;36(1):232–7.
44. Kastritis E, Leleu X, Arnulf B, et al. A randomized phase III trial of melphalan and dexamethasone (MDex) versus bortezomib, melphalan and dexamethasone (BMDex) for untreated patients with AL amyloidosis. Blood. 2016;128(22):646.
45. Manwani R, Cohen O, Sharpley F, et al. A prospective observational study of 915 patients with systemic AL amyloidosis treated with upfront bortezomib. Blood. 2019;134(25):2271–80.
46. Cibeira MT, Blade J. Upfront CyBorD in AL amyloidosis. Blood. 2015;126(5):564–6.
47. Kastritis E, Dialoupi I, Gavriatopoulou M, et al. Primary treatment of light-chain amyloidosis with bortezomib, lenalidomide, and dexamethasone. Blood Adv. 2019;3(20):3002–9.
48. Kastritis E, Leleu X, Arnulf B, et al. Bortezomib, melphalan, and dexamethasone for light-chain amyloidosis. J Clin Oncol. 2020;38(28):3252–60.
49. Cohen OC, Sharpley F, Gillmore JD, et al. Use of ixazomib, lenalidomide and dexamethasone in patients with relapsed amyloid light-chain amyloidosis. Br J Haematol. 2020;189(4):643–9.
50. Milani P, Sharpley F, Schonland SO, et al. Pomalidomide and dexamethasone grant rapid haematologic responses in patients with relapsed and refractory AL amyloidosis: a European retrospective series of 153 patients. Amyloid. 2020;27(4):231–6.
51. Sanchorawala V, Finn KT, Fennessey S, et al. Durable hematologic complete responses can be achieved with lenalidomide in AL amyloidosis. Blood. 2010;116(11):1990–1.
52. Palladini G, Milani P, Foli A, et al. A phase 2 trial of pomalidomide and dexamethasone rescue treatment in patients with AL amyloidosis. Blood. 2017;129(15):2120–3.
53. Dispenzieri A, Kastritis E, Wechalekar AD, et al. A randomized phase 3 study of ixazomib-dexamethasone versus physician's choice in relapsed or refractory AL amyloidosis. Leukemia. 2022;36(1):225–35.
54. Sanchorawala V, Sarosiek S, Schulman A, et al. Safety, tolerability, and response rates of daratumumab in relapsed AL amyloidosis: results of a phase 2 study. Blood. 2020;135(18):1541–7.
55. Emdin M, Morfino P, Crosta L, et al. Monoclonal antibodies and amyloid removal as a therapeutic strategy for cardiac amyloidosis. Eur Heart J Suppl. 2023;25(Suppl. B):B79–84.
56. Renz M, Torres R, Dolan PJ, et al. 2A4 binds soluble and insoluble light chain aggregates from AL amyloidosis patients and promotes clearance of amyloid deposits by phagocytosis (dagger). Amyloid. 2016;23(3):168–77.
57. Gertz MA, Cohen AD, Comenzo RL, et al. Results of the phase 3 VITAL study of NEOD001 (Birtamimab) plus standard of care in patients with light chain (AL) amyloidosis suggest survival benefit for mayo stage IV patients. Blood. 2019;134(Suppl. 1):3166.
58. Gertz MA, Landau H, Comenzo RL, et al. First-in-human phase I/II study of NEOD001 in patients with light chain amyloidosis and persistent organ dysfunction. J Clin Oncol. 2016;34(10):1097–103.
59. Gertz MA, Cohen AD, Comenzo RL, et al. Birtamimab plus standard of care in light chain amyloidosis: the phase 3 randomized placebo-controlled VITAL trial. Blood. 2023;142(14):1208–18.
60. Edwards CV, Rao N, Bhutani D, et al. Phase 1a/b study of monoclonal antibody CAEL-101 (11-1F4) in patients with AL amyloidosis. Blood. 2021;138(25):2632–41.
61. Valent J, Silowsky J, Kurman MR, et al. Cael-101 is well-tolerated in AL amyloidosis patients receiving concomitant Cyclophosphamide-Bortezomib-Dexamethasone (CyborD): a phase 2 dose-finding study (NCT04304144). Blood. 2020;136(Suppl. 1):26–7.
62. Kittleson MM, Ruberg FL, Ambardekar AV, et al. 2023 ACC expert consensus decision pathway on comprehensive multidisciplinary care for the patient with cardiac amyloidosis. J Am Coll Cardiol. 2023;81(11):1076–126.

Treatment of ATTR Amyloidosis: From Stabilizers to Gene Editing

Aldostefano Porcari, Mathew S. Maurer, and Julian D. Gillmore

21.1 Understanding the Amyloidogenic Cascade to Develop Treatments

Transthyretin (TTR), formerly named prealbumin, is a highly conserved 55 kDa protein composed of four monomers that circulates as a homo-tetramer and functions as a carrier protein for thyroxine and retinol-binding protein (RBP) [1]. The native TTR protein is primarily synthesized in the liver and secreted into the blood, with lesser amounts produced by the choroid plexus and retinal pigmented epithelial cells (Fig. 21.1) [2]. Besides its functions as a carrier protein, TTR has a proteolytic activity involved in the cleavage of apoA-I, neuropeptide Y, and Aβ peptide [1].

A. Porcari
National Amyloidosis Centre, Division of Medicine, University College London, London, UK

Center for Diagnosis and Treatment of Cardiomyopathies, Cardiovascular Department, Azienda Sanitaria Universitaria Giuliano-Isontina (ASUGI), University of Trieste, Trieste, Italy

European Reference Network for Rare, Low Prevalence and Complex Diseases of the Heart-ERNGUARD-Heart, Trieste, Italy
e-mail: aldostefano.porcari@nhs.net

M. S. Maurer
Division of Cardiology, Cardiac Amyloidosis Program, Columbia University Irving Medical Center, New York, NY, USA
e-mail: msm10@cumc.columbia.edu

J. D. Gillmore (✉)
National Amyloidosis Centre, Division of Medicine, University College London, London, UK
e-mail: j.gillmore@ucl.ac.uk

M. Emdin et al. (eds.), *Cardiac Amyloidosis*,
https://doi.org/10.1007/978-3-031-51757-0_21

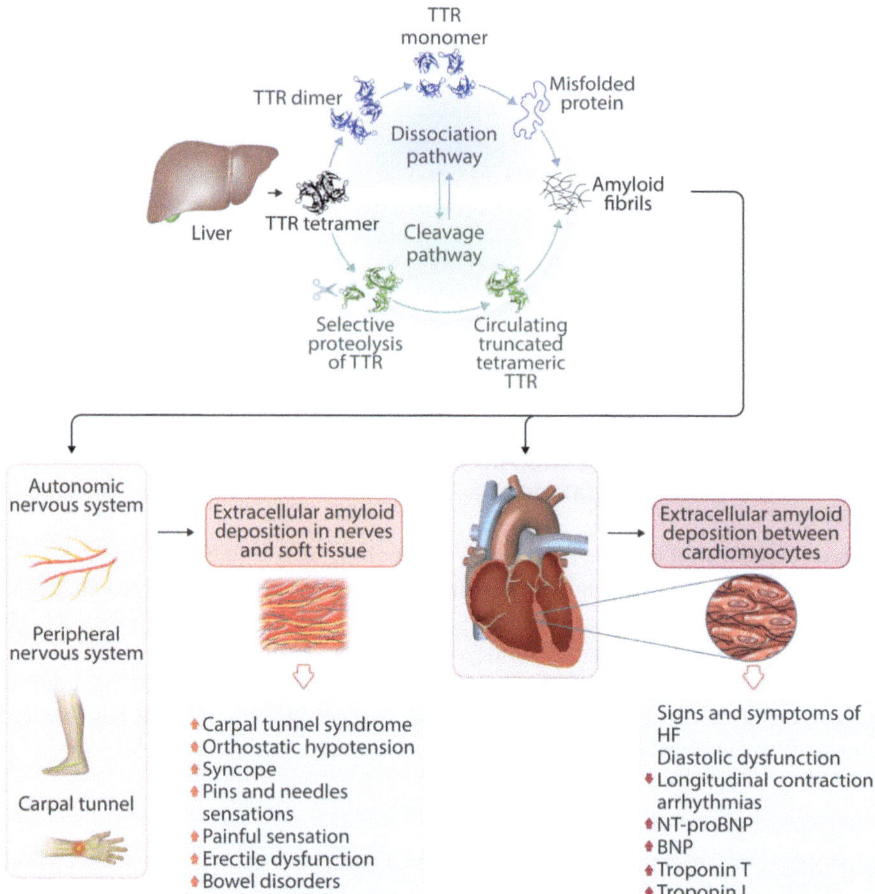

Fig. 21.1 Pathophysiology of transthyretin synthesis with main pathways of the amyloidogenic cascade and consequences of organ involvement. Reproduced from [2] *BNP* brain natriuretic peptide, *HF* heart failure, *NT-proBNP* N-terminal brain natriuretic peptide, *TTR* transthyretin

Transthyretin amyloidosis (ATTR amyloidosis) occurs when TTR misfolds into pathogenic amyloid fibrils. TTR has a native globular structure with a ligand-binding hydrophobic channel at the center of the tetramer, between the dimers [1].

TTR monomers are rich in beta strands and exhibit an intrinsic propensity to aggregate into amyloid fibrils. The amyloidogenic cascade is a complex process, not completely elucidated, and several mechanisms are involved [2]. In vitro, the conversion of TTR into amyloid fibrils starts when the tetrameric form of TTR becomes unstable and the protein dissociates into dimers and monomers that misfold into a non-native conformation. TTR dissociation is the crucial and rate-limiting step in amyloidogenesis under laboratory conditions. TTR instability appears to be promoted by oxidative modifications, age-related failure of homeostatic mechanisms, metal cations, and inherited pathogenic genetic mutations [3]. Misfolded monomers self-assemble in soluble, non-fibrillar oligomers, presumably amyloid fibril precursors, with significant cytotoxic effects on tissues and, later, aggregate and accumulate as amyloid deposits (Fig. 21.1) [2]. Besides TTR tetramer dissociation, a proteolytic pathway for amyloid formation has recently been elucidated using the Ser52Pro TTR variant [4]. This single amino acid substitution promotes susceptibility of the TTR tetramer to selective proteolytic cleavage, resulting in the release of the C-terminal residue 49–127 fragment, which is potently amyloidogenic particularly under conditions of shear stress [4]. This finding strongly suggests that proteolytic cleavage of the native tetrameric TTR variant with formation of the residue 49–127 polypeptide is a distinct pathway of TTR amyloidogenesis in vivo [4]. In the last decade, advances in biological understanding of the mechanisms involved in TTR amyloid formation have led to the development of modern therapeutic strategies (Fig. 21.2) aimed at reducing the deposition of ATTR amyloid in organs or hepatic synthesis of TTR through [5]:

- Targeted stabilization of the TTR tetramer to prevent dissociation into amyloidogenic monomers or cleavage into amyloidogenic fragments [6, 7].
- Disruption of the relevant messenger RNA (mRNA) in the hepatocyte with either small interfering RNA (siRNA) [8] or antisense oligonucleotides (ASOs) [9].
- TTR gene editing to prevent the production of the relevant mRNA [10].
- Recognition of the ATTR fibrils by the immune system and acceleration of their removal from vital organs with monoclonal antibodies [2].

Early diagnosis of ATTR amyloidosis before significant organ dysfunction has ensued, and initiation of disease-modifying therapy is of paramount importance and is associated with reduced morbidity and mortality.

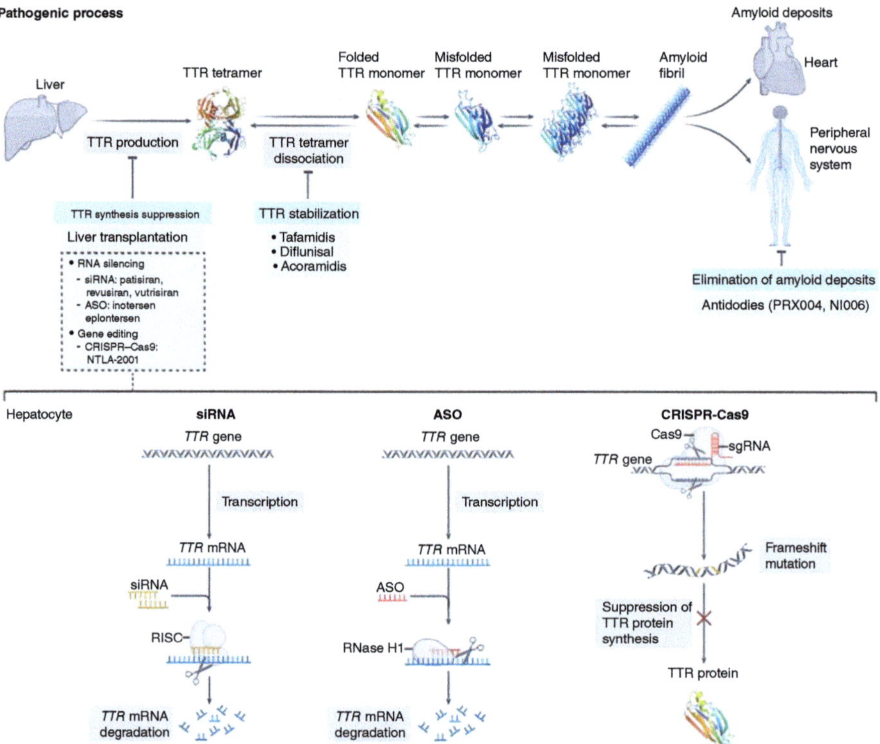

Fig. 21.2 Overview of the treatments available for transthyretin amyloidosis and their mechanism of action

Therapies inhibiting TTR production include liver transplantation, RNA-targeted gene silencing such as small interfering RNAs (siRNAs) (patisiran, revusiran, and vutrisiran) and antisense oligonucleotides (ASOs) (inotersen and eplontersen), and gene editing strategies such as CRISPR–Cas9 technologies (NTLA-2001). siRNAs and ASOs act by binding to complementary TTR mRNA molecules and causing their degradation or silencing. Gene editing with CRISPR-Cas9 induces a double-strand break in the TTR gene, ultimately preventing the production of the protein. Finally, anti-TTR antibodies have been shown to be effective in disrupting amyloid deposits. *RISC*, RNA-induced silencing complex, *sgRNA* single-guide RNA

Notes: PRX 004 is now changed into NNC-6019. There is a phase 1 study of anti-amyloid therapy using antibodies directed toward transthyretin amyloid deposited in various organs

Table 21.1 Therapies for ATTR amyloidosis

Medication	Tafamidis	AG10	Patisiran	Revusiran	Vutrisiran	Inotersen	Eplontersen	NTLA-2001
Mechanism of action	Stabilizer	Stabilizer	siRNA	siRNA	siRNA	ASO	ASO	CRISPR-Cas9
Trial	ATTR-ACT	ATTRIBUTE-CM	APOLLO and APOLLO-B	ENDEAVOUR	HELIOS-A and HELIOS-B	NEURO-TTR	CARDIO-TTRansform and NEURO-TTRansform	NCT04601051
Dosage	80 mg orally once daily	800 mg orally twice daily	80-min intravenous infusion based on body weight every 3 weeks (<100 kg = 0.3 mg/kg; >100 kg = 30 mg)	500 mg subcutaneous injection daily for 5 days, then weekly for 18 months	25 mg subcutaneous injection every 3 months	284 mg subcutaneous injection once weekly	45 mg subcutaneous injection monthly	0.1 mg/kg or 0.3 mg/kg single intravenous infusion
Premedication[a]	Not needed	Not needed	√	–	√	√	Not needed	√
Vitamin A supplementation	Not needed	Not needed	Needed	Needed	Needed	Needed	Needed	Needed
Stage of approval	ESC and FDA approved for ATTRv-PN and ATTR-CM	–	FDA approved for ATTRv-PN	Drug development discontinued	FDA approved for ATTRv-PN	FDA approved for ATTRv-PN	Ongoing evaluation	Ongoing evaluation
Neurological outcomes	Reduced the progression of neuropathy assessed by multiple scales	–	APOLLO: ↓ mNIS+7 ↓ Norfolk QOL-DN ↓ COMPASS-31 ↑ Gait speed	Trial terminated early by DSMB for harm –	HELIOS-A: ↓ mNIS+7 ↓ Norfolk QOL-DN	↓ mNIS+7 ↓ Norfolk QOL-DN ↑ QOL	NEURO-TTRansform ongoing	Awaiting trial

(continued)

Table 21.1 (continued)

Medication	Tafamidis	AG10	Patisiran	Revusiran	Vutrisiran	Inotersen	Eplontersen	NTLA-2001
Cardiological outcomes	↓ All-cause mortality and CV-related hospitalization ↑ KCCQ-OS ↑6MWT	Neutral effect on 6MWT ↑ KCCQ-OS ↓ NT-proBNP ↑ TTR (ongoing trial)	APOLLO cardiac subgroup: ↓ NT-proBNP ↑ Gait speed ↓ LV wall thickness ↑ LVEDV APOLLO-B: ↑6MWT	Trial terminated early by DSMB for harm –	HELIOS-B trial ongoing	Phase 2 trial ongoing	CARDIO-TTRansform trial ongoing	Awaiting trial
Potential adverse effect	–	–	Vitamin A deficiency Infusion-related reactions Peripheral edema	Vitamin A deficiency Increased mortality when compared to placebo	Vitamin A deficiency	Vitamin A deficiency Thrombocytopenia Glomerulonephritis Infusion-related reactions	Vitamin A deficiency Headache	Vitamin A deficiency Headache Nausea Chills Rhinorrhea

ASO antisense oligonucleotide, *ATTR* transthyretin amyloidosis, *ATTR-CM* transthyretin amyloid cardiomyopathy, *CRISPR* clustered regularly interspaced short palindromic repeats, *CV* cardiovascular, *FDA* Food and Drug Administration, *ATTRv-PN* variant ATTR polyneuropathy, *LV* left ventricular, *LVEDV* left ventricular end diastolic volume, *mNIS + 7* modified neuropathy impairment score + 7, *NT-proBNP* N-terminal pro-B-type natriuretic peptide, *QOL-DN* quality of life questionnaire-diabetic neuropathy, *siRNA* small interfering RNA

[a]Premedication may include corticosteroids, paracetamol, ranitidine, and/or antihistamine

21.2 Imitating Nature with Selective TTR Stabilizers

21.2.1 Tafamidis

The benzoxazole tafamidis is a small molecule that stabilizes the circulating TTR tetramer and prevents dissociation in monomers by binding the T4-binding sites [11]. The drug can be orally administered and is generally safe and well tolerated.

In a small open-label, single-arm trial on patients with non-Val30Met ATTR amyloidosis, tafamidis treatment (20 mg daily) achieved TTR tetramer stabilization over 6 weeks [12]. At 12-month follow-up, no deterioration in quality of life and cardiac function, assessed through echocardiographic parameters and serum NT-proBNP, was identified, although there was some worsening of neurological function [12].

In a recent phase 3 multicenter trial, 441 patients with ATTR amyloid cardiomyopathy (ATTR-CM) were randomized in a 2:1:2 ratio to receive tafamidis 80 mg, tafamidis 20 mg, or placebo for 30 months (Table 21.1). ATTR-CM was defined as medical history of HF, LV hypertrophy at echocardiography, or histological demonstration of TTR amyloid deposition in the heart. Patients in NYHA Class IV and estimated glomerular filtration rate < 25 ml/min/m^2 were excluded from the study. When comparing the pooled tafamidis arms (80 mg and 20 mg) with the placebo arm, tafamidis reduced all-cause mortality by 30% (HR 0.70, 95% CI 0.51–0.96) and cardiovascular-related hospitalization with a relative risk ratio of 0.68 (0.48 per year vs. 0.70 per year; 95% CI 0.56–0.81) compared to placebo over the 30-month trial period. Tafamidis was associated with a lower rate of decline in 6-min walking distance and quality of life (measured through the Kansas City Cardiomyopathy Questionnaire-Overall Summary) at 30 months. The consistent mortality benefit was evident after 18–20 months of therapy, when the Kaplan–Meier survival curves diverged for the tafamidis and the placebo arms [6], suggesting that it takes time for therapy to demonstrate efficacy. Across patient subgroups, including ATTRwt vs. ATTRv, New York Heart Association (NYHA) Classes I–II vs. III, and tafamidis dose (80 mg vs. 20 mg), the difference in all-cause mortality and frequency of cardiovascular-related hospitalizations favored tafamidis over placebo. Conversely, patients with NYHA functional Class III had higher hospitalization rates. The reduced benefit with tafamidis in trial patients with NYHA functional Class III was postulated to occur because of a longer survival during a more severe phase of the disease [13]. Longer term data of those with more advanced disease has shown strong trends toward reductions in mortality in baseline NYHA Class III patients (HR 0.65, 95% CI of 0.41–1.01), which was less than in those with baseline Classes I–II (HR 0.56, 95% CI of 0.38–0.82) [14].

Tafamidis has become the first disease-modifying drug to be approved for the treatment of early-stage ATTRv-PN and for ATTRwt- and ATTRv-CM [6, 15, 16]. Based on the results of the ATTR-ACT trial, tafamidis is recommended in Europe for the treatment of patients with ATTR-CM and NYHA Classes I–II (class of recommendation I, level of evidence B) [17], and also in patients with NYHA Class III symptoms in the United States (class of recommendation I, level of evidence B-R) [18].

21.2.2 AG10 (Acoramidis)

The selective TTR stabilizer AG10, also known as acoramidis, binds TTR with greater selectivity than either tafamidis or diflunisal and was designed to mimic the structure of a naturally occurring variant of the TTR gene (T119M), considered as a "rescue mutation" [19]. It has been shown to prevent or slow deposition of ATTR amyloid by stabilizing the TTR tetramer through formation of hydrogen bonds with the same serine residues at position 117 [19]. In a randomized, double-blind, placebo-controlled, phase 2 study on 49 patients with ATTRwt- or ATTRv-CM and symptomatic HF, acoramidis administered at the dose of 400 mg or 800 mg orally twice daily for 28 days was well tolerated and was able to increase circulating TTR levels, resulting in a near-complete stabilization of TTR by in vitro assay [20].

The ATTRibute-CM trial is a phase 3, multicenter, randomized trial designed to assess the efficacy and safety of acoramidis in the treatment of patients with ATTRwt- and ATTRv-CM with NYHA Class I–III symptoms [21]. The study enrolled 632 participants randomized 2:1 between treatment (acoramidis 800 mg) and placebo twice daily. The study is designed as a two-part study with Part A (Month 12) comparing change from baseline in 6MWD and Part B (Month 30) utilizing a hierarchical comparison including all-cause mortality and cardiovascular hospitalizations. At 12 months of follow-up, acoramidis treatment did not result in an improvement in exercise capacity when compared to placebo (primary endpoint) with a median 6-minute walk distance decline of 9 m and 7 m for the treatment and the placebo groups, respectively. The 6MWT has been extensively used as endpoint in previous trials, but this test may not be completely reflective of the changing severity of clinical phenotype and degree of cardiac involvement in ATTR-CM. Older age of patients and presence of multiple comorbidities, specifically orthopedic conditions limiting patients' mobility, might explain, to some extent, the failure to meet the primary study endpoint. Of note, an improvement in KCCQ-OS and a decline in NT-proBNP concentrations as well as an increase in serum TTR concentration were observed in patients receiving acoramidis [22]. The positive results at 30 months have been presented at the 2023 European Society of Cardiology Congress. Acoramidis proved superior to placebo for improving both hard cardiovascular endpoints and quality-of-life endpoints. The primary endpoint, a hierarchical analysis consisting of all-cause mortality, cumulative frequency of cardiovascular-related hospitalization, change from baseline in NT-proBNP, and change from baseline in 6-minute walk distance, had an overall win ratio favoring acoramidis (win ratio 1.77, 95% confidence interval [CI] 1.42–2.22; $p < 0.001$). Acoramidis proved superior to placebo also with respect to all secondary endpoints, namely all-cause mortality (hazard ratio 0.77 [95% CI 0.54–1.10; $p = 0.15$]), change in NT-proBNP from baseline (45% vs. 9%, $p < 0.001$), and improvement from baseline in 6-minute walk distance: 40% vs. 22% ($p < 0.001$). This trial has then proposed acoramidis as a possible effective and safe alternative to tafamidis for the treatment of ATTR-CM.

21.3 Suppressing Protein Production with TTR Silencers

As TTR is a carrier protein of vitamin A, a significant reduction of circulating TTR levels would result in a severe vitamin A depletion. Therefore, daily vitamin A supplementation is recommended in all patients receiving TTR silencers to prevent sequelae from vitamin A deficiency.

21.4 Small Interfering RNAs (siRNAs)

Small interfering RNA (siRNAs) are double-stranded RNA molecules that interfere with TTR gene expression by binding complementary mRNA molecules and inducing degradation [23].

21.4.1 Patisiran

Patisiran is a double-stranded siRNA encapsulated in lipid nanoparticles that blocks the expression of TTR (both wild-type and variant TTR) in the hepatocytes by triggering activation of the Argonaute slicer protein that disrupts the TTR mRNA, hence reducing its hepatic synthesis [24, 25]. Patisiran was the first siRNA developed for ATTR amyloidosis and was approved by the United States Food and Drug Administration (FDA) and the European Commission (EC) in 2018 for the treatment of ATTRv-PN (Table 21.1) [26].

In a phase 1 study of patisiran, single administration of 0.3 mg/kg achieved a maximum reduction in serum TTR concentration of 87.6% [27]. Mild/moderate renal or mild hepatic impairment had no effect on the pharmacokinetics or TTR reduction [25]. Patisiran was well tolerated in ATTRv-PN patients with previous liver transplant [28]. A phase 2 study on 29 patients with ATTRv-PN showed that two doses of patisiran 0.3 mg/kg administered every 3 weeks reduced mean serum TTR levels by about 80% [29].

The randomized, placebo-controlled, double-blind phase 3 APOLLO trial [8] assessed the efficacy and safety of patisiran in 255 patients with ATTRv-PN. Patisiran administered intravenously at the dose of 0.3 mg/kg once every 3 weeks for 18 months met the primary endpoint, which was an improvement from baseline in the modified Neuropathy Impairment Score + 7 (mNIS+7) in the treatment group compared to the placebo group [8]. Patients in the treatment group achieved an improvement in the Norfolk Quality of Life Questionnaire-Diabetic Neuropathy (Norfolk QOL-DN) score and gait speed and autonomic neuropathy assessed with the COMPASS-31 scale compared to placebo group [30].

A post hoc analysis [31] was conducted on 126 patients (56% of the total population) from the APOLLO trial deemed to have CA based on a left ventricular (LV) wall thickness $\geq$ 12 mm in the absence of other causes (i.e., aortic valve stenosis or hypertension) to investigate the impact of patisiran treatment on ATTR-CM. Patisiran promoted favorable myocardial remodeling with reduction in LV wall thickness and relative wall thickness, increase in LV end-diastolic volume, and more favorable change in global longitudinal strain (GLS) on echocardiogram. The treated group also had a significant reduction in NT-proBNP and increase in 10-minute walk test gait speed compared to the placebo group [31]. Results from a recent series of 16 patients with ATTRv-CM and ATTRv-PN receiving patisiran and diflunisal demonstrated a reduction in extracellular volume measured by contrast cardiac magnetic resonance (CMR) accompanied by a reduction in serum TTR and NT-proBNP concentrations and an increase in exercise capacity assessed by 6-minute walk test (6MWT) after 12 months of treatment [32].

The efficacy of patisiran in the treatment of ATTR-CM has been assessed in the phase 3 randomized controlled APOLLO-B trial. This study enrolled patients with ATTRwt-CM or ATTRv-CM, evidence of HF, a serum NT-proBNP between 300 and 8500 ng/L, and a 6MWT $\geq$150 mt followed for 12 months [33]. APOLLO-B met its primary endpoint with a reduction in the rate of decline in 6MWT distance among treated patients compared to those on placebo across 12 months. There was also a reduction in the decline of QoL as assessed with KCCQ among treated patients. From initial reports, there were favorable effects on functional structural and functional echocardiographic parameters. Notably, the study was conducted over a 12-month period, which may not be enough to demonstrate the efficacy of treatment. However, the complete study results are yet to be published, and no formal conclusions can be drawn at this stage [34].

21.4.2 Revusiran

Revusiran is a siRNA conjugated to N-acetylgalactosamine (GalNAc) that facilitates its uptake in the hepatocytes via the asialoglycoprotein receptor on their surface. In a phase 1 trial in healthy volunteers, revusiran was well tolerated and achieved a 50% reduction in serum TTR following a single dose and 90% following multiple doses [35]. Revusiran efficacy in ATTRv-CM was assessed in the phase 3, randomized, placebo-controlled, double-blind ENDEAVOUR trial, which was terminated prematurely due to "an imbalance in mortality observed between patients treated with revusiran and placebo" [2]. During a median follow-up period of 7 months, 13% of patients receiving revusiran died compared with 3% receiving placebo [36]. Although a post hoc safety analysis suggested an imbalance in disease severity at enrolment, a possible mechanism related to revusiran could not be ruled out, and further development of this agent was discontinued [36].

21.4.3 Vutrisiran

Vutrisiran is a second-generation siRNA that utilizes a GalNAc conjugate delivery platform. Due to an enhanced stabilization chemistry, it can be administered subcutaneously with longer dosing intervals compared to revusiran (i.e., every 3 months) and was rapidly absorbed (peak plasma concentrations achieved at 3–5 h) in a phase

1 study of healthy volunteers [37]. The degree of TTR knockdown is dose-dependent with a single 25 mg subcutaneous dose achieving a maximum TTR reduction of 80%, persisting for 90 days [37].

The HELIOS-A trial randomized 164 ATTRv-PN patients to vutrisiran or patisiran and compared outcomes to an external placebo group from the APOLLO trial. At 18 months of follow-up, vutrisiran treatment was associated with an improvement in mNIS+7 and Norfolk QOL-DN scores compared to placebo. Vutrisiran achieved a mean peak TTR knockdown of 88% within 3 weeks and was non-inferior to patisiran [38]. Based on these findings, the FDA and the European Medicines Agency (EMA) approved vutrisiran for the treatment of ATTRv-PN in 2022 [26].

The efficacy and safety of vutrisiran in ATTR-CM (both variant and wild type) are currently undergoing evaluation in the ongoing phase 3, randomized, placebo-controlled, double-blind HELIOS-B trial. The primary endpoint is a composite of all-cause mortality and CV events (CV hospitalizations and urgent HF visits) at 30–36 months. Secondary endpoints include change from baseline in 6MWT, NT-proBNP, mean LV wall thickness, GLS, and KCCQ-OS [26]. The HELIOS-B trial will provide information on the efficacy of combination therapy as up to 30% of patients who are eligible for inclusion can be taking tafamidis.

21.4.4 Antisense Oligonucleotides (ASOs)

Antisense oligonucleotides (ASOs) are a single strand of 16–20 synthetic nucleotides that binds to complementary mRNA to induce degradation of the mRNA [26].

21.4.5 Inotersen

Inotersen is a 2´-O-methoxyethyl-modified ASO that promotes ribonuclease H1-mediated degradation of the complementary mRNA. It is administered at the dose of 300 mg in Europe or 284 mg in the United States by subcutaneous injection once a week. Inotersen was the first ASO developed for ATTR amyloidosis and approved by the FDA and the EMA in 2018 for the treatment of ATTRv-PN [26].

In a randomized, placebo-controlled phase 1 study, inotersen lowered TTR levels in a dose-dependent manner in 65 healthy volunteers, with 300 mg achieving a maximum TTR knockdown of 96%. A long-lasting effect was observed, with trial participants having a mean TTR knockdown of 30% at 10 weeks after administration of their last dose [39].

The phase 3, randomized, placebo-controlled, double-blind NEURO-TTR trial was designed to investigate the efficacy and safety of inotersen in ATTRv-PN (Table 21.1) [9]. The study randomized 172 patients in a 2:1 ratio to weekly subcutaneous injections of inotersen (300 mg) or placebo. The study met its primary endpoints with treated patients achieving a significant reduction in the decline from baseline in mNIS+7 and Norfolk QOL-DN scores compared to placebo patients. At 13 weeks, the mean TTR knockdown from baseline was 84% [9]. Inotersen was discontinued in 14% of patients due to adverse events, most of which were mild or moderate: injection site reactions, nausea, headache, and fever. Thrombocytopenia (platelets <140,000/mm^3) was found in 54% of patients receiving inotersen. The most likely mechanism is thought to be immune mediated as antiplatelet antibodies were identified and patients recovered with glucocorticoid therapy. Biopsy-proven crescentic glomerulonephritis occurred in three patients with ATTR amyloidosis associated with the V30M TTR mutation receiving inotersen and was successfully treated with immunosuppression in two cases (the remaining patients had a late presentation and required dialysis). Therefore, frequent platelet count and renal function monitoring are essential during treatment with inotersen.

One-hundred nine patients from the NEURO-TTR trial participated in an open-label extension study to assess the long-term efficacy and safety of inotersen over 3 years [40]. The inotersen-inotersen group demonstrated sustained benefit, as measured by mNIS+7, Norfolk QOL-DN, and 36-Item Short-Form Health Survey (QoL questionnaire), when compared to the placebo-inotersen group [40]. The placebo-inotersen group demonstrated better neurological outcomes than those predicted by natural history data. However, in this study, 22% of patients discontinued treatment following an adverse event, which was considered related to inotersen only in 4% of cases [40]. No patient had glomerulonephritis.

21.4.6 Eplontersen

Eplontersen is a GalNAc-conjugated ASO with the same primary sequence as inotersen. It is taken up via the high-capacity asialoglycoprotein receptor on hepatocytes [41, 42] where the triantennary GalNAc is metabolized to release the ASO [43]. Eplontersen is 50-fold more potent than inotersen at reducing TTR expression in human hepatocytes [26]. In a randomized, placebo-controlled, phase 1 study of 45 healthy volunteers, a single dose of eplontersen (120 mg) resulted in maximum TTR knockdown of 86%, while multiple doses (45 mg, 60 mg, or 90 mg) resulted in maximum TTR knockdown of 86%, 91%, and 94%, respectively [44]. There were no safety concerns. Eplontersen was well tolerated with no injection-site reactions and no drug discontinuations. The most common adverse events were headache, transient increased ALT, and creatinine kinase. No sequelae associated with vitamin A deficiency were identified, but all patients received vitamin A supplementation [44].

The efficacy and safety of eplontersen in the treatment of ATTRv-PN and ATTRv-CM are currently under evaluation in the ongoing phase 3, multicenter, double-blind, randomized, placebo-controlled NEURO- and CARDIO-TTRansform trials (Table 21.1):

- The NEURO-TTRansform trial enrolled 168 participants randomized to receive eplontersen once every 4 weeks or inotersen once weekly. The NEURO-TTR trial placebo group will serve as an external control group. The co-primary endpoints are the change from baseline in mNIS+7 and percentage change in serum TTR, and the secondary efficacy endpoint is the change from baseline in the Norfolk QOL-DN score. The interim 35-week analysis reported presented at the XVIII International Symposium on Amyloidosis in September 2022 demonstrated that eplontersen slowed the progression of neuropathic disease and improved QoL compared to the external placebo group [45–47]. Results were further confirmed in a subsequent analysis at 66 weeks in which patients treated with eplontersen demonstrated consistent and sustained benefit on the three co-primary endpoints of serum TTR concentration, neuropathy impairment, and QoL. Of note, eplontersen achieved a least squares (LS) mean reduction of 82% in TTR serum concentration from baseline, compared to an 11% reduction from baseline in the external placebo group, and halted disease progression as measured by mNIS+7, resulting in a 0.28 point LS mean increase compared to a 25.06 point increase for the external placebo group from baseline.

- The CARDIO-TTRansform trial aims to recruit 1400 patients who will be randomized to receive eplontersen or placebo. The primary endpoint is a composite of cardiovascular mortality and recurrent cardiovascular events occurring within 140 weeks of follow-up. Secondary endpoints include change in 6MWT and KCCQ-OS at 120 weeks. Eligible patients will be included in a CMR sub-study to assess the effect of eplontersen on amyloid burden as measured by ECV. Additionally, a scintigraphy sub-study will assess the effects of eplontersen on myocardial retention of the isotope indicative of amyloidosis. The CARDIO-TTRansform trial will provide information on the efficacy of combination therapy as patients treated with tafamidis are eligible for inclusion [48].

21.5 Editing the TTR Gene in Hepatocytes

An alternative to TTR stabilizers and mRNA targeting-based gene silencing is the use of the clustered regularly interspaced short palindromic repeats and associated Cas9 endonuclease (CRISPR-Cas9) system to achieve in vivo gene editing. As a monogenic disease, ATTR amyloidosis is the exemplar disease for CRISPR-Cas9-mediated in vivo genome editing therapy. TTR has a specific function of transporting thyroxine and vitamin A. TTR knockdown has only limited additional physiological effects, and vitamin A supplementation appears to be effective in preventing any potential clinical sequelae from vitamin A deficiency [8, 9]. Circulating TTR is exclusively synthesized by the liver, for which targeted hepatocyte delivery of a gene editing therapy can be achieved using lipid nanoparticles. This therapy has the potential to achieve near-complete and permanent knockdown of both wild-type and mutant TTR expression after a single intravenous administration, and thereby prevent or markedly slow ongoing formation of pathogenic ATTR amyloid fibrils.

21.5.1 NTLA-2001

NTLA-2001 is a CRISPR-Cas9-based genome editing therapy, transported by a lipid nanoparticle-mediated delivery system. In animal models, a single administration of NTLA-2001 resulted in significant editing of the mouse TTR gene and 96% reduction in serum TTR levels (persisting for 12 months) [26]. The same results were replicated in other animal models such as cynomolgus monkeys and transgenic mice carrying the human Val30Met TTR variant with no adverse events [49]. A two-part open-label, single-dose, phase 1 multicenter study in patients with ATTRv-PN and ATTR-CM (both wild-type and variant TTR gene) is ongoing to evaluate the safety, tolerability, pharmacokinetics, and pharmacodynamics of NTLA-2001 (Table 21.1).

Interim results from the dose escalation phase of the study in six patients with ATTRv-PN demonstrated that the infusion was completed in all patients, without interruption, and was associated with adverse events of only mild severity: nausea, headache, chills, and rhinorrhea. At 28 days, NTLA-2001 treatment was associated with a dose-dependent effect with a mean reduction from baseline in serum TTR protein concentration of 52% in patients receiving 0.1 mg per kilogram and of 87% in patients receiving 0.3 mg per kilogram. TTR knockdown with NTLA-2001 is expected to be permanent [10]. Although there is a theoretical risk of off-target editing, this risk is expected to be low with NTLA-2001 on the basis of complex computational modeling and biochemical assays, including in vitro with human cells and in vivo in animal models. However, patients who receive this gene editing therapy will require long-term monitoring [10].

Interim results from the cardiomyopathy arm on patients with either ATTRwt-CM or ATTRv-CM and NYHA functional Classes I–III have been presented at the Congress of the American Heart Association 2022 [50]. Part I is a single-ascending dose design, with a minimum of three patients in each of the three cohorts:

- NYHA Class I–II cohort ($n = 3$) administered 0.7 mg/kg.
- NYHA Class III cohort ($n = 3$) administered 0.7 mg/kg.
- NYHA Class I–II cohort ($n = 6$) administered 1.0 mg/kg.

Based on safety and PD profile at 0.7 mg/kg, further dose escalation to 1.0 mg/kg in NYHA functional Class III patients was not undertaken.

The median age of the 12 patients was 75 years, 10 out of 12 patients have ATTRwt-CM, and 50% of all participants were in NYHA functional Class III at the time of enrolment. NTLA-2001 was generally well tolerated across all cohorts through the follow-up period.

Three of 12 patients reported no adverse events, and eight reported only mild or moderate adverse events, commonly infusion-related reaction. All patients received a complete dose of NTLA-2001 and remained on study. A single grade 3 infusion-related reaction was reported at the 0.7 mg/kg dose in a NYHA Class III patient and resolved without any clinical sequelae. The NYHA Class III 0.7 mg/kg cohort was expanded per protocol to six patients, and no additional patients in this cohort reported a treatment-related adverse event higher than grade 1 (mild). No clinically significant laboratory finding was observed.

At 6 months of follow-up, all patients with NYHA Class I–II symptoms receiving NTLA-2001 at the dose of 0.7 mg/kg achieved a consistent, sustained response with a mean 93% reduction in circulating TTR. In the NYHA Class III 0.7 mg/kg and NYHA Class I/II 1.0 mg/kg cohorts, mean reductions of 94% and 92%, respectively, were observed at 4 months of follow-up. By day 28, all 12 patients achieved at least 90% TTR reduction. The deep and sustained TTR reduction observed in the interim analyses has the potential to bring about not only clinical stability, but also genuine clinical improvement in patients with ATTR-CM.

The dose expansion phase in both the polyneuropathy and cardiomyopathy arms of the trial is ongoing [51]. Longer follow-up of patients is necessary to assess long-term safety and clinical efficacy in terms of clinically meaningful outcome measures.

21.6 Conclusion

Major advances in the treatment of ATTR amyloidosis with cardiomyopathy and polyneuropathy have completely transformed the therapeutic landscape of this progressive and universally fatal condition. Tafamidis has become the first ever treatment to improve survival in ATTR-CM and has been recommended in guidelines from the International Societies of Cardiology worldwide. The TTR stabilizer acoramidis has recently emerged as a possible safe and effective alternative to tafamidis. Novel gene silencing and gene editing therapies have rapidly expanded the armamentarium of treatments available for ATTR amyloidosis. Targeting TTR production has resulted in tremendous improvements in patient outcomes without any clinical consequences in the short to medium term of depletion of circulating TTR. Simultaneous targeting of gene silencing and stabilization of circulating TTR might even have a synergistic effect. Whether combining these agents (i.e., gene silencers with TTR stabilizer) could augment their therapeutic efficacy requires further large-scale studies in the future.

References

1. Kelly J, Colon W, Lai Z, Lashuel H, McCulloch J, McCutchen S, et al. Transthyretin quaternary and tertiary structural changes facilitate misassembly into amyloid. In: Advances in protein chemistry. Elsevier; 1997. p. 161–81. Available from: https://linkinghub.elsevier.com/retrieve/pii/S0065323308603216.
2. Porcari A, Fontana M, Gillmore JD. Transthyretin cardiac amyloidosis. Cardiovasc Res. 2023;118(18):3517–35. https://doi.org/10.1093/cvr/cvac119.
3. Zhao L, Buxbaum JN, Reixach N. Age-related oxidative modifications of transthyretin modulate its amyloidogenicity. Biochemistry. 2013;52(11):1913–26.
4. Mangione PP, Porcari R, Gillmore JD, Pucci P, Monti M, Porcari M, et al. Proteolytic cleavage of Ser52Pro variant transthyretin triggers its amyloid fibrillogenesis. Proc Natl Acad Sci U S A. 2014;111(4):1539–44.

5. Emdin M, Aimo A, Rapezzi C, Fontana M, Perfetto F, Seferović PM, et al. Treatment of cardiac transthyretin amyloidosis: an update. Eur Heart J. 2019;40(45):3699–706.
6. Maurer MS, Schwartz JH, Gundapaneni B, Elliott PM, Merlini G, Waddington-Cruz M, et al. Tafamidis treatment for patients with transthyretin amyloid cardiomyopathy. N Engl J Med. 2018;379(11):1007–16.
7. Berk JL, Suhr OB, Obici L, Sekijima Y, Zeldenrust SR, Yamashita T, et al. Repurposing diflunisal for familial amyloid polyneuropathy: a randomized clinical trial. JAMA. 2013;310(24):2658–67.
8. Adams D, Gonzalez-Duarte A, O'Riordan WD, Yang CC, Ueda M, Kristen AV, et al. Patisiran, an RNAi therapeutic, for hereditary transthyretin amyloidosis. N Engl J Med. 2018;379(1):11–21.
9. Benson MD, Waddington-Cruz M, Berk JL, Polydefkis M, Dyck PJ, Wang AK, et al. Inotersen treatment for patients with hereditary transthyretin amyloidosis. N Engl J Med. 2018;379(1):22–31.
10. Gillmore JD, Gane E, Taubel J, Kao J, Fontana M, Maitland ML, et al. CRISPR-Cas9 in vivo gene editing for transthyretin amyloidosis. N Engl J Med. 2021;385(6):493–502.
11. Bulawa CE, Connelly S, Devit M, Wang L, Weigel C, Fleming JA, et al. Tafamidis, a potent and selective transthyretin kinetic stabilizer that inhibits the amyloid cascade. Proc Natl Acad Sci U S A. 2012;109(24):9629–34.
12. Merlini G, Planté-Bordeneuve V, Judge DP, Schmidt H, Obici L, Perlini S, et al. Effects of tafamidis on transthyretin stabilization and clinical outcomes in patients with non-Val30Met transthyretin amyloidosis. J Cardiovasc Transl Res. 2013;6(6):1011–20.
13. Rapezzi C, Kristen AV, Gundapaneni B, Sultan MB, Hanna M. Benefits of tafamidis in patients with advanced transthyretin amyloid cardiomyopathy. Eur Heart J. 2020;41(Suppl. 2):ehaa946.2115.
14. Elliott P, Drachman BM, Gottlieb SS, Hoffman JE, Hummel SL, Lenihan DJ, et al. Long-term survival with tafamidis in patients with transthyretin amyloid cardiomyopathy. Circ Heart Fail. 2022;15(1):e008193.
15. Coelho T, Maia LF, Martins da Silva A, Waddington Cruz M, Plante-Bordeneuve V, Lozeron P, et al. Tafamidis for transthyretin familial amyloid polyneuropathy: a randomized, controlled trial. Neurology. 2012;79(8):785–92.
16. Lozeron P, Théaudin M, Mincheva Z, Ducot B, Lacroix C, Adams D. Effect on disability and safety of Tafamidis in late onset of Met30 transthyretin familial amyloid polyneuropathy. Eur J Neurol. 2013;20(12):1539–45.
17. McDonagh TA, Metra M, Adamo M, Gardner RS, Baumbach A, Böhm M, et al. 2021 ESC Guidelines for the diagnosis and treatment of acute and chronic heart failure. Eur Heart J. 2021;42(36):3599–726.
18. Heidenreich PA, Bozkurt B, Aguilar D, Allen LA, Byun JJ, Colvin MM, et al. 2022 AHA/ACC/HFSA guideline for the management of heart failure: a report of the American College of Cardiology/American Heart Association Joint Committee on Clinical Practice Guidelines. Circulation. 2022;145(18):e895–1032.
19. Quarta CC, Fontana M, Damy T, Catini J, Simoneau D, Mercuri M, et al. Changing paradigm in the treatment of amyloidosis: from disease-modifying drugs to anti-fibril therapy. Front Cardiovasc Med. 2022;9:1073503.
20. Yadav JD, Othee H, Chan KA, Man DC, Belliveau PP, Towle J. Transthyretin amyloid cardiomyopathy-current and future therapies. Ann Pharmacother. 2021;55(12):1502–14.
21. Gillmore JD, Garcia-Pavia P, Grogan M, Hanna MA, Heitner SB, Jacoby D, et al. Abstract 14214: ATTRibute-CM: a randomized, double-blind, placebo-controlled, multi-center, global phase 3 study of AG10 in patients with transthyretin amyloid cardiomyopathy (ATTR-CM). Circulation. 2019;140(Suppl. 1):A14214.
22. Cannata' A, Merlo M, Artico J, Gentile P, Camparini L, Cristallini J, et al. Cardiovascular aging. J Cardiovasc Med. 2018;19(10):517–26. Available from: http://europepmc.org/abstract/med/30024423

23. Porcari A, Merlo M, Rapezzi C, Sinagra G. Transthyretin amyloid cardiomyopathy: an uncharted territory awaiting discovery. Eur J Intern Med. 2020;82:7–15.
24. Setten RL, Rossi JJ, Han SP. The current state and future directions of RNAi-based therapeutics. Nat Rev Drug Discov. 2019;18(6):421–46.
25. Urits I, Swanson D, Swett MC, Patel A, Berardino K, Amgalan A, et al. A review of Patisiran (ONPATTRO®) for the treatment of polyneuropathy in people with hereditary transthyretin amyloidosis. Neurol Ther. 2020;9(2):301–15.
26. Ioannou A, Fontana M, Gillmore JD. RNA Targeting and gene editing strategies for transthyretin amyloidosis. BioDrugs. 2023;37(2):127–42.
27. Coelho T, Adams D, Silva A, Lozeron P, Hawkins PN, Mant T, et al. Safety and efficacy of RNAi therapy for transthyretin amyloidosis. N Engl J Med. 2013;369(9):819–29.
28. Schmidt HH, Wixner J, Planté-Bordeneuve V, Muñoz-Beamud F, Lladó L, Gillmore JD, et al. Patisiran treatment in patients with hereditary transthyretin-mediated amyloidosis with polyneuropathy after liver transplantation. Am J Transplant. 2022;22(6):1646–57.
29. Suhr OB, Coelho T, Buades J, Pouget J, Conceicao I, Berk J, et al. Efficacy and safety of patisiran for familial amyloidotic polyneuropathy: a phase II multi-dose study. Orphanet J Rare Dis. 2015;10(1):109. Available from: http://www.ojrd.com/content/10/1/109
30. González-Duarte A, Berk JL, Quan D, Mauermann ML, Schmidt HH, Polydefkis M, et al. Analysis of autonomic outcomes in APOLLO, a phase III trial of the RNAi therapeutic patisiran in patients with hereditary transthyretin-mediated amyloidosis. J Neurol. 2020;267(3):703–12.
31. Solomon SD, Adams D, Kristen A, Grogan M, González-Duarte A, Maurer MS, et al. Effects of patisiran, an RNA interference therapeutic, on cardiac parameters in patients with hereditary transthyretin-mediated amyloidosis. Circulation. 2019;139(4):431–43. https://doi.org/10.1161/CIRCULATIONAHA.118.035831.
32. Fontana M, Martinez-Naharro A, Chacko L, Rowczenio D, Gilbertson JA, Whelan CJ, et al. Reduction in CMR derived extracellular volume with patisiran indicates cardiac amyloid regression. JACC Cardiovasc Imaging. 2021;14(1):189–99.
33. Geyer H, Caracciolo G, Abe H, Wilansky S, Carerj S, Gentile F, et al. Assessment of myocardial mechanics using speckle tracking echocardiography: fundamentals and clinical applications. J Am Soc Echocardiogr. 2010;23(4):351–69.
34. Nieminen MS, Brutsaert D, Dickstein K, Drexler H, Follath F, Harjola VP, et al. EuroHeart Failure Survey II (EHFS II): a survey on hospitalized acute heart failure patients: description of population. Eur Heart J. 2006;27(22):2725–36.
35. Zimmermann TS, Karsten V, Chan A, Chiesa J, Boyce M, Bettencourt BR, et al. Clinical proof of concept for a novel hepatocyte-targeting GalNAc-siRNA conjugate. Mol Ther. 2017;25(1):71–8.
36. Judge DP, Kristen AV, Grogan M, Maurer MS, Falk RH, Hanna M, et al. Phase 3 multicenter study of revusiran in patients with hereditary transthyretin-mediated (hATTR) amyloidosis with cardiomyopathy (ENDEAVOUR). Cardiovasc Drugs Ther. 2020;34(3):357–70.
37. Habtemariam BA, Karsten V, Attarwala H, Goel V, Melch M, Clausen VA, et al. Single-dose pharmacokinetics and pharmacodynamics of transthyretin targeting N-acetylgalactosamine-small interfering ribonucleic acid conjugate, vutrisiran, in healthy subjects. Clin Pharmacol Ther. 2021;109(2):372–82.
38. Adams D, Tournev IL, Taylor MS, Coelho T, Planté-Bordeneuve V, Berk JL, et al. Efficacy and safety of vutrisiran for patients with hereditary transthyretin-mediated amyloidosis with polyneuropathy: a randomized clinical trial. Amyloid. 2023;30(1):18–26. https://doi.org/10.1080/13506129.2022.2091985.
39. Ackermann EJ, Guo S, Benson MD, Booten S, Freier S, Hughes SG, et al. Suppressing transthyretin production in mice, monkeys and humans using 2nd-Generation antisense oligonucleotides. Amyloid Int J Exp Clin Investig Off J Int Soc Amyloidosis. 2016;23(3):148–57.
40. Brannagan TH, Coelho T, Wang AK, Polydefkis MJ, Dyck PJ, Berk JL, et al. Long-term efficacy and safety of inotersen for hereditary transthyretin amyloidosis: NEURO-TTR open-label extension 3-year update. J Neurol. 2022;269(12):6416–27.

41. Tanowitz M, Hettrick L, Revenko A, Kinberger GA, Prakash TP, Seth PP. Asialoglycoprotein receptor 1 mediates productive uptake of N-acetylgalactosamine-conjugated and unconjugated phosphorothioate antisense oligonucleotides into liver hepatocytes. Nucleic Acids Res. 2017;45(21):12388–400.

42. Prakash TP, Yu J, Migawa MT, Kinberger GA, Wan WB, Østergaard ME, et al. Comprehensive structure-activity relationship of triantennary N-acetylgalactosamine conjugated antisense oligonucleotides for targeted delivery to hepatocytes. J Med Chem. 2016;59(6):2718–33.

43. Shemesh CS, Yu RZ, Gaus HJ, Greenlee S, Post N, Schmidt K, et al. Elucidation of the biotransformation pathways of a Galnac3-conjugated antisense oligonucleotide in rats and monkeys. Mol Ther Nucleic Acids. 2016;5(5):e319.

44. Viney NJ, Guo S, Tai LJ, Baker BF, Aghajan M, Jung SW, et al. Ligand conjugated antisense oligonucleotide for the treatment of transthyretin amyloidosis: preclinical and phase 1 data. ESC Hear Fail. 2021;8(1):652–61.

45. Coelho T, Ando Y, Benson MD, Berk JL, Waddington-Cruz M, Dyck PJ, et al. Design and rationale of the global phase 3 NEURO-TTRansform study of antisense oligonucleotide AKCEA-TTR-L(Rx) (ION-682884-CS3) in hereditary transthyretin-mediated amyloid polyneuropathy. Neurol Ther. 2021;10(1):375–89.

46. AstraZeneca. Press release. Eplontersen met co-primary and secondary endpoints in interim analysis of the NEURO-TTRansform Phase III trial for hereditary transthyretin-mediated amyloid polyneuropathy (ATTRv-PN) (last accessed 16 March 2023). Available from: https://www.astrazeneca.com/media-centre/press-releases/2022/eplontersen-phase-iii-trial-met-co-primary-endpoints.html.

47. NEURO-TTRansform: A Study to Evaluate the Efficacy and Safety of Eplontersen (Formerly Known as ION-682884, IONIS- TTR-LRx and AKCEA-TTR-LRx) in Participants With Heredi- tary Transthyretin-Mediated Amyloid Polyneuropathy. ClinicalTrials.gov. https://www.clinicaltrials.gov/ct2/show/NCT04 136184. Accessed 11 Sep 2022.

48. Ionis presents positive results from Phase 3 NEURO-TTRans- form study at International Symposium on Amyloidosis | Ionis Pharmaceuticals, Inc. https://ir.ionispharma.com/news-releases/news-release-details/ionis-presents-positive-results-phase-3-neuro-ttransform-study. Accessed 22 Dec 2022.

49. Finn JD, Smith AR, Patel MC, Shaw L, Youniss MR, van Heteren J, et al. A single administration of CRISPR/Cas9 lipid nanoparticles achieves robust and persistent in vivo genome editing. Cell Rep. 2018;22(9):2227–35.

50. https://www.acc.org/education-and-meetings/image-and-slide-gallery/media-detail?id=44bd7ca7119744aab5305f8f67fbb10c.

51. Study to Evaluate Safety, Tolerability, Pharmacokinetics, and Pharmacodynamics of NTLA-2001 in Patients With Hereditary Transthyretin Amyloidosis With Polyneuropathy (ATTRv-PN) and Patients With Transthyretin Amyloidosis-Related Cardio- myopathy (ATTR-CM). ClinicalTrials.gov. https://www.clinicaltr ials.gov/ct2/show/NCT04601051. Accessed 19 Sep 2022.

Treatment of Cardiac Complications

22

Claudio Passino and Alberto Aimo

Abbreviations

ACEi/ARB	Angiotensin-converting enzyme inhibitor or angiotensin receptor blocker
AF	Atrial fibrillation
AL	Amyloid light chain
AS	Aortic stenosis
ATTR	Amyloid transthyretin (v, variant; wt, wild type)
AV	Atrioventricular
CA	Cardiac amyloidosis
CI	Confidence interval
CrCl	Creatinine clearance
CRT	Cardiac resynchronization therapy
CT	Computed tomography
DCCV	Direct-current cardioversion
ECV	Extracellular volume
ESC	European Society of Cardiology
HF	Heart failure
HR	Hazard ratio
HT	Heart transplantation
LA(A)	Left atrial (appendage)
LV	Left ventricular
NOAC	Non-vitamin K antagonist anticoagulant

C. Passino (✉) · A. Aimo
Interdisciplinary Center for Health Sciences, Scuola Superiore Sant'Anna, Pisa, Italy

Cardiology Division, Fondazione Toscana Gabriele Monasterio, Pisa, Italy
e-mail: passino@ftgm.it; aimoalb@ftgm.it

M. Emdin et al. (eds.), *Cardiac Amyloidosis*,
https://doi.org/10.1007/978-3-031-51757-0_22

NT-proBNP	N-terminal pro-B-type natriuretic peptide
PM	Pacemaker
PVI	Pulmonary vein isolation
RV	Right ventricular
TAVR	Transcatheter aortic valve replacement
TEE	Transesophageal echocardiogram
TIA	Transient ischemic attack
VKA	Vitamin K antagonist

Therapies targeting the amyloidogenic cascade can modify the natural history of the disease, albeit only after a period of latency following treatment initiation (for example, around 18 months for tafamidis) [1]. In the meantime, cardiac involvement remains a crucial determinant of morbidity and mortality, and its evolution is partially independent from the underlying disorder. The guidelines and similar documents on the management of cardiac amyloidosis (CA) provide several recommendations that are usually based on weak evidence or simple expert opinions [2]. In this chapter, we will discuss the six topics identified by the European Society of Cardiology (ESC) position statement (aortic stenosis [AS], atrial fibrillation [AF], thromboembolism, conduction disorders, ventricular arrhythmias, heart failure [HF]) [3], plus orthostatic hypotension, which is specifically considered in the 2022 guideline on variant transthyretin amyloidosis (ATTRv) [4].

22.1 Severe Aortic Stenosis

The coexistence of calcific AS and CA increases with age, and their association is not uncommon in the elderly. The identification of CA is particularly challenging in patients with AS because these two conditions share several features [5]. The prevalence of CA in the general population and in patients with AS is likely underestimated because of the lack of a systematic screening. In a meta-analysis of studies where CA was searched in all patients with AS (usually severe AS referred to surgical or transcatheter aortic valve replacement [TAVR]), the median prevalence was 8% (with a 95% confidence interval [CI] from 5% to 13%). Men accounted for 67% of patients with AS and CA, the median age was 84 years, and almost all patients (98%) had ATTR-CA [6]. A multicenter study on 407 patients evaluated for TAVR tried to identify red flags for AS-CA. A scoring system was created exploring carpal tunnel syndrome, disproportionate electrical remodeling, disproportionate myocardial remodeling, chronic myocardial injury, and age (Fig. 22.1). Scores of ≥ 2 and ≥ 3 points had high sensitivity and fair specificity for the presence of CA [7].

When CA is diagnosed, AS severity should be assessed according to current guidelines [5]. Around 50% of patients are with CA and a paradoxical low-flow, low-gradient pattern, i.e., low-flow, low-gradient AS with preserved LV ejection fraction [5]. The high prevalence of low-flow state in patients with CA may be

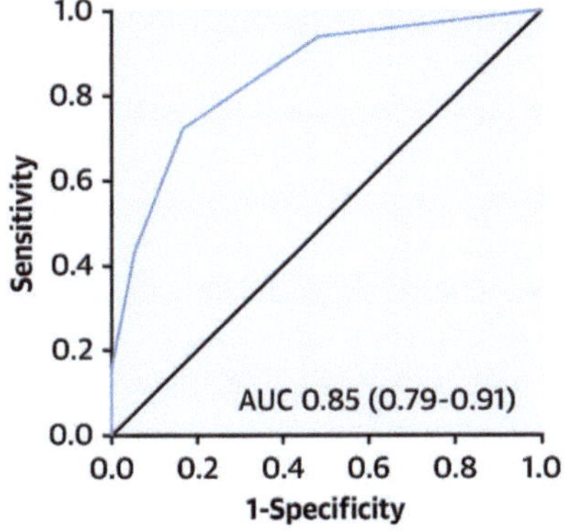

Parameter	Points
CTS	3
RBBB	2
Age ≥85 years	1
Hs-TnT >20 ng/l	1
IVS ≥18 mm	1
If in SR*: E/A ratio >1.4	1
If no BBB or PM: Sokolow index <1.9 mV	1

* AUC for AFib sub-cohort: 0.83

Score	Specificity	Sensitivity
≥6 points	100%	14.9%
≥5 points	98.9%	23.4%
≥4 points	95.0%	42.6%
≥3 points	83.6%	72.3%
≥2 points	52.1%	93.6%
≥1 point	16.7%	97.9%

Fig. 22.1 Scoring system to discriminate lone aortic stenosis (AS) from combined AS and cardiac amyloidosis*AFib* atrial fibrillation, *AS* aortic stenosis, *AUC* area under the curve, *BBB* bundle branch block, *CA* cardiac amyloidosis, *CTS* carpal tunnel syndrome, *hs-TnT* high-sensitivity troponin T, *IVS* interventricular septum, *PM* pacemaker, *RBBB* right bundle branch block, *SR* sinus rhythm. Reprinted with permission from Nitsche et al. [7]

explained by the following factors: severe LV concentric remodeling, impairment of diastolic filling, LA remodeling and dysfunction, markedly reduced LV longitudinal systolic function, and right ventricular (RV) remodeling and dysfunction [5]. The assessment of AS severity is more challenging in patients with low-flow, low-gradient AS, and additional imaging tests are required to differentiate a true-severe versus a pseudo-severe AS. Dobutamine stress echocardiography may be used to confirm AS severity, but often fails to significantly increase LV outflow and thus provides inconclusive results [5]. Therefore, the quantitation of aortic valve calcium burden using non-contrast computed tomography (CT) is often crucial to confirm AS severity in patients with CA [5]. Nonetheless, the aortic valves of patients with AS and CA are less calcified than those of patients with AS alone [8]. This may point to a different pathophysiology of AS in patients with coexisting CA; more importantly, from a clinical perspective, this may lead to an underestimation of AS severity when the same cutoffs as in the general population are used (i.e., >2000 Agatston units in men, >1200 in women), as previously proposed [5].

Patients with severe AS and (ATTR-)CA have a similar outcome than those with AS alone when maximum LV thickness is <16 mm, while they have a worse prognosis when LV wall thickness is higher [9]. TAVR improves survival to a similar extent in patients with or without CA [7]. In patients undergoing TAVR, major adverse events occurred at the same rate as in those with lone AS and AS-CA: stroke (2.7% vs. 2.9%), vascular complication (4.7% vs. 2.9%), acute kidney injury (7.5% vs. 6.1%), and pacemaker (PM) implantation (6.4% vs. 14.7%) (p for all >0.05) [7].

CT angiography is an essential element of TAVR planning. A possible integration of CT angiography is the calculation of myocardial extracellular volume (ECV). ECV values correlate with the amount of myocardial amyloid and then with disease severity [10]. Unsurprisingly, there is an inverse relationship between ECV and the likelihood of early recovery of systolic function after TAVR [11], or long-term outcome [10]. Even more importantly, ECV is significantly higher in patients with CA than those with lone AS, and particularly high in those with ATTR-CA [10], who account for the vast majority of patients with AS-CA, as stated above. This finding may disclose the intriguing perspective of a systematic screening of CA among patients referred to TAVR.

22.2 Atrial Fibrillation: Rhythm and Rate Control

No evidence on the prognostic benefit of keeping sinus rhythm vs. controlling the heart rate is available, and the consensus documents do not provide any specific recommendation [2]. A pragmatic approach is to pursue a rhythm control strategy when the atria are not extensively remodeled, i.e., enlarged and dysfunctional.

All patients with AF, atrial flutter, or tachycardia should undergo a transesophageal echocardiogram (TEE) before an elective cardioversion to exclude atrial thrombosis. In a retrospective analysis of the Mayo Clinic registries, all patients with CA referred for elective direct-current cardioversion (DCCV) for atrial arrhythmias ($n = 58$; AF in 58%, atrial flutter in 41%, and atrial tachycardia in 1%) and 114 matched controls were examined. Patients with CA had more often a thrombus in the left atrium (LA) or the LA appendage (LAA; 28% vs. 3%; $p < 0.001$). As a result, the CA group had a much higher cancellation rate (28% vs. 7%; $p < 0.001$) (Fig. 22.2). Notably, among the CA patients with an intracardiac thrombus, 15% had AF from less than 48 h, and 29% had an international normalized ratio in the therapeutic range for ≥ 3 weeks. No differences were noted between patients with amyloid light-chain (AL) vs. ATTR amyloidosis, or those with AF vs. atrial flutter [12].

In the same study, among patients with CA proceeding to DCCV, the success rate (90%), the proportion of patients requiring >1 shock (33%), and median energy required (110 J) were not significantly different than the other patients [12]. Complications (ventricular tachycardia/fibrillation, need for PM implantation, acute hypoxemia, stroke) occurred in very low percentages of patients [12]. Elective DCCV performed after TEE thus emerged as an effective and safe procedure.

Evidence on pulmonary vein isolation (PVI) for AF is very limited. The success rate in patients with CA seems lower than in the general population (75% at 1 year and 60% at 3 years) [13]. Only the Japanese guideline provides specific recommendations on PVI, stating that patients with paroxysmal AF without LA dilatation or LV hypertrophy (i.e., those without extensively remodeled atria) may be candidates

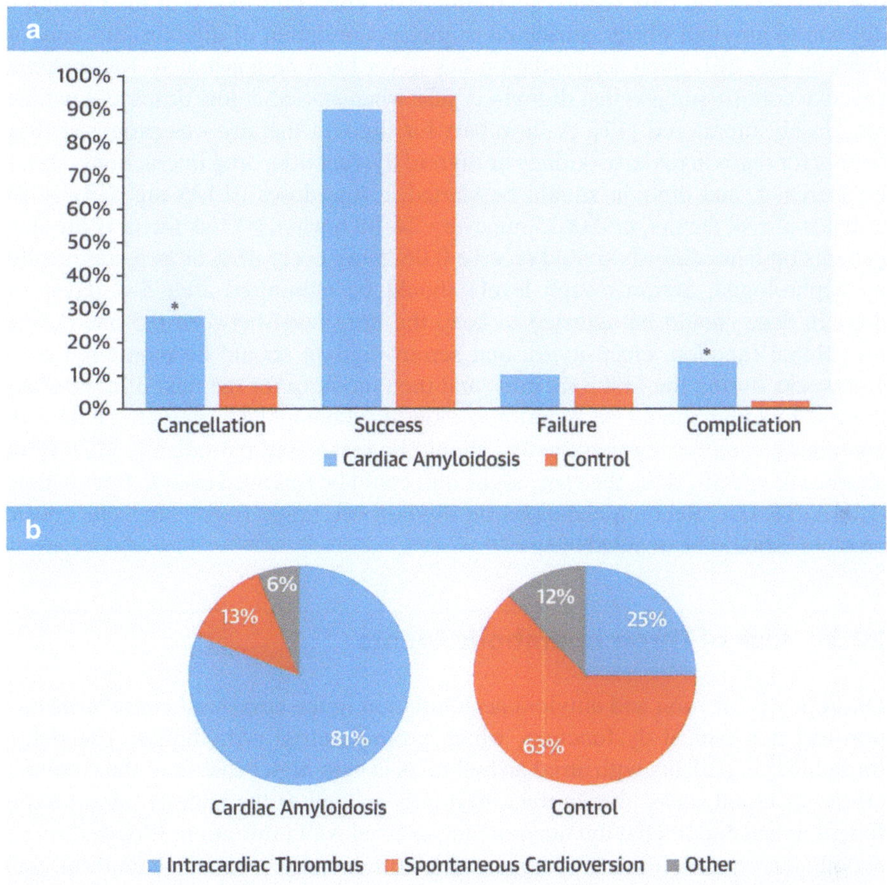

Fig. 22.2 Outcomes of transesophageal echocardiography and cardioversionTransesophageal and direct-current cardioversion procedural outcomes (**a**) and reasons for cancelling planned cardioversion (**b**) in patients with cardiac amyloidosis (CA) compared with control patients ($^*p < 0.05$ cases vs. control patients). Reprinted with permission from El-Am et al. [12]

for PVI (class IIb, level C) [2, 14]. Conversely, PVI is contraindicated for patients with AL amyloidosis, poor prognosis and severe LA dilatation, and LV hypertrophy (class III, level C) [14].

Among antiarrhythmic drugs, non-dihydropyridine calcium channel blockers (verapamil and diltiazem) should be avoided or used with extreme caution because of the risk to precipitate HF decompensation [2]. The Japanese guideline allows the use of these drugs, on a case-by-case basis, in patients with ATTR-CA and preserved ejection fraction. Beta-blockers should be avoided or used cautiously, as discussed more extensively in the section about HF management. Amiodarone is presented as the first-choice antiarrhythmic drug basically because of concerns about the other drugs [2]; its adverse effects, particularly during long-term administration, are well known. Digoxin was traditionally contraindicated in patients with

CA because of old case reports reporting toxic effects attributed to the binding of digoxin to amyloid fibrils, attributed to the accumulation of digoxin into amyloid deposits [15, 16]. Such accumulation has never been demonstrated. Recent retrospective cohorts suggest that digoxin is safe when started at low doses and patients are closely monitored [17]. A flowchart for digoxin therapy was proposed. Risk factors for digoxin toxicity (kidney or thyroid dysfunction, drug interactions) should be searched, and digoxin should be started at low doses (0.125 mg daily in the absence of risk factors, or 0.0625 mg every 24–48 h when ≥ 1 risk factor is present); patients on hemodialysis should receive 0.0625 mg every 48 h or as recommended by nephrologist. Serum trough levels should be monitored after 5–7 days, and digoxin dose should be adjusted to keep the drug level between 0.5 and 0.8 ng/mL. Renal function, electrolytes, and serum digoxin should be monitored every 1–2 weeks during the first 3 months, and then monthly for the next 3 months, and thyroid function should be monitored monthly. Potential adverse effects and the continuing need for digoxin therapy should be reassessed periodically [17]. In the absence of specific data, the same algorithm could be followed even to treat patients with ATTR-CA. Recommendations on digoxin use range from "might be considered" to "should be avoided" [2].

22.3 Risk of Thromboembolic Events

Diastolic dysfunction and amyloid accumulation in the atrial wall cause atrial dilation and mechanical dysfunction, which promote atrial arrhythmias. The risk of thrombosis in patients with atrial arrhythmias is very high because of the combined effects of blood stasis (due to the arrhythmia as well as the underlying atrial dysfunction) and endothelial dysfunction due to atrial wall infiltration. Blood stasis and endothelial dysfunction may trigger atrial thrombosis even in patients in sinus rhythm [18].

A retrospective series of 116 autopsy or explanted cases of CA reported intracardiac thrombosis in 38 hearts (33%), with 2–5 thrombi. Patients with AL-CA had significantly more intracardiac thrombus (51% vs. 16%, $p < 0.001$) and more fatal embolic events (26% vs. 8%, $p < 0.03$) than the other 61 patients (55 with wild-type [wt] ATTR) [19]. Another retrospective case series of the Mayo Clinic reported that intracardiac thrombi were present in 42 out of 156 patients (27%) undergoing a transesophageal echocardiogram for any reason [20]. Most thrombi were found in the LAA (32/58, 55%). The risk of intracardiac thrombosis was particularly high in patients with AL-CA and in those with AF, but LV diastolic dysfunction emerged as a predictor of intracardiac thrombosis independent from AF [20]. In a more recent series of 324 patients with CA from 2 European centers (79% men, 51% with ATTR-CA, 31% with AF or flutter), the prevalence of intracardiac thrombi was 6.2% (95% CI 3.5–8.8%) in the overall population, 5.2% (95% CI 1.6–8.7%) in AL, and 7.2% (95% CI 3.3–11.2%) in ATTR ($p = 0.45$) [21]. Of the patients with intracardiac thrombi ($n = 20$), 13 were in AF and 7 in sinus rhythm. The prevalence of thrombi in patients in AF/flutter was high (13.1%), 9.1% in AL, and 14.3% in ATTR ($p = 0.52$). All the patients with intracardiac thrombi in AF were under long-term anticoagulation (46% with warfarin and 54% with direct oral anticoagulants), suggesting that even anticoagulation might not be sufficient to prevent thrombus formation. The prevalence of intracardiac thrombi in patients in sinus rhythm and AL amyloidosis was 4.5%, whereas in ATTR, it was 1.1% ($p = 0.11$). Most of the intracardiac thrombi were found in the LAA (90%), but 6 patients had thrombi in other locations (30%); 2 of them had in isolation (without thrombi in the LAA), and 4 patients had thrombi in other locations as well as in the LAA (2 patients in the right atrial appendage, 1 in the LA, 1 patient had multiple thrombi). The presence of intracardiac thrombi was significantly higher in patients with more severe biventricular systolic dysfunction, atrial dilatation (LA, $p < 0.05$; right atrium, $p < 0.01$), more extensive amyloid infiltration (as estimated through the extracellular volume; $p < 0.01$), and higher levels of N-terminal pro-B-type natriuretic peptide (NT-proBNP; $p < 0.01$) and AF ($p < 0.05$) [21].

Intracardiac thrombosis may cause systemic embolic events, manifesting as stroke, transient ischemic attack (TIA), or extracranial embolic events in the lower extremities, visceral-mesenteric district, or upper extremities [22]. A multicenter retrospective study evaluated 406 patients with CA (134 AL, 73 ATTRv, and 199 ATTRwt), followed up for a median of 19 months. Thirty-one patients (7.6%) had an event (ischemic stroke, TIA, or peripheral embolism), with 10 events representing the first manifestation of CA, and the other 21 occurring over the follow-up. Ten patients experiencing an event (32.2%) were in sinus rhythm and had no history of AF. Across different CA etiologies, a consistent proportion of events occurred in the absence of documented AF (33.3% AL, 16.7% ATTRv, 37.5% ATTRwt) [23]. In another retrospective cohort of patients with CA, "no ischemic, thromboembolic, or major bleeding events" were recorded during follow-up in the 38 patients with AF (all on warfarin), and only one patient in sinus rhythm had a TIA. Eighty-one patients died (52 AL, 21 ATTRv, 8 ATTRwt) because of HF in 70 and sudden cardiac death in 6, with a similar survival in patients with or without AF [24].

Based on these premises, there is a general consensus that anticoagulation should be prescribed to patients with any atrial arrhythmia, also regardless of the CHA_2DS_2-VASc score, and may be considered also for some patients in sinus rhythm when the atria are enlarged and dysfunctional [2]. To our knowledge, the only proposed criterion for empiric anticoagulation in patients in sinus rhythm is "decreased A-wave amplitude and LA appendage velocities on echocardiography," according to the American Heart Association document [25].

In the absence of any specific evidence about the relative safety and efficacy of the possible anticoagulation strategies in patients with CA, both vitamin K antagonists (VKAs) or oral non-vitamin K antagonist anticoagulants (NOACs) can be prescribed, taking into account the same contraindications and criteria for dose reductions as the other disease settings. An interaction between dexamethasone, a drug frequently used in patients with AL amyloidosis, and VKAs has been reported, with prolongation of the international normalized ratio [26]. In patients receiving NOACs, particular attention should be paid to renal function. Dabigatran and edoxaban are excreted by 80% and 50% by kidneys, respectively, and cannot be prescribed when creatinine clearance (CrCl) is <30 mL/min [27]. Rivaroxaban must be prescribed at a lower dose (15 mg daily) when CrCl is 15–29 mL/min and cannot be prescribed when CrCl is <15 mL/min. By contrast, it has been proposed that the dose of apixaban should not be reduced in patients with advanced chronic kidney disease (including those on dialysis) unless there are at least two criteria for dose reduction: creatinine ≥1.5 mg/dL, age ≥ 80 years, and weight < 60 kg [27]. Nonetheless, therapy with VKA is the most common approach to anticoagulation when CrCl is <30 mL/min or the patient is on dialysis [27].

22.4 Conduction Disturbances

Many patients with CA develop atrioventricular (AV) conduction disturbances due to the extrinsic compression or infiltration of the atrioventricular node and His bundle. Interestingly, the basal segments of the septum are thought to be among the first sites of amyloid deposition [28]. The right atrium is less severely affected than the interventricular septum; accordingly, sinus node disease is less common than AV conduction disturbances [29, 30].

Fragmented data exist on the prevalence of AV conduction disturbances in patients with CA, and in those with ATTR- vs. AL-CA. In a small cohort of 25 patients with AL-CA, infra-His conduction times were prolonged in 92%, while sinus node function was normal in 88% [29]. In 18 patients with ATTR- or AL-CA, the HV interval was prolonged (>55 ms) in all patients [30]. In a larger cohort of patients with ATTR-CA (ATTRwt-CA, $n = 261$; ATTRv-CA, $n = 108$), 9.5% of patients had high-grade AV block requiring PM implantation at the time of diagnosis of ATTR-CA. The most common conduction abnormality was a wide QRS complex, present in 51% with ATTRwt-CA and 48% with ATTRv-CA, followed by first-degree AV block, which was present in 49% with ATTRwt-CA and 43% with ATTRv-CA. During follow-up, high-grade AV block developed in 10% of those with ATTRv-CA and 12% of patients with ATTRwt-CA and did not independently predict mortality. In a multicenter study on 405 patients (AL-CA, 29%; ATTRv-CA, 15%; ATTRwt-CA, 56%) without a PM at baseline, 9% received a PM within 3 years. History of AF (hazard ratio [HR] 3.80, $p = 0.002$), PR interval (HR 1.013, $p = 0.002$), and QRS >120 ms (HR 4.7, $p = 0.001$) on baseline ECG were independently associated with the need for PM implantation. The combined presence of these elements was associated with a sixfold higher risk of PM implantation (HR 6.26, 95% CI 1.90–20.60), while the absence of these three factors had a negative predictive value of 92% over the first 6 months. According to the authors, a specific follow-up is not needed for 6 months if no risk factor is present; otherwise, the need for PM implantation must be checked more closely, e.g., by repeating ECG Holter monitoring with less than 6-month interval to detect AV conduction disturbances [31]. In a study by Algalarrondo et al., prophylactic PM implantation was performed in patients with ATTRv polyneuropathy and some possible risk factors for AV conduction disturbances: His-ventricular interval ≥ 70 ms, His-ventricular interval > 55 ms associated with a fascicular block, a first-degree AV block, or a Wenckebach anterograde point ≤100 beats/min. Over 45 ± 35 months, a high-degree AV block was documented in 25% of these patients [32].

According to 4 out of 5 consensus documents, PM implantation might be considered according to standard indications (advanced AV block, bradycardic AF, symptomatic sinus sick syndrome) [2]. The Japanese guideline opens to prophylactic PM implantation when the risk factors considered by Algalarrondo et al. are present [32] (class IIb, level C) [14]. PM implantation should be avoided in patients with a life expectancy lower than 1 year. An abstract raised the concern of an increase in the thresholds of ventricular catheters over time, following tissue amyloid deposition [33]. This point requires further investigation.

22.5 Ventricular Arrhythmias and Dyssynchrony

In the absence of dedicated studies, all consensus documents agree that an implantable cardioverter-defibrillator should be offered to patients with standard indications for secondary prevention, with the partial exception of the Japanese guideline, which does not give a class I indication for secondary prevention because of the lack of demonstrated prognostic benefit and the frequency of pulseless electric activity as the ultimate cause of death [2, 14]. The attitude toward implantable cardioverter-defibrillator for primary prevention ranges from the "rather generous (primary prophylactic) indication" (German document) [34] to the "usually not recommended" (ESC document) [3]. The general consensus is that defibrillator implantation should be avoided in patients with a life expectancy lower than 1 year [2].

As for cardiac resynchronization therapy (CRT), all documents refer to the recommendations by the corresponding national and international societies [2]. Nonetheless, the indications to CRT were established in patients with non-amyloidotic HF, which warrants further investigations in the specific setting of CA. The ESC statement is the only one recommending that CRT be considered in patients requiring PM implantation if the paced burden is predicted to be high [3], likely based on the finding that a higher RV pacing burden is associated with deleterious remodeling and congestive HF in patients with ATTR-CA, while biventricular pacing is associated with improvements in LV ejection fraction, New York Heart Association class, and degree of mitral regurgitation [35].

22.6 Heart Failure

Patients with CA usually have dyspnea and tissue edema because of increased pressures in the pulmonary vessels and the venous system. Diuretics (loop diuretics and mineralocorticoid receptor antagonists) are often needed in high doses, are well tolerated, and may be combined. Care should be taken to avoid worsening renal function, electrolyte disturbances, and excessive preload reduction.

Beta-blockers may be poorly tolerated or contraindicated, for example because of low blood pressure levels or orthostatic hypotension, conduction disturbances, or impossibility of adequately increasing cardiac output, especially in cases with overt restrictive pathophysiology, when cardiac output becomes critically dependent on heart rate [36]. Angiotensin-converting enzyme inhibitors or angiotensin receptor blockers (ACEi/ARBs) may be poorly tolerated as well, particularly in hypotensive patients. Several consensus documents advise against the prescription of beta-blockers or ACEi/ARBs, and the ESC document even suggests discontinuing beta-blockers even if well tolerated. On the other hand, almost 30% of patients in the ATTR-ACT trial were on beta-blockers or ACEi/ARBs [1], and we have reported that the vast majority of patients may tolerate these therapies (e.g., beta-blockers in as many as 87%), with no major adverse events, if these drugs are started at a low dose and slowly up-titrated, and patients are monitored quite closely [37]. A retrospective study found no evidence of a survival benefit from beta-blocker or ACEi/ARB therapy in patients with ATTR-CA, which may challenge the need for neurohormonal antagonists in CA [38]. Nonetheless, patients with CA have a greater neurohormonal activation than those with HF [39], and such activation might contribute over time to the progression of cardiac disease. Additionally, endomyocardial biopsies of patients with CA have a large amount of fibrosis [40], which may contribute to the final manifestations of heart disease and could be blunted by antifibrotic drugs such as ACEi/ARB.

Sodium-glucose cotransporter 2 inhibitors have been shown to improve the outcome of patients with HF and either preserved or reduced EF, but patients with CA have been excluded from all phase 3 trials on empagliflozin and dapagliflozin [41–44]. The slight diuretic effect and multiple proposed cardiac protective mechanisms [45] may prove beneficial even in patients with CA. A small, single-center, retrospective study compared patients with ATTR-CA and on tafamidis ($n = 40$) with patients on tafamidis and also starting dapagliflozin ($n = 17$); both tafamidis and dapagliflozin were started at the discretion of treating physicians. Over 3 months, dapagliflozin was well tolerated, but changes in NT-proBNP did not differ between the two groups ($p = 0.557$) [46].

The evidence about inotropic therapy is very limited. In a small, retrospective cohort of patients with CA receiving levosimendan during an episode of acute HF, according to clinical indication, levosimendan proved to be well tolerated and safe, but seemed to have a limited impact on in-hospital and post-discharge outcome [47]. Even in patients with cardiogenic shock, inotrope therapy does not seem to be able to improve patient outcome. In a single-center, retrospective study, 26 patients with CA were admitted to the intensive care unit because of cardiogenic shock. Dobutamine was administered to 21 patients, with norepinephrine added in 10 patients, with progressive increase in infusion doses over the first 48 h; 2 patients were switched from dobutamine to levosimendan. The response to inotrope therapy was poor, with 17 patients (81%) dying during hospitalization, and other 4 (15%) within 3 months [48].

The small LV cavity size and restrictive physiology make CA patients poor candidates to LV assist device implantation [49]. There is evidence from retrospective cohort studies of the feasibility of intra-aortic balloon pump as a bridge to transplantation and total artificial heart implantation [50].

Heart transplantation (HT) is an option for patients with ATTRv (either as a stand-alone procedure or combined with liver transplantation), for the few patients with ATTRw who are younger than 65 years, and for selected patients with AL amyloidosis. In patients with ATTRv-CA, a multidisciplinary team including cardiologists, hepatologists, and neurologists is recommended to assess the need for combined heart and liver transplantation (class IIA, level of evidence B, in the International Society for Heart and Lung Transplantation guidelines) [51]. The Stanford cardiac transplantation evaluation guidelines may be usefully considered for screening candidates to HT [52]. In patients with AL-CA, HT should be considered only after initial chemotherapy has led to successful control of the blood dyscrasia; in selected cases, when disease-specific treatments are contraindicated because of HF, autologous stem cell transplantation should be planned as soon as clinically feasible (class IIA, level of recommendation B). Severe extracardiac amyloid organ dysfunction is a contraindication to HT (class IIA, level of evidence B) [51]. Even in this case, the Stanford evaluation guidelines may help screen candidates to HT [52]. No document provides guidance on disease-modifying therapy after HT, either alone or together with liver transplantation, or in a recipient of a transplanted heart after a domino transplantation [2].

22.7 Orthostatic Hypotension

The most common cause of orthostatic hypotension in AL and ATTRv is autonomic neuropathy. A cautious increase in salt and water intake (while avoiding HF decompensation), physical exercise, specific counter-maneuvers, compression stockings, smaller and more frequent meals, and reduced alcohol intake may all prove useful [53]. When additional pharmacological management is needed, the oral α1-adrenoreceptor agonist midodrine has been advocated in both AL [54] and ATTRv amyloidosis [53], despite the absence of dedicated studies. It has been reported that patients with AL amyloidosis do not develop supine hypertension in response to midodrine; thus, the drug can be used even at high doses [54]; conversely, supine hypertension is common in patients with ATTRv on midodrine; therefore, they should take this drug more than 3–4 h before bedtime [53]. Patients with CA can also develop hypotension during exercise, which should be distinguished from light-headedness during exercise despite normal supine and standing blood pressures, possibly because of a fixed cardiac output [54]. Treadmill testing might aid in the differential diagnosis; the first condition often responds to pre-exercise midodrine [54].

The synthetic mineralocorticoid fludrocortisone should be preferably avoided in patients with cardiac involvement [53]. Droxidopa, an oral synthetic amino acid that is converted to norepinephrine, has been proposed as an approach to orthostatic hypotension in ATTRv but is not approved in Europe [53].

22.8 Conclusions

CA requires a tailored treatment that is not less important than therapies targeting the amyloidogenic cascade. Guideline recommendations, summarized in Tables 22.1 and 22.2, do not rely on a solid body of evidence, and the process of clinical

Table 22.1 Drug therapies for heart failure and atrial fibrillation

Setting	Drug	ESC (1)	DGK (2)	CCS/CHFS (3)	AHA (5)	JCS (6)
HF	Loop or thiazide diuretics	Recommended ***	Recommended ***	Recommended ***	Recommended, but avoid underfilling and worsening renal function from restrictive physiology ***	Recommended ***
	Nitrates or carperitide (AHF)	No recommendation	No recommendation	No recommendation	No recommendation	Might be considered ***
	Catecholamines, PDEi (AHF)	No recommendation	No recommendation	No recommendation	No recommendation	Might be considered ***
	Beta-blockers	Not recommended, deprescribe ***	Avoid or very cautious use ***	Avoid or very cautious use ***	No data for benefit; may not be tolerated given fixed stroke volume ***	Tolerated dosing might be considered ***
	ACEi/ARB	Not recommended ***	Avoid or very cautious use ***	Avoid or very cautious use ***	No data for benefit; may exacerbate amyloid-related hypotension from autonomic dysfunction ***	Tolerated dosing might be considered ***
	Sacubitril/valsartan	No recommendation	No recommendation	No recommendation	No data for benefit; may exacerbate amyloid-related hypotension from autonomic dysfunction ***	No recommendation
	MRA	No recommendation	No recommendation	Recommended ***	Might be considered in conjunction with loop diuretics if adequate blood pressure and renal function ***	Tolerated dosing might be considered ***
AF/flutter/ tachycardia	Digoxin	Might be considered **	Avoid or very cautious use **	Avoid or very cautious use **	Might be considered; use cautiously **	Not recommended **
	Amiodarone	Might be considered (1st choice) ***	No recommendation	Might be considered (1st choice) ***	Might be considered (1st choice) ***	No recommendation
	Beta-blockers	Not recommended ***	Avoid or very cautious use ***	Avoid or very cautious use ***	Might be considered ***	Case-by-case decision ***
	Non-DHP CCB: ATTR-CA, preserved LV function	No recommendation	Avoid or very cautious use ***	Avoid or very cautious use ***	Avoid whenever possible ***	Case-by-case decision ***
	Non-DHP CCB: ATTR-CA, reduced LV function					Not recommended ***
	Non-DHP CCB: AL-CA				Not recommended ***	Not recommended ***
	Anticoagulation regardless of CHA$_2$DS$_2$-VASc score?	Yes ***	No recommendation	Yes ***	Yes ***	No recommendation
	Anticoagulation in SR?	Might be considered ***	No recommendation	No recommendation	Might be considered ***	No recommendation

Recommended treatments are highlighted in green, those that may be considered in yellow, and those that should be avoided in red. The levels of evidence are classified as follows: *evidence from a clinical trial in this specific population; **evidence from a subgroup analysis, retrospective studies, or case series; ***expert consensus opinion. *ACEi/ARB* angiotensin-converting enzyme inhibitor/angiotensin receptor blocker, *AF* atrial fibrillation, *AHA* American Heart Association, *AHF* acute heart failure, *AT* atrial tachycardia, *AL-CA* amyloid light-chain cardiac amyloidosis, *ATTR-CA* amyloid transthyretin cardiac amyloidosis; CCB, calcium channel blocker, *CCS/CHFS* Canadian Cardiovascular Society/Canadian Heart Failure Society, *DHP* dihydropyridine, *DOAC* direct oral anticoagulant, *DGK Deutsche Gesellschaft für Kardiologie* (German Cardiac Society), *ESC* European Society of Cardiology, *JCS* Japanese Circulation Society, *LOE* level of evidence, *LV* left ventricle, *MRA* mineralocorticoid receptor antagonist, *PDEi* phosphodiesterase inhibitor, *SR* sinus rhythm, *VKA* vitamin K antagonist. Modified with permission from Rapezzi et al. [2]

Table 22.2 Summary of statements about catheter ablation, device therapies, and heart transplantation

Strategy	ESC (1)	DGK (2)	CCS/CHFS (3)	AHA (5)	JCS (6)
AF ablation	Scarce and controversial data	*No recommendation*	Uncertain efficacy	Might be considered in selected cases **	Might be considered in patients with paroxysmal AF without LA dilatation or LV hypertrophy ** Is contraindicated for patients with AL amyloidosis, poor prognosis and severe LA dilatation, and LV hypertrophy ***
PM	Might be considered according to standard indications **	Might be considered according to standard indications ** Is contraindicated in patients with a median life expectancy <1 year ***	Might be considered according to standard indications **	Might be considered according to standard indications **	Might be considered in patients with risk factors (1st degree block, Wenckebach rate <100 bpm, AH >70 ms, HV >55 ms, bundle branch block), symptomatic sinus sick syndrome or bradycardic AF **
ICD	Is recommended for secondary prevention ** Is usually not recommended for primary prevention **	Is recommended for secondary prevention ** Might be considered in primary prevention (especially with an increased mortality risk according to serum or imaging parameters and/or documented nsVTs) ** Is contraindicated in patients with a median life expectancy <1 year ***	Is recommended for secondary prevention ** An individualized approach should be used for primary prevention **	Is recommended for secondary prevention (aborted SCD with expected survival >1 year or significant ventricular arrhythmias) ** Questionable benefit for primary prevention **	Might be considered in patients with mild hypertrophy preserved systolic/diastolic function, a good prognosis after adequate therapy ** Is contraindicated in patients with a poor prognosis (<1 year) ***
CRT	Might be considered if high pacing burden expected ***	Might be considered according to the general indications ***	No specific evidence	Might be considered in PM-dependent patients ***	Might be considered in patients with LBBB and an expected survival >1 year *** Is contraindicated for patients with a poor prognosis (<1 year), QRS <150 ms, conduction disturbances other than LBBB ***
Heart transplantation	Might be considered in selected cases **	*No recommendation*	Might be considered for select patients with advanced HF, in whom significant extracardiac manifestations are absent and the risk of disease progression is considered low and/or amenable to disease-modifying therapy **	Might be considered in patients with stage D HF **	*No recommendation*
MCS	LVAD not suitable for most patients **	*No recommendation*	Uncertain role	Limited data	*No recommendation*

Recommended treatments are highlighted in green, those that may be considered in yellow, and those that should be avoided in red. The levels of evidence are classified as follows: *evidence from a clinical trial in this specific population; **evidence from a subgroup analysis, retrospective studies, or case series; ***expert consensus opinion. *AHA* American Heart Association, *AL* amyloid light chain, *CCS/CHFS* Canadian Cardiovascular Society/Canadian Heart Failure Society, *CRT* cardiac resynchronization therapy, *DGK Deutsche Gesellschaft für Kardiologie* (German Cardiac Society), *ESC* European Society of Cardiology, *HF* heart failure, *ICD* implantable cardioverter defibrillator, *JCS* Japanese Circulation Society, *LA* left atrial, *LV* left ventricular, *LBBB* left bundle branch block, *LOE* level of evidence, *LVAD* left ventricular assist device, *MCS* mechanical circulatory support, *PM* pacemaker, *SCD* sudden cardiac death. Modified with permission from Rapezzi et al. [2]

decision-making must integrate these recommendations with a careful assessment of the individual phenotype, a multidisciplinary evaluation, the request for advice from specialized centers, and also active engagement of patients and their families in therapeutic choices.

References

1. Maurer MS, Schwartz JH, Gundapaneni B, Elliott PM, Merlini G, Waddington-Cruz M, Kristen AV, Grogan M, Witteles R, Damy T, Drachman BM, Shah SJ, Hanna M, Judge DP, Barsdorf AI, Huber P, Patterson TA, Riley S, Schumacher J, Stewart M, Sultan MB, Rapezzi C. Tafamidis treatment for patients with transthyretin amyloid cardiomyopathy. N Engl J Med. 2018;379:1007–16.
2. Rapezzi C, Aimo A, Serenelli M, Barison A, Vergaro G, Passino C, Panichella G, Sinagra G, Merlo M, Fontana M, Gillmore J, Quarta CC, Maurer MS, Kittleson MM, Garcia-Pavia P, Emdin M. Critical comparison of documents from scientific societies on cardiac amyloidosis: JACC state-of-the-art review. J Am Coll Cardiol. 2022;79:1288–303.
3. Garcia-Pavia P, Rapezzi C, Adler Y, Arad M, Basso C, Brucato A, Burazor I, Caforio ALP, Damy T, Eriksson U, Fontana M, Gillmore JD, Gonzalez-Lopez E, Grogan M, Heymans S, Imazio M, Kindermann I, Kristen AV, Maurer MS, Merlini G, Pantazis A, Pankuweit S, Rigopoulos AG, Linhart A. Diagnosis and treatment of cardiac amyloidosis. A position statement of the European Society of Cardiology Working Group on Myocardial and Pericardial Diseases. Eur J Heart Fail. 2021;23:512–26.
4. Ando Y, Adams D, Benson MD, Berk JL, Planté-Bordeneuve V, Coelho T, Conceição I, Ericzon BG, Obici L, Rapezzi C, Sekijima Y, Ueda M, Palladini G, Merlini G. Guidelines and new directions in the therapy and monitoring of ATTRv amyloidosis. Amyloid. 2022;29:143–55.
5. Ternacle J, Krapf L, Mohty D, Magne J, Nguyen A, Galat A, Gallet R, Teiger E, Côté N, Clavel MA, Tournoux F, Pibarot P, Damy T. Aortic stenosis and cardiac amyloidosis: JACC review topic of the week. J Am Coll Cardiol. 2019;74:2638–51.
6. Aimo A, Merlo M, Porcari A, Georgiopoulos G, Pagura L, Vergaro G, Sinagra G, Emdin M, Rapezzi C. Redefining the epidemiology of cardiac amyloidosis. A systematic review and meta-analysis of screening studies. Eur J Heart Fail. 2022;24:2342–51.
7. Nitsche C, Scully PR, Patel KP, Kammerlander AA, Koschutnik M, Dona C, Wollenweber T, Ahmed N, Thornton GD, Kelion AD, Sabharwal N, Newton JD, Ozkor M, Kennon S, Mullen M, Lloyd G, Fontana M, Hawkins PN, Pugliese F, Menezes LJ, Moon JC, Mascherbauer J, Treibel TA. Prevalence and outcomes of concomitant aortic stenosis and cardiac amyloidosis. J Am Coll Cardiol. 2021;77:128–39.
8. Hussain M, Hanna M, Griffin BP, Conic J, Patel J, Fava AM, Watson C, Phelan DM, Jellis C, Grimm RA, Rodriguez LL, Schoenhagen P, Hachamovitch R, Jaber WA, Cremer PC, Collier P. Aortic valve calcium in patients with transthyretin cardiac amyloidosis: a propensity-matched analysis. Circ Cardiovasc Imaging. 2020;13:e011433.
9. Ricci F, Ceriello L, Khanji MY, Dangas G, Bucciarelli-Ducci C, Di Mauro M, Fedorowski A, Zimarino M, Gallina S. Prognostic significance of cardiac amyloidosis in patients with aortic stenosis: a systematic review and meta-analysis. JACC Cardiovasc Imaging. 2021;14:293–5.
10. Gama F, Rosmini S, Bandula S, Patel KP, Massa P, Tobon-Gomez C, Ecke K, Stroud T, Condron M, Thornton GD, Bennett JB, Wechelakar A, Gillmore JD, Whelan C, Lachmann H, Taylor SA, Pugliese F, Fontana M, Moon JC, Hawkins PN, Treibel TA. Extracellular volume fraction by computed tomography predicts long-term prognosis among patients with cardiac amyloidosis. JACC Cardiovasc Imaging. 2022;15:2082–94.
11. Han D, Tamarappoo B, Klein E, Tyler J, Chakravarty T, Otaki Y, Miller R, Eisenberg E, Park R, Singh S, Shiota T, Siegel R, Stegic J, Salseth T, Cheng W, Dey D, Thomson L, Berman D, Makkar R, Friedman J. Computed tomography angiography-derived extracellular volume

fraction predicts early recovery of left ventricular systolic function after transcatheter aortic valve replacement. Eur Heart J Cardiovasc Imaging. 2021;22:179–85.

12. El-Am EA, Dispenzieri A, Melduni RM, Ammash NM, White RD, Hodge DO, Noseworthy PA, Lin G, Pislaru SV, Egbe AC, Grogan M, Nkomo VT. Direct current cardioversion of atrial arrhythmias in adults with cardiac amyloidosis. J Am Coll Cardiol. 2019;73:589–97.

13. Tan NY, Mohsin Y, Hodge DO, Lacy MQ, Packer DL, Dispenzieri A, Grogan M, Asirvatham SJ, Madhavan M, Mc LC. Catheter ablation for atrial arrhythmias in patients with cardiac amyloidosis. J Cardiovasc Electrophysiol. 2016;27:1167–73.

14. Kitaoka H, Izumi C, Izumiya Y, Inomata T, Ueda M, Kubo T, Koyama J, Sano M, Sekijima Y, Tahara N, Tsukada N, Tsujita K, Tsutsui H, Tomita T, Amano M, Endo J, Okada A, Oda S, Takashio S, Baba Y, Misumi Y, Yazaki M, Anzai T, Ando Y, Isobe M, Kimura T, Fukuda K. JCS 2020 guideline on diagnosis and treatment of cardiac amyloidosis. Circ J. 2020;84:1610–71.

15. Cassidy JT. Cardiac amyloidosis. Two cases with digitalis sensitivity. Ann Int Med. 1961;55:989–94.

16. Rubinow A, Skinner M, Cohen AS. Digoxin sensitivity in amyloid cardiomyopathy. Circulation. 1981;63:1285–8.

17. Muchtar E, Gertz MA, Kumar SK, Lin G, Boilson B, Clavell A, Lacy MQ, Buadi FK, Hayman SR, Kapoor P, Dingli D, Rajkumar SV, Dispenzieri A, Grogan M. Digoxin use in systemic light-chain (AL) amyloidosis: contra-indicated or cautious use? Amyloid. 2018;25:86–92.

18. Vergaro G, Aimo A, Rapezzi C, Castiglione V, Fabiani I, Pucci A, Buda G, Passino C, Lupón J, Bayes-Genis A, Emdin M, Braunwald E. Atrial amyloidosis: mechanisms and clinical manifestations. Eur J Heart Fail. 2022;24:2019–28.

19. Feng D, Edwards WD, Oh JK, Chandrasekaran K, Grogan M, Martinez MW, Syed IS, Hughes DA, Lust JA, Jaffe AS, Gertz MA, Klarich KW. Intracardiac thrombosis and embolism in patients with cardiac amyloidosis. Circulation. 2007;116:2420–6.

20. Feng D, Syed IS, Martinez M, Oh JK, Jaffe AS, Grogan M, Edwards WD, Gertz MA, Klarich KW. Intracardiac thrombosis and anticoagulation therapy in cardiac amyloidosis. Circulation. 2009;119:2490–7.

21. Martinez-Naharro A, Gonzalez-Lopez E, Corovic A, Mirelis JG, Baksi AJ, Moon JC, Garcia-Pavia P, Gillmore JD, Hawkins PN, Fontana M. High prevalence of intracardiac thrombi in cardiac amyloidosis. J Am Coll Cardiol. 2019;73:1733–4.

22. Bekwelem W, Connolly SJ, Halperin JL, Adabag S, Duval S, Chrolavicius S, Pogue J, Ezekowitz MD, Eikelboom JW, Wallentin LG, Yusuf S, Hirsch AT. Extracranial systemic embolic events in patients with nonvalvular atrial fibrillation: incidence, risk factors, and outcomes. Circulation. 2015;132:796–803.

23. Cappelli F, Tini G, Russo D, Emdin M, Del Franco A, Vergaro G, Di Bella G, Mazzeo A, Canepa M, Volpe M, Perfetto F, Autore C, Di Mario C, Rapezzi C, Musumeci MB. Arterial thrombo-embolic events in cardiac amyloidosis: a look beyond atrial fibrillation. Amyloid. 2021;28:12–8.

24. Longhi S, Quarta CC, Milandri A, Lorenzini M, Gagliardi C, Manuzzi L, Bacchi-Reggiani ML, Leone O, Ferlini A, Russo A, Gallelli I, Rapezzi C. Atrial fibrillation in amyloidotic cardiomyopathy: prevalence, incidence, risk factors and prognostic role. Amyloid. 2015;22:147–55.

25. Kittleson MM, Maurer MS, Ambardekar AV, Bullock-Palmer RP, Chang PP, Eisen HJ, Nair AP, Nativi-Nicolau J, Ruberg FL. Cardiac amyloidosis: evolving diagnosis and management: a scientific statement from the American Heart Association. Circulation. 2020;142:e7–e22.

26. Sellam J, Costedoat-Chalumeau N, Amoura Z, Aymard G, Choquet S, Trad S, Vignes BL, Hulot JS, Berenbaum F, Lechat P, Cacoub P, Ankri A, Mariette X, Leblond V, Piette JC. Potentiation of fluindione or warfarin by dexamethasone in multiple myeloma and AL amyloidosis. Joint Bone Spine. 2007;74:446–52.

27. Chan KE, Giugliano RP, Patel MR, Abramson S, Jardine M, Zhao S, Perkovic V, Maddux FW, Piccini JP. Nonvitamin K anticoagulant agents in patients with advanced chronic kidney disease or on dialysis with AF. J Am Coll Cardiol. 2016;67:2888–99.

28. Grigoratos C, Aimo A, Rapezzi C, Genovesi D, Barison A, Aquaro GD, Vergaro G, Pucci A, Passino C, Marzullo P, Gimelli A, Emdin M. Diphosphonate single-photon emission computed tomography in cardiac transthyretin amyloidosis. Int J Cardiol. 2020;307:187–92.
29. Reisinger J, Dubrey SW, Lavalley M, Skinner M, Falk RH. Electrophysiologic abnormalities in AL (primary) amyloidosis with cardiac involvement. J Am Coll Cardiol. 1997;30:1046–51.
30. Barbhaiya CR, Kumar S, Baldinger SH, Michaud GF, Stevenson WG, Falk R, John RM. Electrophysiologic assessment of conduction abnormalities and atrial arrhythmias associated with amyloid cardiomyopathy. Heart Rhythm. 2016;13:383–90.
31. Porcari A, Rossi M, Cappelli F, Canepa M, Musumeci B, Cipriani A, Tini G, Barbati G, Varrà GG, Morelli C, Fumagalli C, Zampieri M, Argirò A, Vianello PF, Sessarego E, Russo D, Sinigiani G, De Michieli L, Di Bella G, Autore C, Perfetto F, Rapezzi C, Sinagra G, Merlo M. Incidence and risk factors for pacemaker implantation in light-chain and transthyretin cardiac amyloidosis. Eur J Heart Fail. 2022;24:1227–36.
32. Algalarrondo V, Dinanian S, Juin C, Chemla D, Bennani SL, Sebag C, Planté V, Le Guludec D, Samuel D, Adams D, Slama MS. Prophylactic pacemaker implantation in familial amyloid polyneuropathy. Heart Rhythm. 2012;9:1069–75.
33. Wang JQ, Yang DY, Fang Q. Stability of pacemaker parameters in cardiac amyloidosis patients. Eur Heart J. 2021;42(Suppl. 1):ehab724-0678.
34. Yilmaz A, Bauersachs J, Bengel F, Büchel R, Kindermann I, Klingel K, Knebel F, Meder B, Morbach C, Nagel E, Schulze-Bahr E, Aus dem Siepen F, Frey N. Diagnosis and treatment of cardiac amyloidosis: position statement of the German Cardiac Society (DGK). Clin Res Cardiol. 2021;110:479–506.
35. Donnellan E, Wazni OM, Saliba WI, Baranowski B, Hanna M, Martyn M, Patel D, Trulock K, Menon V, Hussein A, Aagaard P, Jaber W, Kanj M. Cardiac devices in patients with transthyretin amyloidosis: impact on functional class, left ventricular function, mitral regurgitation, and mortality. J Cardiovasc Electrophysiol. 2019;30:2427–32.
36. Milani P, Dispenzieri A, Scott CG, Gertz MA, Perlini S, Mussinelli R, Lacy MQ, Buadi FK, Kumar S, Maurer MS, Merlini G, Hayman SR, Leung N, Dingli D, Klarich KW, Lust JA, Lin Y, Kapoor P, Go RS, Pellikka PA, Hwa YL, Zeldenrust SR, Kyle RA, Rajkumar SV, Grogan M. Independent prognostic value of stroke volume index in patients with immunoglobulin light chain amyloidosis. Circ Cardiovasc Imaging. 2018;11:e006588.
37. Aimo A, Vergaro G, Castiglione V, Rapezzi C, Emdin M. Safety and tolerability of neurohormonal antagonism in cardiac amyloidosis. Eur J Int Med. 2020;80:66–72.
38. Cheng RK, Vasbinder A, Levy WC, Goyal P, Griffin JM, Leedy DJ, Maurer MS. Lack of association between neurohormonal blockade and survival in transthyretin cardiac amyloidosis. J Am Heart Assoc. 2021;10:e022859.
39. Vergaro G, Aimo A, Campora A, Castiglione V, Prontera C, Masotti S, Musetti V, Chianca M, Valleggi A, Spini V, Emdin M, Passino C. Patients with cardiac amyloidosis have a greater neurohormonal activation than those with non-amyloidotic heart failure. Amyloid. 2021;28:252–8.
40. Pucci A, Aimo A, Musetti V, Barison A, Vergaro G, Genovesi D, Giorgetti A, Masotti S, Arzilli C, Prontera C, Pastormerlo LE, Coceani MA, Ciardetti M, Martini N, Palmieri C, Passino C, Rapezzi C, Emdin M. Amyloid deposits and fibrosis on left ventricular endomyocardial biopsy correlate with extracellular volume in cardiac amyloidosis. J Am Heart Assoc. 2021;10:e020358.
41. Anker SD, Butler J, Filippatos G, Ferreira JP, Bocchi E, Böhm M, Brunner-La Rocca HP, Choi DJ, Chopra V, Chuquiure-Valenzuela E, Giannetti N, Gomez-Mesa JE, Janssens S, Januzzi JL, Gonzalez-Juanatey JR, Merkely B, Nicholls SJ, Perrone SV, Piña IL, Ponikowski P, Senni M, Sim D, Spinar J, Squire I, Taddei S, Tsutsui H, Verma S, Vinereanu D, Zhang J, Carson P, Lam CSP, Marx N, Zeller C, Sattar N, Jamal W, Schnaidt S, Schnee JM, Brueckmann M, Pocock SJ, Zannad F, Packer M. Empagliflozin in heart failure with a preserved ejection fraction. N Engl J Med. 2021;385:1451–61.
42. Packer M, Anker SD, Butler J, Filippatos G, Pocock SJ, Carson P, Januzzi J, Verma S, Tsutsui H, Brueckmann M, Jamal W, Kimura K, Schnee J, Zeller C, Cotton D, Bocchi E, Böhm M, Choi DJ, Chopra V, Chuquiure E, Giannetti N, Janssens S, Zhang J, Gonzalez Juanatey JR,

Kaul S, Brunner-La Rocca HP, Merkely B, Nicholls SJ, Perrone S, Pina I, Ponikowski P, Sattar N, Senni M, Seronde MF, Spinar J, Squire I, Taddei S, Wanner C, Zannad F. Cardiovascular and renal outcomes with empagliflozin in heart failure. N Engl J Med. 2020;383:1413–24.

43. McMurray JJV, Solomon SD, Inzucchi SE, Køber L, Kosiborod MN, Martinez FA, Ponikowski P, Sabatine MS, Anand IS, Bělohlávek J, Böhm M, Chiang CE, Chopra VK, de Boer RA, Desai AS, Diez M, Drozdz J, Dukát A, Ge J, Howlett JG, Katova T, Kitakaze M, Ljungman CEA, Merkely B, Nicolau JC, O'Meara E, Petrie MC, Vinh PN, Schou M, Tereshchenko S, Verma S, Held C, DeMets DL, Docherty KF, Jhund PS, Bengtsson O, Sjöstrand M, Langkilde AM. Dapagliflozin in patients with heart failure and reduced ejection fraction. N Engl J Med. 2019;381:1995–2008.

44. Solomon SD, McMurray JJV, Claggett B, de Boer RA, DeMets D, Hernandez AF, Inzucchi SE, Kosiborod MN, Lam CSP, Martinez F, Shah SJ, Desai AS, Jhund PS, Belohlavek J, Chiang CE, Borleffs CJW, Comin-Colet J, Dobreanu D, Drozdz J, Fang JC, Alcocer-Gamba MA, Al Habeeb W, Han Y, Cabrera Honorio JW, Janssens SP, Katova T, Kitakaze M, Merkely B, O'Meara E, Saraiva JFK, Tereshchenko SN, Thierer J, Vaduganathan M, Vardeny O, Verma S, Pham VN, Wilderäng U, Zaozerska N, Bachus E, Lindholm D, Petersson M, Langkilde AM. Dapagliflozin in heart failure with mildly reduced or preserved ejection fraction. N Engl J Med. 2022;387:1089–98.

45. Packer M. Critical reanalysis of the mechanisms underlying the cardiorenal benefits of sglt2 inhibitors and reaffirmation of the nutrient deprivation signaling/autophagy hypothesis. Circulation. 2022;146:1383–405.

46. Dobner S, Bernhard B, Asatryan B, Windecker S, Stortecky S, Pilgrim T, Gräni C, Hunziker L. SGLT2 inhibitor therapy for transthyretin amyloid cardiomyopathy: early tolerance and clinical response to dapagliflozin. ESC Heart Fail. 2023;10(1):397–404.

47. Aimo A, Rapezzi C, Arzilli C, Vergaro G, Emdin M. Safety and efficacy of levosimendan in patients with cardiac amyloidosis. Eur J Int Med. 2020;80:114–6.

48. d'Humières T, Fard D, Damy T, Roubille F, Galat A, Doan HL, Oliver L, Dubois-Randé JL, Squara P, Lim P, Ternacle J. Outcome of patients with cardiac amyloidosis admitted to an intensive care unit for acute heart failure. Arch Cardiovasc Dis. 2018;111:582–90.

49. Fine NM, Davis MK, Anderson K, Delgado DH, Giraldeau G, Kitchlu A, Massie R, Narayan J, Swiggum E, Venner CP, Ducharme A, Galant NJ, Hahn C, Howlett JG, Mielniczuk L, Parent MC, Reece D, Royal V, Toma M, Virani SA, Zieroth S. Canadian Cardiovascular Society/ Canadian Heart Failure Society joint position statement on the evaluation and management of patients with cardiac amyloidosis. Can J Cardiol. 2020;36:322–34.

50. Witteles RM. Cardiac transplantation and mechanical circulatory support in amyloidosis. JACC CardioOncol. 2021;3:516–21.

51. Mehra MR, Canter CE, Hannan MM, Semigran MJ, Uber PA, Baran DA, Danziger-Isakov L, Kirklin JK, Kirk R, Kushwaha SS, Lund LH, Potena L, Ross HJ, Taylor DO, Verschuuren EA, Zuckermann A. The 2016 International Society for Heart Lung Transplantation listing criteria for heart transplantation: a 10-year update. J Heart Lung Transplant. 2016;35:1–23.

52. Varr BC, Liedtke M, Arai S, Lafayette RA, Schrier SL, Witteles RM. Heart transplantation and cardiac amyloidosis: approach to screening and novel management strategies. J Heart Lung Transplant. 2012;31:325–31.

53. Palma JA, Gonzalez-Duarte A, Kaufmann H. Orthostatic hypotension in hereditary transthyretin amyloidosis: epidemiology, diagnosis and management. Clin Auton Res. 2019;29:33–44.

54. Falk RH, Alexander KM, Liao R, Dorbala S. AL (light-chain) cardiac amyloidosis: a review of diagnosis and therapy. J Am Coll Cardiol. 2016;68:1323–41.

Monitoring Disease Progression and Response to Disease-Modifying Treatments

23

Giuseppe Vergaro, Gabriele Buda, and Marianna Fontana

23.1 Disease Monitoring in Transthyretin Cardiac Amyloidosis

ATTR amyloidosis is a progressive disorder related to the deposition into amyloid fibrils of misfolded mutated (variant ATTR, vATTR) or non-mutated (wild-type ATTR, wtATTR) transthyretin. In wtATTR, heart and soft tissues are typically involved, while the extent of cardiac and nervous system involvement depends on the pathogenic *TTR* mutation in vATTR [1].

In clinical practice, several variables from different domains can be considered to assess disease course and progression during individual patient follow-up. Among clinical variables, the heart failure (HF)-related hospitalization is likely the more meaningful, as it reflects a clinical worsening of the patients and the need for intravenous diuretic therapy [2]. Other clinical variables that are also frequently adopted as end points in clinical trials [3] are changes in New York Heart Association (NYHA) functional class, quality-of-life questionnaires (e.g., the Kansas City Cardiomyopathy Questionnaire or the Short Form 36 Health Survey), and changes in the distance walked at 6-minute walking test (6MWT). Although widely adopted,

G. Vergaro (✉)
Health Science Interdisciplinary Center, Scuola Superiore Sant'Anna and Fondazione Toscana Gabriele Monasterio, Pisa, Italy
e-mail: giuseppe1.vergaro@santannapisa.it

G. Buda
Hematology Department, University of Pisa, Pisa, Italy
e-mail: g.buda@ao-pisa.toscana.it

M. Fontana
National Amyloidosis Centre, University College London, London, UK
e-mail: m.fontana@ucl.ac.uk

both NYHA class and quality-of-life questionnaires are subjective and should be used together with other objective measures to confirm stability or progression of the disease. 6MWT distance can be a valuable tool for disease monitoring, as it is a simple, cheap, and widely available measure of functional capacity [4].

Circulating biomarkers are useful to raise initial suspicion of the disease and to support and confirm the diagnosis [5], but they also hold a relevant prognostic value. B-type natriuretic peptides (BNP and N-terminal fraction of proBNP, NT-proBNP) and troponins increase in CA due to volume overload, cardiac remodeling following amyloid infiltration, and direct cytotoxicity of amyloid precursors [6]. Natriuretic peptides and/or troponins have been incorporated into several risk stratification scores such as the Mayo staging systems [7], the National Amyloidosis Centre (NAC) staging system for ATTR-CA [8], or the score proposed by Cheng and Colleagues [9] (Table 23.1). Still, caution should be used in patients with atrial fibrillation, which is known to increase circulating concentration of natriuretic peptides [10], and in patients with impaired or fluctuating glomerular filtration rate, as clearance of natriuretic peptide (NT-proBNP more than BNP) and of troponin is dependent on renal function.

Electrocardiogram (ECG) is frequently abnormal at diagnosis in patients with ATTR-CA [11], but the appearance of new-onset supraventricular arrhythmias, in particular atrial fibrillation, and of atrioventricular or intraventricular conduction disorders can determine a clinical decompensation and may require a device implantation [12]. They are therefore often considered as indices of disease progression in patients with ATTR-CA.

Imaging tools are also frequently used to assess and to monitor cardiac involvement in patients with either wtATTR or vATTR. Echocardiography can provide a measure of left ventricular (LV) mass, as well as of LV systolic and diastolic function, of valvular diseases, and of four-chamber deformation (with speckle tracking imaging) [13]. Echocardiography is easily available and can be serially repeated during a patient follow-up, but intra- and inter-operator variability should be considered. Based on clinical trial data showing that 8% of patients experienced ≥ 2 mm increase in LV wall thickness, this threshold is considered to be suggestive of disease progression [14, 15]. Notably, different echocardiographic variables may be more indicative of disease progression at different stages of disease. For example,

Table 23.1 Staging systems for transthyretin amyloid cardiomyopathy

Mayo [7]	National Amyloidosis Centre [8]	Cheng [9]
Troponin T > 0.05 ng/mL NT-proBNP >3000 pg/mL	eGFR <45 mL/min NT-proBNP >3000 pg/mL	Mayo or NAC score (0–2 points) Daily dose of furosemide or equivalent: 0 mg/kg (0 points), >0–0.5 mg/kg (1 point), >0.5–1 mg/kg (2 points), and > 1 mg/kg (3 points) NYHA class I–IV (1–4 points)

eGFR estimated glomerular filtration rate, *NAC* National Amyloidosis Centre, *NYHA* New York Heart Association, *NT-proBNP* N-terminal fragment of B-type natriuretic peptide deformation analysis and diastolic dysfunction may be more informative in patients at earlier stages, while changes on LV mass and systolic function may occur later.

Cardiac magnetic resonance (CMR) can provide more accurate measures of cardiac structure and function, and with the use of native T1 mapping and of T1 with late gadolinium enhancement (LGE) can provide a myocardial tissue characterization as well as the measurement of extracellular volume (ECV) [16]. The potential for CMR in the monitoring of disease is enormous, but its cost and availability limit its serial use during patients' follow-up.

Finally, cardiac scintigraphy with bone-avid tracers has an established role in the diagnostic flowchart of CA and can confirm the diagnosis of ATTR-CA without the need for a tissue confirmation in selected cases [17]. Assessment of amyloid burden with single-photon emission computed tomography (SPECT) is of potential utility in patients with ATTR-CA, but there is currently no recommendation about serial SPECT imaging.

An expert consensus has been published in 2021 on the monitoring of patients with ATTR-CA, proposing a multivariable approach. The authors have included some of the previously mentioned variables and have proposed that, to define a clinically meaningful progression of the disease, a worsening in at least one item from each of the three relevant domains ("clinical and functional," "laboratory biomarkers," and "imaging and ECG") has to be observed [14] (Fig. 23.1). The authors

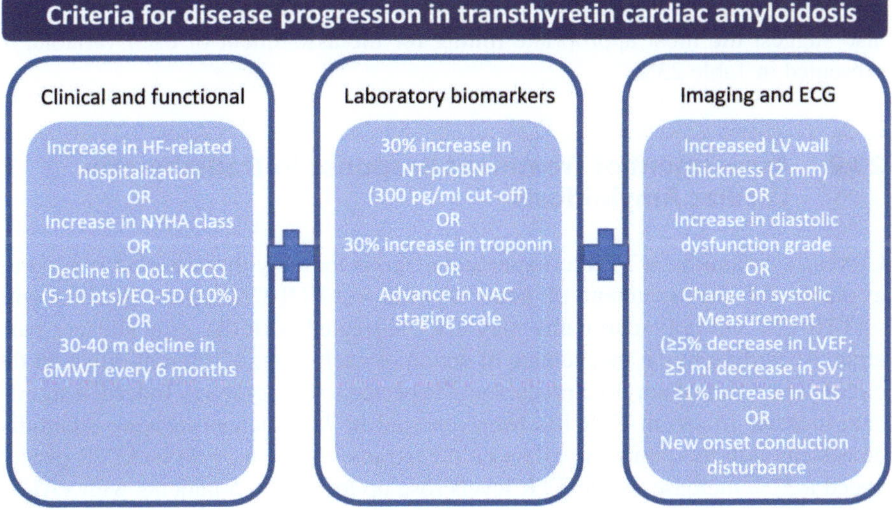

Fig. 23.1 Criteria for disease progression in patients with transthyretin cardiac amyloidosisAt least one marker from each domain is required to define disease progression. *6MWT* 6-minute walking test, *ECG* electrocardiogram, *EQ-5D* EuroQol five dimensions, *GLS* global longitudinal strain, *HF* heart failure, *KCCQ* Kansas City Cardiomyopathy Questionnaire, *LV* left ventricular, *LVEF, LV* left ventricular ejection fraction, *NAC* UK National Amyloidosis Centre, *NT-proBNP* N-terminal pro-B-type natriuretic peptide, *NYHA* New York Heart Association, *QoL* quality of life. Modified from Garcia-Pavia et al. [14]

Table 23.2 Timing for measurement of items for the assessment of disease progression

Item and domain	Tool	Recommended frequency of measurement
Clinical and functional		
Clinical and medical history	Cardiovascular-related hospitalizations	6 months
HF class: NYHA class	Stepwise class change	6 months
QoL: EQ-5D tool and KCCQ	Description of measurements	6–12 months
Functional capacity	6MWT	6 months
Biomarkers and laboratory markers		
Biomarkers and laboratory markers	NT-proBNP	6 months
	Troponin (high-sensitivity) assay	6 months
	Clinical staging system	6 months
Imaging parameters and ECG		
Echocardiography	LV measures wall thickness/mass	6–12 months
	Systolic function measurements	12 months
	Diastolic dysfunction worsening	12 months
ECG/Holter ECG	New onset of arrhythmic/ conduction disturbances	6 months

6MWT 6-minute walking test, *ECG* electrocardiogram, *EQ-5D* EuroQol five dimensions, *HF* heart failure, *KCCQ*, Kansas City Cardiomyopathy Questionnaire, *LV* left ventricular, *LVEF LV* left ventricular ejection fraction, *NT-proBNP* N-terminal pro-B-type natriuretic peptide, *NYHA* New York Heart Association, *QoL* quality of life. Modified from Garcia-Pavia et al. [14]

also suggest the most appropriate timing for the assessment of each variable, as presented in Table 23.2.

23.2 Assessment of Treatment Response in Transthyretin Cardiac Amyloidosis

Currently, tafamidis, a TTR tetramer stabilizer, is the only disease-modifying drug available for the treatment of patients with wtATTR-CA, while patients with vATTR-CA and polyneuropathy may also be treated with the gene silencer patisiran. According to the mechanism of action of each drug, a different effect on the circulating levels of amyloid precursor is expected to be observed. Indeed, a significant increase in serum TTR has been reported in 72 patients receiving tafamidis, consistent with its stabilizing effect on the tetramer; patients with wtATTR experienced a 32% increase, while TTR levels rose up to 71% in 5 patients with vATTR [18]. Among patients with vATTR enrolled in the APOLLO trial (A Phase 3 Multicenter, Multinational, Randomized, Double-blind, Placebo-controlled Study to Evaluate the Efficacy and Safety of Patisiran in Transthyretin-Mediated Polyneuropathy), half of them presenting with cardiomyopathy, treatment with patisiran was instead associated with a decrease in serum TTR compared to the placebo group as early as 3 weeks after treatment initiation [19]. Finally, there is initial evidence that the analysis of circulating forms of TTR (e.g., dimers, trimers, tetramers complexed with 1 or 2 retinol-binding protein) may be helpful in identifying responders to disease-modifying treatments in ATTR-CA [20].

Further to the amyloidogenic precursor, other biohumoral markers of cardiac involvement may reflect the extent of organ damage and track response to therapy. Both natriuretic peptides and troponins hold a relevant role for the diagnosis and risk stratification in ATTR-CA, but their potential for the assessment of therapeutic response has been poorly investigated. There is data from the phase III Transthyretin Amyloidosis Cardiomyopathy Clinical Trial (ATTR-ACT) trial reporting a smaller increase in NT-proBNP at 12 and 30 months among patients on tafamidis compared to those randomized to placebo (least squares mean difference, −735 [95% CI, −1249 to −221] at 12 months) [3]. Such evidence is consistent with a stabilizing effect of tafamidis on different clinical markers and features of ATTR-CA.

Echocardiography is a safe, cheap, and widely available technique. Echocardiographic findings can be influenced, at different extents and at different timings, by treatments for ATTR-CA. In a retrospective analysis of 45 patients with ATTR-CA (23 treated with tafamidis, 22 untreated), absolute global longitudinal strain (GLS), myocardial work index, and efficiency deteriorated more in the untreated group compared to the tafamidis group, while no difference was observed in LV ejection fraction (LVEF) [21]. In the cardiac subpopulation ($n = 126$) of the APOLLO trial, patisiran reduced mean LV wall thickness and septal and posterior wall thickness at month 18 versus placebo [15].

Compared to echocardiography, CMR can provide an advanced myocardial tissue characterization with native T1 mapping and measurement of extracellular volume (ECV), both indicating cardiac amyloid burden and predicting outcome [22, 23]. In a study performed at the UK National Amyloid Center in London, serial CMR studies showed a reduction in ECV (adjusted mean difference between groups: −6.2% [95% confidence interval [CI]: −9.5% to −3.0%]; $p = 0.001$) in patients treated with patisiran, consistent with a regression of cardiac amyloid burden at least in a subset of treated patients (Fig. 23.2) [24]. Interestingly, in the same

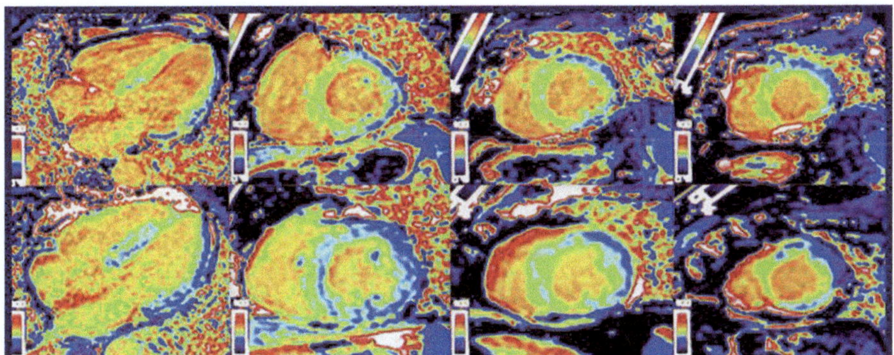

Fig. 23.2 Cardiac magnetic resonance showing reduction in extracellular volume with treatment in transthyretin cardiac amyloidosis

ECV maps (left-to-right: four-chamber, basal, mid, and apical short axis) of a patient at baseline (upper panels) and 12 months after treatment with patisiran (lower panels). *ECV* extracellular volume. Modified from Fontana et al. [24]

study, most of treated patients had a reduction in cardiac uptake of 99mTc-3,3-diphosphono-1,2-propanodicarboxylic acid (DPD) scintigraphy. The use of scintigraphy with bone tracer is currently not supported for the monitoring of response to treatment, but quantitative assessment of global and regional myocardial uptake may be promising [25].

23.3   Disease Monitoring in Light-Chain Cardiac Amyloidosis

Light-chain (AL) amyloidosis is a systemic disorder caused by an abnormal production of monoclonal immunoglobulin light chain, which misfolds and deposits in the interstitial space of different tissues. In AL amyloidosis, organ dysfunction is related to both amyloid deposition and tissue disruption and to a direct toxic effect of free light chains (FLCs). Each FLC has a specific organ tropism, but heart and kidney are the most commonly involved organs.

Disease monitoring in AL amyloidosis is much better defined than in ATTR amyloidosis and is strictly related to the assessment of response to the hematological treatment aimed at suppressing the plasma cell clone. The hematological response to treatment is based on the assay of FLC and classified into:

- Amyloid complete response (aCR): negative serum and urine immunofixation, and normal FLC ratio.
- Very good partial response (VGPR): difference between involved minus uninvolved serum FLC (dFLC) <40 mg/L.
- Partial response (PR): dFLC decrease >50%.
- No response (NR): all the other categories [26].

In patients with low baseline dFLC (20–50 mg/L), a dFLC <10 mg/L has been proposed as a criterion for hematologic response [27]. Conversely, hematological disease progression is defined as:

- In case of previous complete response, any detectable monoclonal protein or abnormal κ/λ ratio (FLCs must double).
- In case of previous partial response, 50% increase in serum M protein to values >0.5 g/dL or 50% increase in urine M protein to values >200 mg/die.
- 50% increase in FLC up to values >100 mg/dL.

The disease is considered stable in the absence of treatment response or disease progression.

Although hematological response is an important determinant of outcome, it is not invariably associated with organ response, due to established, irreversible target organ damage and due to the persistence of amyloid deposits. Criteria for the definition of organ response have been established during the tenth International Symposium on Amyloid and Amyloidosis in 2014 [28]. In patients with cardiac involvement, progression of disease was defined as ≥ 2 mm increase in interventricular septum thickness or an increase in NYHA class by 1 grade with a decrease in LVEF of $\geq 10\%$. Conversely, cardiac response was defined as a ≥ 2 mm decrease in mean interventricular septal thickness, 20% improvement in ejection fraction, improvement by 2 NYHA classes without modification in diuretic use, and no increase in wall thickness. Notably, these criteria did not include cardiac biomarkers such as natriuretic peptides and troponins.

Several studies have demonstrated that a >30% or a >300 ng/L NT-proBNP reduction after treatment in patients with baseline NT-proBNP >650 ng/L predicts survival in patients with AL-CA [29], while a >30% or >300 ng/L increase in NT-proBNP, as well as a >33% increase in troponin T/I or a LVEF reduction $\geq 10\%$ has been proposed as indicators of progression of cardiac involvement and has been endorsed by the International Society of Amyloidosis [30]. BNP has also been proposed as a tool for the assessment of cardiac response, as a reduction >30% and >50 ng/L from baseline was reported to be associated with improved outcome [31].

Circulating biomarkers of cardiac involvement should be used cautiously in patients receiving certain therapeutic regimens including drugs with cardiotoxic potential, such as the immunomodulatory drugs lenalidomide and pomalidomide, as an increase in natriuretic peptide and/or troponin may not be reflecting a cardiac damage primarily related to the progression of the underlying disease. Moreover, a reduction in circulating concentration of natriuretic peptides is not invariably associated with an improvement in echocardiographic parameters. In a study performed on 51 patients treated for AL-CA, among the 20 patients in whom NT-proBNP improved after chemotherapy, only 3 displayed a ≥ 2 mm decrease in mean left ventricular wall thickness [32], suggesting that each class of biological marker may have a different trajectory after treatment initiation.

Finally, a graded response classification, encompassing hematological and organ (cardiac, renal, and liver) response, has been proposed [33], including four categories:

- Complete organ response (nadir NT-proBNP ≤ 400 ng/L; nadir proteinuria ≤ 0.2 g/24 h; nadir alkaline phosphatase ≤ 2 times institutional lower limit of normal).
- Very good partial organ response (target biomarker reduction >60% from baseline, not meeting complete organ response definition).
- Partial organ response (target biomarker reduction 31–60% from baseline).
- No response (target biomarker reduction $\leq 30\%$ from baseline).

Although biohumoral markers are the most widely used tools for disease monitoring in AL amyloidosis, some echocardiographic parameters may also detect response to therapeutic regimens, including chemotherapy and stem cell transplantation. In a retrospective analysis of 61 patients with AL-CA treated with high-dose melphalan or bortezomib-based regimens, a complete response (normal FLC ratio and negative serum/urine immunofixation) was associated with improved longitudinal strain (LS), while no changes were observed in wall thickness, LVEF, or diastolic function [34]. These findings were later confirmed in a larger series of 915 newly diagnosed patients with AL-CA (69% with cardiac involvement), in whom improvement in LS was seen in patients achieving a hematological complete response during follow-up, suggesting that a deep response is required to detect improvement in cardiac deformation [35]. Evidence on the effects of stem cell transplantation on conventional echocardiographic findings is limited and controversial. In a study performed on 187 patients treated with high-dose melphalan and peripheral blood stem cell transplantation, those showing a hematological response were more likely to present also a cardiac response, defined as reduction in interventricular septal wall thickness ≥2 mm and improvement in LVEF ≥20% [36]. In a smaller study, patients with a complete hematological response after autologous stem cell transplantation did not show improvement in wall thickness and systolic or diastolic function at 1-year follow-up [37].

There is limited evidence on the potential role of CMR for tracking changes over time in AL-CA. It is known that the T2 is higher in patients with AL amyloidosis before initiation of chemotherapy compared to treated patients and is a predictor of prognosis [38].

ECV is also lower in treated patients, although to a lesser extent, possibly reflecting a reduction in myocardial edema, rather than only in amyloid burden. A retrospective study performed at the UK NAC has demonstrated that serial CMR examinations can disclose the regression of cardiac amyloid following a substantial response to chemotherapy in patients with AL amyloidosis. A reduction in ECV by at least 2 standard deviations occurred in 13/31 patients and was more commonly observed in patients with complete response/very good partial response versus patients in partial response/no response (Fig. 23.3). Further, reduction in amyloid burden was consistent with improvement in NT-proBNP, left ventricular mass, left atrial area, and diastolic function parameters [22]. The tissue characterization provided by CMR imaging may therefore track the cardiac structural changes following disease-modifying treatments that are likely missed by echocardiography.

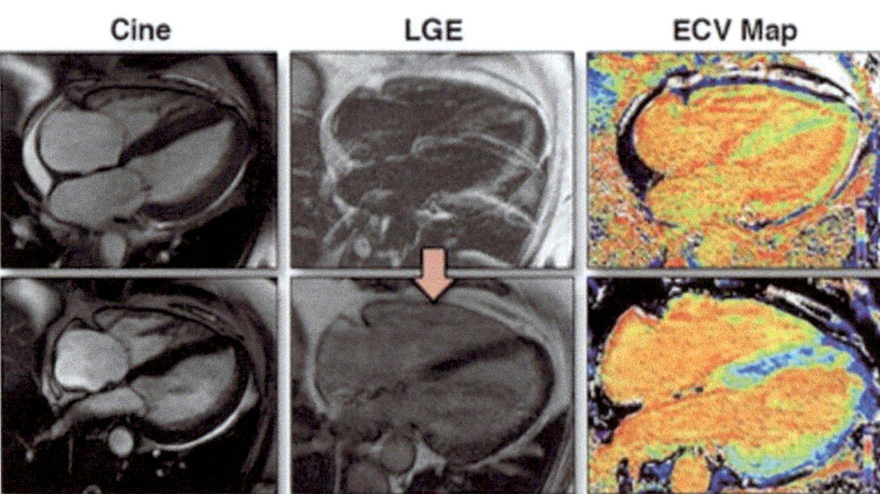

Fig. 23.3 Cardiac magnetic resonance showing regression of cardiac amyloid
Four-chamber cine (left), corresponding LGE (middle), and ECV (right) mapping before and after chemotherapy in a responder patient with immunoglobulin light-chain cardiac amyloidosis. *ECV* extracellular volume, *LGE* late gadolinium enhancement. Modified from Martinez-Naharro et al. [22]

23.4 Perspectives

Recent advances have increased our ability to diagnose and treat CA and have improved patient outcome, but strategies for disease monitoring and for the assessment of response to disease-modifying treatments need to be standardized, especially in ATTR-CA. Information from advanced imaging, namely CMR, may effectively track those changes in cardiac structure and in tissue characteristics related to the progression or regression of CA or to therapeutic interventions, possibly demonstrating resorption of amyloid deposits. This potential of CMR may be of enormous importance with the use of some monoclonal antibodies targeting amyloid deposits currently under investigation for both AL and ATTR-CA [39, 40].

Nuclear medicine techniques have an established role in the diagnosis in ATTR-CA and will be likely useful also in patients with suspected AL-CA [41]. The assessment of changes in regional and global myocardial uptake with SPECT and CT-PET imaging may, in the next future, inform the clinician on the course of myocardial involvement and organ-specific response to therapies.

23.5 Conclusions

Monitoring of disease and assessment of response to treatment require a multi-marker approach in patients with CA. While there is consensus on the criteria for the assessment of hematological and organ response in AL-CA, evidence is more limited in ATTR-CA. Circulating biomarkers, ECG, and echocardiography are widely available, cheap, and safe tools, but advanced imaging, including CMR and nuclear medicine techniques, can provide earlier, specific, and more accurate information on the disease course (Table 23.3).

Table 23.3 Characteristic of different measures for the assessment of disease progression and response to therapy in cardiac amyloidosis

Monitoring tool	Cost	Potential for serial assessment	Sensitivity to early changes	Disease specificity
Signs/Symptoms				
QoL questionnaires				
Circulating biomarkers				
ECG				
Echocardiography				
Cardiac magnetic resonance				
Nuclear medicine				

Green = positive characteristics; yellow = intermediate characteristics; red = negative characteristics; *ECG* electrocardiogram, *QoL* quality of life

References

1. Sipe JD, Benson MD, Buxbaum JN, Ikeda SI, Merlini G, Saraiva MJM, et al. Amyloid fibril proteins and amyloidosis: chemical identification and clinical classification International Society of Amyloidosis 2016 Nomenclature Guidelines. Amyloid. 2016;23:209–13.
2. Cotter G, Metra M, Davison BA, Senger S, Bourge RC, Cleland JG, Jondeau G, Krum H, O'Connor CM, Parker JD, Torre-Amione G, van Veldhuisen DJ, Milo O, Kobrin I, Rainisio M, McMurray JJ, Teerlink JR, Investigators VERITAS. Worsening heart failure, a critical event during hospital admission for acute heart failure: results from the VERITAS study. Eur J Heart Fail. 2014;16:1362–71.
3. Maurer MS, Schwartz JH, Gundapaneni B, Elliott PM, Merlini G, Waddington-Cruz M, Kristen AV, Grogan M, Witteles R, Damy T, Drachman BM, Shah SJ, Hanna M, Judge DP, Barsdorf AI, Huber P, Patterson TA, Riley S, Schumacher J, Stewart M, Sultan MB, Rapezzi C, ATTR-ACT Study Investigators. Tafamidis treatment for patients with transthyretin amyloid cardiomyopathy. N Engl J Med. 2018;379:1007–16.
4. Hanna M, Fine N, Stewart M, Gundapaneni B, Sultan MB, Witteles R. Functional capacity, health-related quality-of-life and cardiac biomarker improvement with tafamidis in the Tafamidis in Transthyretin Cardiomyopathy Clinical Trial (ATTR-ACT). J Card Fail. 2020;26(10):S65.
5. Vergaro G, Castiglione V, Aimo A, Prontera C, Masotti S, Musetti V, Nicol M, Cohen Solal A, Logeart D, Georgiopoulos G, Chubuchny V, Giannoni A, Clerico A, Buda G, Patel KN, Razvi Y, Patel R, Wechalekar A, Lachmann H, Hawkins PN, Passino C, Gillmore J, Emdin M, Fontana M. N-terminal pro-B-type natriuretic peptide and high-sensitivity troponin T hold diagnostic value in cardiac amyloidosis. Eur J Heart Fail. 2023;25(3):335–46. https://doi.org/10.1002/ejhf.2769.
6. Castiglione V, Franzini M, Aimo A, Carecci A, Lombardi CM, Passino C, Rapezzi C, Emdin M, Vergaro G. Use of biomarkers to diagnose and manage cardiac amyloidosis. Eur J Heart Fail. 2021;23(2):217–30. https://doi.org/10.1002/ejhf.2113.
7. Grogan M, Scott CG, Kyle RA, Zeldenrust SR, Gertz MA, Lin G, Klarich KW, Miller WL, Maleszewski JJ, Dispenzieri A. Natural history of wild-type transthyretin cardiac amyloidosis and risk stratification using a novel staging system. J Am Coll Cardiol. 2016;68:1014–20.
8. Gillmore JD, Damy T, Fontana M, Hutchinson M, Lachmann HJ, Martinez-Naharro A, Quarta CC, Rezk T, Whelan CJ, Gonzalez-Lopez E, Lane T, Gilbertson JA, Rowczenio D, Petrie A, Hawkins PN. A new staging system for cardiac transthyretin amyloidosis. Eur Heart J. 2018;39:2799–806.
9. Cheng RK, Levy WC, Vasbinder A, Teruya S, De Los SJ, Leedy D, Maurer MS. Diuretic dose and NYHA functional class are independent predictors of mortality in patients with transthyretin cardiac amyloidosis. JACC CardioOncol. 2020;2:414–24.
10. Eckstein J, Potocki M, Murray K, Breidthardt T, Ziller R, Mosimann T, Klima T, Hoeller R, Moehring B, Sou SM, Rubini Gimenez M, Morgenthaler NG, Mueller C. Direct comparison of mid-regional pro-atrial natriuretic peptide with N-terminal pro B-type natriuretic peptide in the diagnosis of patients with atrial fibrillation and dyspnoea. Heart. 2012;98(20):1518–22. https://doi.org/10.1136/heartjnl-2012-302260.
11. Merlo M, Pagura L, Porcari A, Cameli M, Vergaro G, Musumeci B, Biagini E, Canepa M, Crotti L, Imazio M, Forleo C, Cappelli F, Perfetto F, Favale S, Di Bella G, Dore F, Girardi F, Tomasoni D, Pavasini R, Rella V, Palmiero G, Caiazza M, Carella MC, Igoren Guaricci A, Branzi G, Caponetti AG, Saturi G, La Malfa G, Merlo AC, Andreis A, Bruno F, Longo F, Rossi M, Varrà GG, Saro R, Di Ienno L, De Carli G, Giacomin E, Arzilli C, Limongelli G, Autore C, Olivotto I, Badano L, Parati G, Perlini S, Metra M, Emdin M, Rapezzi C, Sinagra G. Unmasking the prevalence of amyloid cardiomyopathy in the real world: results from Phase 2 of the AC-TIVE study, an Italian nationwide survey. Eur J Heart Fail. 2022;24(8):1377–86. https://doi.org/10.1002/ejhf.2504.

12. Porcari A, Rossi M, Cappelli F, Canepa M, Musumeci B, Cipriani A, Tini G, Barbati G, Varrà GG, Morelli C, Fumagalli C, Zampieri M, Argirò A, Vianello PF, Sessarego E, Russo D, Sinigiani G, De Michieli L, Di Bella G, Autore C, Perfetto F, Rapezzi C, Sinagra G, Merlo M. Incidence and risk factors for pacemaker implantation in light-chain and transthyretin cardiac amyloidosis. Eur J Heart Fail. 2022;24(7):1227–36. https://doi.org/10.1002/ejhf.2533.

13. Aimo A, Fabiani I, Giannoni A, Mandoli GE, Pastore MC, Vergaro G, Spini V, Chubuchny V, Pasanisi EM, Petersen C, Poggianti E, Taddei C, Castiglione V, Latrofa S, Panichella G, Sciaccaluga C, Georgiopoulos G, Passino C, Cameli M, Emdin M. Multi-chamber speckle tracking imaging and diagnostic value of left atrial strain in cardiac amyloidosis. Eur Heart J Cardiovasc Imaging. 2022;24(1):130–41. https://doi.org/10.1093/ehjci/jeac057.

14. Garcia-Pavia P, Bengel F, Brito D, Damy T, Duca F, Dorbala S, Nativi-Nicolau J, Obici L, Rapezzi C, Sekijima Y, Elliott PM. Expert consensus on the monitoring of transthyretin amyloid cardiomyopathy. Eur J Heart Fail. 2021;23(6):895–905. https://doi.org/10.1002/ejhf.2198.

15. Solomon SD, Adams D, Kristen A, Grogan M, González-Duarte A, Maurer MS, Merlini G, Damy T, Slama MS, Brannagan TH 3rd, Dispenzieri A, Berk JL, Shah AM, Garg P, Vaishnaw A, Karsten V, Chen J, Gollob J, Vest J, Suhr O. Effects of patisiran, an RNA interference therapeutic, on cardiac parameters in patients with hereditary transthyretin-mediated amyloidosis. Circulation. 2019;139(4):431–43. https://doi.org/10.1161/CIRCULATIONAHA.118.035831.

16. Fontana M, Chung R, Hawkins PN, Moon JC. Cardiovascular magnetic resonance for amyloidosis. Heart Fail Rev. 2015;20(2):133–44. https://doi.org/10.1007/s10741-014-9470-7.

17. Gillmore JD, Maurer MS, Falk RH, Merlini G, Damy T, Dispenzieri A, Wechalekar AD, Berk JL, Quarta CC, Grogan M, Lachmann HJ, Bokhari S, Castano A, Dorbala S, Johnson GB, Glaudemans AW, Rezk T, Fontana M, Palladini G, Milani P, Guidalotti PL, Flatman K, Lane T, Vonberg FW, Whelan CJ, Moon JC, Ruberg FL, Miller EJ, Hutt DF, Hazenberg BP, Rapezzi C, Hawkins PN. Nonbiopsy diagnosis of cardiac transthyretin amyloidosis. Circulation. 2016;133(24):2404–12. https://doi.org/10.1161/CIRCULATIONAHA.116.021612.

18. Falk RH, Haddad M, Walker CR, Dorbala S, Cuddy SAM. Effect of tafamidis on serum transthyretin levels in non-trial patients with transthyretin amyloid cardiomyopathy. JACC CardioOncol. 2021;3(4):580–6. https://doi.org/10.1016/j.jaccao.2021.08.007.

19. Adams D, Gonzalez-Duarte A, O'Riordan WD, Yang CC, Ueda M, Kristen AV, Tournev I, Schmidt HH, Coelho T, Berk JL, Lin KP, Vita G, Attarian S, Planté-Bordeneuve V, Mezei MM, Campistol JM, Buades J, Brannagan TH 3rd, Kim BJ, Oh J, Parman Y, Sekijima Y, Hawkins PN, Solomon SD, Polydefkis M, Dyck PJ, Gandhi PJ, Goyal S, Chen J, Strahs AL, Nochur SV, Sweetser MT, Garg PP, Vaishnaw AK, Gollob JA, Suhr OB. Patisiran, an RNAi therapeutic, for hereditary transthyretin amyloidosis. N Engl J Med. 2018;379(1):11–21. https://doi.org/10.1056/NEJMoa1716153.

20. Sanguinetti C, Minniti M, Panichella G, Vergaro G, Aimo A, Castiglione V, Caponi L, Paolicchi A, Emdin M, Ma F. 276 Circulating forms of plasma transthyretin in patients with wild-type transthyretin amyloidosis and effects of treatment with tafamidis. Eur Heart J Suppl. 2022;24(Suppl. K):suac121.578. https://doi.org/10.1093/eurheartjsupp/suac121.578.

21. Giblin GT, Cuddy SAM, González-López E, Sewell A, Murphy A, Dorbala S, Falk RH. Effect of tafamidis on global longitudinal strain and myocardial work in transthyretin cardiac amyloidosis. Eur Heart J Cardiovasc Imaging. 2022;23(8):1029–39. https://doi.org/10.1093/ehjci/jeac049.

22. Martinez-Naharro A, Abdel-Gadir A, Treibel TA, Zumbo G, Knight DS, Rosmini S, Lane T, Mahmood S, Sachchithanantham S, Whelan CJ, Lachmann HJ, Wechalekar AD, Kellman P, Gillmore JD, Moon JC, Hawkins PN, Fontana M. CMR-verified regression of cardiac AL amyloid after chemotherapy. JACC Cardiovasc Imaging. 2018;11(1):152–4. https://doi.org/10.1016/j.jcmg.2017.02.012.

23. Martinez-Naharro A, Kotecha T, Norrington K, Boldrini M, Rezk T, Quarta C, Treibel TA, Whelan CJ, Knight DS, Kellman P, Ruberg FL, Gillmore JD, Moon JC, Hawkins PN, Fontana M. Native T1 and extracellular volume in transthyretin amyloidosis. JACC Cardiovasc Imaging. 2019;12(5):810–9. https://doi.org/10.1016/j.jcmg.2018.02.006.

24. Fontana M, Martinez-Naharro A, Chacko L, Rowczenio D, Gilbertson JA, Whelan CJ, Strehina S, Lane T, Moon J, Hutt DF, Kellman P, Petrie A, Hawkins PN, Gillmore JD. Reduction in CMR derived extracellular volume with patisiran indicates cardiac amyloid regression. JACC Cardiovasc Imaging. 2021;14(1):189–99. https://doi.org/10.1016/j.jcmg.2020.07.043.
25. Rettl R, Wollenweber T, Duca F, Binder C, Cherouny B, Dachs TM, Luciana CL, Schrutka L, Dalos D, Beitzke D, Loewe C, Eslam RB, Kastner J, Hacker M, Bonderman D. Monitoring tafamidis treatment with quantitative SPECT/CT in transthyretin amyloid cardiomyopathy. Eur Heart J Cardiovasc Imaging. 2023;24(8):1019–30. https://doi.org/10.1093/ehjci/jead030.
26. Palladini G, Dispenzieri A, Gertz MA, Kumar S, Wechalekar A, Hawkins PN, Schönland S, Hegenbart U, Comenzo R, Kastritis E, Dimopoulos MA, Jaccard A, Klersy C, Merlini G. New criteria for response to treatment in immunoglobulin light chain amyloidosis based on free light chain measurement and cardiac biomarkers: impact on survival outcomes. J Clin Oncol. 2012;30(36):4541–9. https://doi.org/10.1200/JCO.2011.37.7614.
27. Milani P, Basset M, Russo F, Foli A, Merlini G, Palladini G. Patients with light-chain amyloidosis and low free light-chain burden have distinct clinical features and outcome. Blood. 2017;130(5):625–31. https://doi.org/10.1182/blood-2017-02-767467.
28. Gertz MA, Comenzo R, Falk RH, Fermand JP, Hazenberg BP, Hawkins PN, Merlini G, Moreau P, Ronco P, Sanchorawala V, Sezer O, Solomon A, Grateau G. Definition of organ involvement and treatment response in immunoglobulin light chain amyloidosis (AL): a consensus opinion from the 10th International Symposium on Amyloid and Amyloidosis, Tours, France, 18–22 April 2004. Am J Hematol. 2005;79(4):319–28. https://doi.org/10.1002/ajh.20381.
29. Palladini G, Barassi A, Klersy C, Pacciolla R, Milani P, Sarais G, Perlini S, Albertini R, Russo P, Foli A, Bragotti LZ, Obici L, Moratti R, Melzi d'Eril GV, Merlini G, Vico G, Merlini G, Melzi d'Eril GV, Merlini G. The combination of high-sensitivity cardiac troponin T (hs-cTnT) at presentation and changes in N-terminal natriuretic peptide type B (NT-proBNP) after chemotherapy best predicts survival in AL amyloidosis. Blood. 2016;116:3426–31.
30. Comenzo RL, Reece D, Palladini G, Seldin D, Sanchorawala V, Landau H, Falk R, Wells K, Solomon A, Wechalekar A, Zonder J, Dispenzieri A, Gertz M, Streicher H, Skinner M, Kyle RA, Merlini G. Consensus guidelines for the conduct and reporting of clinical trials in systemic light-chain amyloidosis. Leukemia. 2012;26:2317–25.
31. Lilleness B, Doros G, Ruberg FL, Sanchorawala V. Establishment of brain natriuretic peptide-based criteria for evaluating cardiac response to treatment in light chain (AL) amyloidosis. Br J Haematol. 2020;188(3):424–7. https://doi.org/10.1111/bjh.16198.
32. Palladini G, Lavatelli F, Russo P, Perlini S, Perfetti V, Bosoni T, Obici L, Bradwell AR, D'Eril GM, Fogari R, Moratti R, Merlini G. Circulating amyloidogenic free light chains and serum N-terminal natriuretic peptide type B decrease simultaneously in association with improvement of survival in AL. Blood. 2006;107:3854–8.
33. Muchtar E, Dispenzieri A, Leung N, Lacy MQ, Buadi FK, Dingli D, Grogan M, Hayman SR, Kapoor P, Hwa YL, Fonder A, Hobbs M, Chakraborty R, Gonsalves W, Kourelis TV, Warsame R, Russell S, Lust JA, Lin Y, Go RS, Zeldenrust S, Kyle RA, Rajkumar SV, Kumar SK, Gertz MA. Depth of organ response in AL amyloidosis is associated with improved survival: grading the organ response criteria. Leukemia. 2018;32(10):2240–9. https://doi.org/10.1038/s41375-018-0060-x.
34. Salinaro F, Meier-Ewert HK, Miller EJ, Pandey S, Sanchorawala V, Berk JL, et al. Longitudinal systolic strain, cardiac function improvement, and survival following treatment of light-chain (AL) cardiac amyloidosis. Eur Heart J Cardiovasc Imaging. 2017;18:1057–64.
35. Cohen OC, Ismael A, Pawarova B, Manwani R, Ravichandran S, Law S, Foard D, Petrie A, Ward S, Douglas B, Martinez-Naharro A, Chacko L, Quarta CC, Mahmood S, Sachchithanantham S, Lachmann HJ, Hawkins PN, Gillmore JD, Fontana M, Falk RH, Whelan CJ, Wechalekar AD. Longitudinal strain is an independent predictor of survival and response to therapy in patients with systemic AL amyloidosis. Eur Heart J. 2022;43(4):333–41. https://doi.org/10.1093/eurheartj/ehab507.
36. Madan S, Kumar SK, Dispenzieri A, Lacy MQ, Hayman SR, Buadi FK, Dingli D, Rajkumar SV, Hogan WJ, Leung N, Grogan M, Gertz MA. High-dose melphalan and peripheral blood

stem cell transplantation for light-chain amyloidosis with cardiac involvement. Blood. 2012;119(5):1117–22. https://doi.org/10.1182/blood-2011-07-370031.

37. Pun SC, Landau HJ, Riedel ER, Jordan J, Yu AF, Hassoun H, Chen CL, Steingart RM, Liu JE. Prognostic and added value of two-dimensional global longitudinal strain for prediction of survival in patients with light chain amyloidosis undergoing autologous hematopoietic cell transplantation. J Am Soc Echocardiogr. 2018;31(1):64–70. https://doi.org/10.1016/j. echo.2017.08.017.

38. Kotecha T, Martinez-Naharro A, Treibel TA, Francis R, Nordin S, Abdel-Gadir A, Knight DS, Zumbo G, Rosmini S, Maestrini V, Bulluck H, Rakhit RD, Wechalekar AD, Gilbertson J, Sheppard MN, Kellman P, Gillmore JD, Moon JC, Hawkins PN, Fontana M. Myocardial edema and prognosis in amyloidosis. J Am Coll Cardiol. 2018;71(25):2919–31. https://doi. org/10.1016/j.jacc.2018.03.536.

39. Prothena Biosciences Ltd. A study to evaluate the efficacy and safety of Birtamimab in Mayo stage IV patients with AL amyloidosis (AFFIRM-AL); 2023. clinicaltrials.gov/ct2/show/ NCT04973137

40. Michalon A, Hagenbuch A, Huy C, Varela E, Combaluzier B, Damy T, Suhr OB, Saraiva MJ, Hock C, Nitsch RM, Grimm J. A human antibody selective for transthyretin amyloid removes cardiac amyloid through phagocytic immune cells. Nat Commun. 2021;12(1):3142. https:// doi.org/10.1038/s41467-021-23274-x.

41. Genovesi D, Vergaro G, Giorgetti A, Marzullo P, Scipioni M, Santarelli MF, Pucci A, Buda G, Volpi E, Emdin M. [18F]-Florbetaben PET/CT for differential diagnosis among cardiac immunoglobulin light chain, transthyretin amyloidosis, and mimicking conditions. JACC Cardiovasc Imaging. 2021;14(1):246–55. https://doi.org/10.1016/j.jcmg.2020.05.031.

Michele Emdin, Giuseppe Vergaro, Alberto Aimo, Marianna Fontana, and Giampaolo Merlini

Abbreviations

AL	Amyloid light chain
ASO	Antisense oligonucleotide
ATTR	Amyloid transthyretin (v, variant; wt, wild type)
CA	Cardiac amyloidosis
ECV	Extracellular volume
GLS	Global longitudinal strain
LGE	Late gadolinium enhancement
mNIS+7	Modified Neuropathy Impairment Score +7
NT-proBNP	N-terminal pro-B-type natriuretic peptide
PET	Positron-emission tomography
siRNA	Small interfering RNA
TTR	Transthyretin
VGPR	Very good partial response

M. Emdin (✉) · G. Vergaro · A. Aimo
Interdisciplinary Center for Health Sciences, Scuola Superiore Sant'Anna, Pisa, Italy

Cardiothoracic Department, Fondazione Toscana Gabriele Monasterio, Pisa/Massa, Italy
e-mail: m.emdin@santannapisa.it; vergaro@ftgm.it; aimoalb@ftgm.it

M. Fontana
National Amyloidosis Centre, University College London, London, UK
e-mail: marianna.fontana@nhs.net

G. Merlini
Amyloidosis Research and Treatment Center, Fondazione IRCCS,
Policlinico San Matteo, Italy
e-mail: gmerlini@smatteo.pv.it

Over the last 10 years, the advancement of knowledge has profoundly transformed the clinical approach in cardiac amyloidosis (CA) [1]. The heart is often affected by amyloid deposition, and its involvement drives the outcome of CA patients [2]. Our approach to CA has been influenced by advances in diagnostics, namely in the use of biomarkers and multimodal noninvasive cardiac imaging, as well as by the introduction of new, effective therapies. However, many aspects of pathophysiology, epidemiology, and patient management still remain unexplored. In this section, we will identify the unsolved issues and the possible perspectives for future studies.

24.1 Mechanisms of Amyloid Formation and Tissue Infiltration

Amyloid fibrils are long and unbranched structures resulting from the abnormal polymerization of monomeric peptides, with a typical width of 7.5–20 nm and length of micrometers. Amyloid fibrils consist of multiple subunits, defined as protofilaments, twisted together. The formation of fibrils requires that misfolded monomers pathologically assemble with each other into a nucleus, which then forms oligomers and higher order species through a nucleated elongation process until reaching stability [3]. Amyloid fibrils also bind to other fibrils, proteins (e.g., serum amyloid P-component), and extracellular matrix components.

The dissociation of transthyretin (TTR) tetramer is the starting point and rate-limiting step in amyloid fibrillogenesis. Disease-causing mutations promote the disassembling of TTR tetramers into monomers that then misfold and form amyloid fibers in tissues, differently from protective mutations which favor the tetramer conformation. In the context of wild-type (wt) TTR amyloidosis (ATTR), the tetramer becomes kinetically unstable likely because of aging-associated decrease in protein quality control mechanisms. Many years are required before this process causes clinical manifestations. This long latency period has been explained by postulating a two-step process: a phase of formation of the first nuclei of amyloid fibrils ("seeding" or "nesting"), requiring many years, and then a far more rapid phase of further aggregation [4]. This hypothesis may account for the rapid progression of disease (particularly cardiac involvement) even after liver transplantation, which effectively removes all mutated TTR, but does not affect the production of wild-type (wt) TTR [5]. The very long time needed for amyloid seeding has been explained by the existence of protective mechanisms that wane over time, or the development of some determinants of instability of TTR tetramers. With respect to the last mechanisms, some groups have focused on the mechanisms of protein cleavage, which change over time and promote protein misfolding and fibril formation. Some experiments have identified plasmin as the most important of these cleavage mechanisms [6].

With respect to amyloid light-chain (AL) amyloidosis, the presence of an abnormal plasma cell clone producing monoclonal and abnormal light chains is the underlying cause of the disease. Some somatic mutations in the gene coding for the variable region of immunoglobulin light chains are associated with low fold stability and high protein dynamics [7, 8].

The phenotypic variability of systemic amyloidosis is huge. In ATTR and AL amyloidosis, both central and peripheral factors (i.e., related to protein synthesis or tissue deposition, respectively) have been postulated. As for central factors, a few variants in the genes coding for the light chain (*IGKV1-16, IGLV6-57, IGLV2-14, IGLV3-1*) account for two-thirds of cases of cardiac involvement in AL amyloidosis [9], and *TTR* gene mutations are crucial determinants of clinical manifestations, thus being classified as neurological, cardiologic, or mixed phenotypes [10]. The molecular mechanisms underlying the amyloid tropism remain to be elucidated, but some structural or genetic mutations may be key drivers in amyloid deposition. Other sources of phenotypic heterogeneity have been identified in the last years: age, geographical area, transmission pattern of mutations, and patient sex. This last factor plays an important role in determining the features of cardiac involvement. An analysis of the Transthyretin Amyloidosis Outcomes Survey registry shows that female sex is associated with a lower prevalence and severity of cardiac disease, at least until the sixth or seventh decade of life [11]. With respect to peripheral factors, the accumulation of full-length or fragmented ATTR molecules influences the clinical presentation and response to some therapies, even in patients with the same TTR gene mutation [12].

The relative contribution of circulating precursors or fibrils to tissue damage has not been clarified yet, also because of few available animal models. Exceptions are represented by zebrafish as a transgene model of AL amyloidosis [13] and *Clostridium elegans* in the study of cardiotoxic potential of the amyloidogenic light chains [14]. As reported at the 2023 Symposium of the International Society of Amyloidosis, although transgenic mouse models for ATTR and AL amyloidosis have been developed [15, 16], the deposition of amyloid was observed in both models only after the injection of preformed amyloid fibrils, which served as seed. Notably, both mouse models showed no cardiac functional impairment, with normal life span, despite conspicuous cardiac amyloid deposition. This finding indicates that cardiac dysfunction cannot be solely ascribed to the deposition of the fibrils. The main evidence supporting a role of prefibrillar species in organ damage is indirect and derives from the clinical response to disease-modifying therapies. It is known that the benefit of an effective chemotherapy in AL cardiomyopathy manifests well before the (possible) reduction of left ventricular wall thickness, while it is accompanied by a marked reduction in circulating levels of N-terminal pro-B-type natriuretic peptide (NT-proBNP) and free light chains [17]. Furthermore, the recent evidence that the quality of cardiac response strictly depends on the depth of the reduction of free light-chain concentrations reaching more than 90% in patients with negative residual disease further supports the previous observation [18]. In ATTR amyloidosis, the first data on the effects on cardiac morphology and function of patisiran, a drug blocking *TTR* gene expression, show a very limited reduction of wall thickness, a more prominent improvement of strain values (particularly in the basal region of the left ventricle), and a moderate decrease in NT-proBNP [20, 21], in line with the hypothesis of a relief from direct toxicity more than infiltrative damage.

24.2 Towards a Completely Noninvasive Diagnostic Algorithm of Cardiac Amyloidosis

The new radiopharmaceuticals for positron-emission tomography (PET) for the search for cerebral amyloid deposits in suspected Alzheimer's disease are proving to have good affinity also for systemic amyloid deposits, particularly at the cardiac level, and represent a promising tool for *in vivo* non-biopsy diagnosis of AL amyloidosis. A recent study has demonstrated that a PET/computed tomography scan carried out between 50 and 60 min after the injection of ^{18}F-florbetaben allows to identify an uptake in the cardiac region in patients with AL-CA, but not in those with ATTR-CA or with other mimicking conditions [22]. This method could therefore represent the first noninvasive diagnostic tool in patients with suspected AL-CA, significantly reducing the need to perform an endomyocardial biopsy in subjects with suspected CA and a monoclonal protein. The ongoing multicenter PETAL study coordinated by the Fondazione Monasterio (Pisa, Italy) will hopefully define the role of this new tracer in the diagnosis of CA.

24.3 Open Issues in the Management of AL-CA

The main unmet medical need in cardiac AL amyloidosis is an effective therapy for patients with advanced cardiac damage, in stage IIIb. The survival of this population is 4–6 months, and stage IIIb patients represent 20% of the whole AL amyloidosis population. Unfortunately, this percentage has not changed throughout the last decade [23], indicating the need to improve the diagnostic approach through enhanced awareness, use of sensitive biomarkers of amyloid cardiac involvement (NT-proBNP and cardiac troponin) [24], and advanced imaging [25]. Anticlone therapies can produce a complete or very good partial response (VGPR) in 1 month in approximately one-fifth of patients translating into a survival benefit [26]. A recent study reported treatment outcomes with novel agents, and despite VGPR or better response rate at 1 month of 52.6%, using daratumumab, the median survival was only 6 months [27]. In this poor prognosis patients, it is even possible to achieve a cardiac VGPR response; however, this was obtained in only 8% of the patients [28]. Clearly, new drugs targeting other critical steps of the amyloid cascade are needed. Preliminary results indicate that treatment with the anti-amyloid monoclonal antibody, anselamimab, in patients previously successfully treated with anti-clone therapy, produced a good cardiological response rate [29]. Therefore, there is great expectation for the outcome of the two ongoing phase III studies evaluating the benefits of adding anselamimab to standard of care in patients in stage IIIa or IIIb CA [30].

24.4 Impact of Earlier Diagnosis

Anticipating the end-stage amyloid cardiac damage is the prerequisite to improving AL amyloidosis care. Waiting for cardiac symptoms is a much less effective approach, as documented by the lack of reduction of the proportions of patients in stage IIIb in the newly diagnosed population during the last decade [23]. Ideally, patients with AL amyloidosis cardiac involvement should be identified before the symptoms develop. Several years ago, the Pavia group proposed the use of sensitive biomarkers of amyloid organ involvement, NT-proBNP for the heart, albuminuria for the kidney, and alkaline phosphatase for the liver, to screen patients with MGUS and abnormal FLC periodically, to detect amyloid organ involvement early, in the presymptomatic stage. This approach was prospectively applied to all 1375 new patients diagnosed with MGUS in Pavia from 2012 to 2020. Twenty-two presymptomatic, biopsy-proven AL amyloidosis patients were identified, and 5 had asymptomatic cardiac involvement. Early treatment resulted in a 100% VGPR or better hematologic response with a 100% cardiac response with normalization of cardiac biomarkers (manuscript in preparation). The outcome of the Pavia approach suggests that early diagnosis is the prerequisite to cure AL amyloidosis. Sensitive imaging methods can also help improve the time of diagnosis in the presence of clinical suspicion; however, this is usually based on symptoms.

Advances in cardiac imaging, alongside the increased awareness among clinicians, have contributed to early diagnosis of ATTR-CA. To date, undiagnosed patients experience a shorter duration of symptoms and display a milder disease stage at the time of diagnosis [31]. The less severe cardiac phenotype has translated into improved survival from the time of diagnosis, even when accounting for the impact of disease-modifying therapy. Early administration of gene silencing and gene editing therapies early in the natural history of ATTR-CA may prevent the development of overt heart failure and result in improved clinical outcomes, but more data are needed to guide decisions on when and in whom to initiate treatment. Importantly, changes in the clinical phenotype of patients diagnosed with ATTR-CA will influence the design of future clinical trials and will likely result in a requirement for greater cohorts and longer follow-up to ensure adequate power [31].

24.5 Comparisons Between Different Gene Silencers and Gene Editing Therapies

The last decade has seen incredible advances in the treatment for ATTR-CA. The first strategies sought to achieve TTR stabilization and resulted in the introduction of tafamidis for ATTR-CA [32]. Although clinical trials demonstrated efficacy in slowing disease progression, tafamidis does not reach complete TTR stabilization in vivo, and the disease continues to slowly progress despite treatment. The advent of gene silencers has transformed the treatment landscape. These novel therapeutic agents target TTR production and reduce the amount of circulating TTR. Patisiran is the first siRNA approved for the treatment of ATTR polyneuropathy, since it improves neurological outcomes [33], while early data suggest that it may not only be able to stabilize cardiac disease, and possibly even induce disease regression [34]. Further research led to the development of vutrisiran, a siRNA that can be administered subcutaneously every 3 months without premedication, as opposed to the 3-weekly intravenous infusions of patisiran. Following publication of the HELIOS-A trial results, vutrisiran was licensed for treatment of ATTR polyneuropathy and actually represents a convenient but equally alternative to patisiran [35, 36]. The HELIOS-B trial results will shed further light on the efficacy of vutrisiran for treatment of ATTR-CA (NCT04153149). The evidence for ASO-based treatments is limited to the NEURO-TTR trial, which assessed the use of weekly inotersen administration for treatment of ATTR polyneuropathy. Although effective, inotersen was not superior to patisiran in decreasing circulating TTR levels and was poorly tolerated with a significant proportion of patients discontinuing therapy due to adverse effects (e.g., thrombocytopenia and glomerulonephritis) [37]. Importantly, the modified Neuropathy Impairment Score +7 (*mNIS+7*) composite scores differ between siRNA and ASO trials [33, 37]. While siRNAs initially seemed more promising than ASO therapy because of a better safety profile, the introduction of eplontersen may change this premise. Eplontersen is an ASO injected subcutaneously once a month. Initial phase 1 results have confirmed a favorable safety profile, with no reports of serious toxicities, and demonstrated an amplified potency compared to inotersen [38]. The large-scale phase 3 NEURO-TTRansform (NCT04136184) and CARDIO-TTRansform (NCT04136171) trials are ongoing and are designed to assess the efficacy of eplontersen in ATTR polyneuropathy and CA, respectively. The most promising treatment under development is probably the CRISPR/Cas9 in vivo gene editing, capable to specifically and effectively target the TTR gene. The perspective of a single-dose treatment for ATTR amyloidosis may be the first step towards a "one and done" cure for ATTR amyloidosis [39].

Gene silencers and editing therapies effectively achieve an 80–95% knockdown of circulating TTR, although residual TTR maintains the potential to misfold into pathogenic fibrils. More data are required to establish whether combining these agents with a TTR stabilizer such as tafamidis or acoramidis could affect their therapeutic efficacy. It is conceivable that simultaneously targeting both TTR production and TTR stabilization could have a synergistic effect and result in improved clinical outcomes, but only the combination of patisiran with diflunisal demonstrated amyloid regression in ATTR-CA [34]. The intriguing finding that anti-TTR monoclonal antibodies may promote amyloid regression [40] allows speculating that the future approach to ATTR-CA will include the combination of TTR silencers and anti-TTR monoclonal antibodies to block TTR synthesis and promote amyloid regression.

24.6 Monitoring the Cardiac Response to Treatment

The majority of large clinical trials have assessed the efficacy of gene silencers in ATTR polyneuropathy, and primary end points have been changes in standardized measures of neuropathic disease severity such as mNIS+7 and Norfolk QOL-DN scores [33, 37]. There is growing interest in the use of gene silencers to treat ATTR-CA, and hence an increasing need to develop standardized measures of cardiac response. The ATTR-ACT trial of tafamidis used a composite hierarchical primary end point of all-cause mortality and cardiovascular hospitalizations and secondary end points of change in 6-minute walking time and KCC-QS score [32]. Although this trial did meet its primary end point, none of the changes assessed were a direct measure of change in CA burden, and all were subject to other confounders.

Natriuretic peptides, particularly NT-proBNP, have long been used in heart failure to monitor treatment response and have been validated in a large international study as a powerful tool to monitor cardiac response in AL amyloidosis [41]. This biomarker has been extensively utilized in monitoring chemotherapy response in cardiac AL amyloidosis [17], consistently predicting survival. Although changes in NT-proBNP represent the final common pathway of several mechanisms such as renal impairment, fluid status, or neurohormonal activation [42], the effect of cardiotoxic light chains on NT-proBNP concentration overwhelms all other confounding factors. This biomarker is presently the most accurate tool to evaluate the quality of cardiac response and to predict survival. Its international standardization and analytical robustness, operator independent, represent additional advantages of this biomarker. The possibility to accurately grade the quality of the cardiac response to chemotherapy using solely NT-proBNP concentrations has been recently validated in a large international study [19]. Patients achieving complete cardiac response based on NT-proBNP below 350 ng/L present a life expectancy overlapping that of the normal matched population. Therefore, reaching a complete cardiac response according to NT-proBNP equals curing AL amyloidosis using anticlone therapy. Data obtained with the anti-amyloid antibody anselamimab indicate that NT-proBNP can also be used to monitor cardiac response in anti-amyloid therapy [29]. Data on cardiac response of ATTR cardiac amyloidosis to tafamidis, patisiran, and anti-amyloid antibody NI006 indicate that NT-proBNP can be useful also in these settings, although not to the same extent as in AL amyloidosis [21, 32, 40]. High-sensitivity troponins, which accurately measure ongoing myocyte damage in various acute conditions such as myocardial infarction and myocarditis [43], contribute to the risk stratification of patients with AL-CA [44]. However, the use of high-sensitivity troponins in monitoring cardiac treatment response has never been validated.

The advent of anti-amyloid therapy has ignited the interest in evaluating the changes in the mass of the amyloid deposits and hence in cardiac imaging. Echocardiography remains the most widely available and inexpensive imaging modality and has demonstrated utility in cardiac AL amyloidosis patients, whereby global longitudinal strain (GLS) has been associated with the CA burden [45], so that improvements in GLS, in response to chemotherapy, independently predict survival [46]. GLS has also been utilized in patients with ATTR-CA, showing stabilization following treatment with diflunisal [47] and improvement following treatment with patisiran [21]. However, echocardiographic measures are subject to significant intra- and inter-observer variability, which is an important limitation when only small measurement variations are expected [48]. Improvements in precision could play a central role in monitoring treatment response and may be assisted by the emergence of data science [49]. The utility of artificial intelligence and more specifically convolutional neural networks has shown great promise in cardiovascular imaging [50, 51]. Elimination of manual operator contouring results in robust measures, with a significant improvement in precision medicine [50, 52]. These advances in automation may enable more accurate measurement of cardiac response to treatment by echocardiography. However, so far, echocardiography has not been validated in large studies.

CMR with the utilization of multi-parametric mapping techniques is rapidly emerging as an important tool in the assessment of ATTR-CA. Late gadolinium enhancement (LGE) demonstrates the continuity of CA, from subendocardial LGE to increasing transmurality as the disease develops [53]. Extracellular volume (ECV) measurement enables myocyte and extracellular compartment to be independently investigated. Since amyloidosis is an exemplar interstitial disease resulting in extracellular expansion, myocardial ECV quantification is an accurate surrogate measure of CA burden [54–56]. In AL-CA, ECV accurately measured disease severity and improved risk stratification [42, 57], while changes in ECV following treatment accurately predicted outcome even after adjusting for known predictors, such as changes in NT-proBNP and GLS [58]. ECV mapping allows detection of changes in tissue characterization that are likely to occur, ahead of changes in conventional structural and functional echocardiographic parameters. To our knowledge, only three studies have reported evidence of ATTR amyloid regression in the heart, two of them employing antibodies targeting TTR fibrils [34, 40, 59]. If large-scale studies will replicate and validate previous findings, ECV mapping may become the gold standard to monitor the effects of treatment on amyloid burden. It is noteworthy that reduced cardiac uptake has been reported on bone scintigraphy following combination treatment with patisiran and diflunisal on single-photon emission computed tomography. However, changes in cardiac uptake can be influenced by modifications in both the dynamics and kinetics of bone tracers that bind to several other "compartments," including bones, soft tissues, and myocardium. In fact, two recent well-documented case reports showed marked regression of cardiac bone tracer uptake following therapy with tafamidis and patisiran, despite evidence of persistent, substantial cardiac amyloid deposits [60, 61]. Therefore, bone scintigraphy alone cannot be used as a reliable measure of the cardiac response to treatment [34].

PET is another imaging technique with diagnostic potential in ATTR-CA. Several PET tracers, such as ^{18}F-florbetapir, ^{18}F-florbetaben, ^{18}F-flutemetamol, and ^{11}C-Pittsburgh B, have been successfully used to diagnose CA, with tracers binding to amyloid fibrils with high affinity and potentially allowing quantification of amyloid burden. There is a lack of robust data to support its use in tracking treatment response, but future PET developments may lead to novel promising measures of cardiac response [22, 62–67].

24.7 Long-Term Safety of TTR Depletion

Although in the short to medium term TTR knockdown through gene silencing and editing approaches appears safe, further research is needed to establish the long-term effects of TTR deficiency [68]. Traditionally, it was thought that the physiological role of TTR was confined to the transport of vitamin A and thyroxine. However, there is some evidence that TTR may have other functions in the central nervous system. Studies from preclinical models suggest that complete TTR knockdown in 5-month-old mice results in memory impairment compared with age-matched mice [69], and the absence of TTR in rats accelerates the decline in cognitive performance associated with aging [70]. Such findings led to the hypothesis that TTR may protect against neurodegeneration, particularly towards Alzheimer's disease. TTR may also have a role in metabolism. Animal models demonstrated that central TTR plays a role in modulating food intake and body weight through its anorectic properties [71]. Circulating TTR also plays a role in maintaining serum levels of retinol-binding protein 4, an adipokine linked to metabolic syndrome, by preventing its renal clearance [72]. Interestingly, obese mice treated with a TTR silencer showed decreased insulin levels and increased insulin sensitivity [73]. However, there is no evidence of cognitive decline or metabolic abnormalities in patients receiving gene silencers for more than 5 years and, importantly, TTR in the cerebrospinal fluid, and it is unaffected by NTLA-2001 therapy.

Specific concerns regarding off-target gene editing and unintended gene sequence deletions or insertions with CRISPR/Cas9 therapy have been raised [74, 75]. However, complex computational modeling and biochemical assays, including in vitro with human cells and in vivo in animal models, have shown no evidence of off-target editing with NTLA-2001 [39].

ATTR amyloidosis remains a progressive, debilitating, and ultimately fatal disease, for which gene silencers and gene editing therapies show great promise, but long-term safety remains unknown.

24.8 Organization of Diagnosis, Management of Cardiac Amyloidosis, and Treatment Issues

In the past, diagnosis of amyloidosis was based only on tissue biopsy, and this condition was known to a small group of specialists. At present, an algorithm for non-invasive diagnosis of cardiac ATTR amyloidosis is commonly employed. Imaging techniques including diphosphonate scintigraphy and cardiovascular magnetic resonance are becoming increasingly available, and disease awareness is spreading even among nonspecialists [76]. Collaboration between centers and multiple specialists remains crucial for a timely diagnosis and proper treatment [77]. The best setting for this collaboration is probably a network where most centers can do at least some parts of the diagnostic workup, exchange opinions and consults, and send patients to a regional/national referral center for selected procedures or particularly complex decisions.

The core message of the whole book is that it is critical to (a) promote collaborative research to increase our knowledge on the pathophysiology and epidemiology of diverse CA forms, (b) increase knowledge among clinicians on the disease allowing earlier suspicion, (c) improve differential diagnosis tools and identify their appropriate use at a peripheral as well as at referral center level, (d) facilitate the access to experts for speeding therapeutical decision-making, (e) define the criteria for identifying clinical improvement or worsening at follow-up, and (f) improve and tailor individual treatment testing new drugs and their combination: for this last goal, it is of critical importance that patients participate in clinical trials.

As novel evidence indicates that CA may be no more considered as a rare disease, and more and more patients are diagnosed and need an effective treatment, either tafamidis or new drugs present significant financial toxicity, and drug accessibility represents a real problem [78, 79].

Pharmaceutical companies, policy makers, and regulatory agencies must follow the clinicians' and researchers' advise, in order to make vital drugs available to those in need, which is an ethical imperative [80, 81].

References

1. Maurer MS, Elliott P, Comenzo R, Semigran M, Rapezzi C. Addressing common questions encountered in the diagnosis and management of cardiac amyloidosis. Circulation. 2017;135:1357–77.
2. Ravichandran S, Lachmann HJ, Wechalekar AD. Epidemiologic and survival trends in amyloidosis, 1987–2019. N Engl J Med. 2020;382:1567–8.
3. Iadanza MG, Jackson MP, Hewitt EW, Ranson NA, Radford SE. A new era for understanding amyloid structures and disease. Nat Rev Mol Cell Biol. 2018;19:755–73.
4. Saelices L, Chung K, Lee JH, Cohn W, Whitelegge JP, Benson MD, et al. Amyloid seeding of transthyretin by ex vivo cardiac fibrils and its inhibition. Proc Natl Acad Sci U S A. 2018;115:E6741–E50.
5. Liepnieks JJ, Benson MD. Progression of cardiac amyloid deposition in hereditary transthyretin amyloidosis patients after liver transplantation. Amyloid. 2007;14:277–82.
6. Mangione PP, Verona G, Corazza A, Marcoux J, Canetti D, Giorgetti S, et al. Plasminogen activation triggers transthyretin amyloidogenesis in vitro. J Biol Chem. 2018;293:14192–9.
7. Morgan GJ, Kelly JW. The kinetic stability of a full-length antibody light chain dimer determines whether endoproteolysis can release amyloidogenic variable domains. J Mol Biol. 2016;428:4280–97.
8. Oberti L, Rognoni P, Barbiroli A, Lavatelli F, Russo R, Maritan M, et al. Concurrent structural and biophysical traits link with immunoglobulin light chains amyloid propensity. Sci Rep. 2017;7:16809.
9. Merlini G, Dispenzieri A, Sanchorawala V, Schonland SO, Palladini G, Hawkins PN, et al. Systemic immunoglobulin light chain amyloidosis. Nat Rev Dis Primers. 2018;4:38.
10. Ruberg FL, Grogan M, Hanna M, Kelly JW, Maurer MS. Transthyretin amyloid cardiomyopathy: JACC state-of-the-art review. J Am Coll Cardiol. 2019;73:2872–91.
11. Caponetti AG, Rapezzi C, Gagliardi C, Milandri A, Dispenzieri A, Kristen AV, et al. Sex-related risk of cardiac involvement in hereditary transthyretin amyloidosis: insights from THAOS. JACC Heart Fail. 2021;9:736–46.
12. Suhr OB, Lundgren E, Westermark P. One mutation, two distinct disease variants: unravelling the impact of transthyretin amyloid fibril composition. J Int Med. 2017;281:337–47.

13. Mishra S, Joshi S, Ward JE, Buys EP, Mishra D, Mishra D, et al. Zebrafish model of amyloid light chain cardiotoxicity: regeneration versus degeneration. Am J Physiol Heart Circ Physiol. 2019;316:H1158–H66.
14. Diomede L, Rognoni P, Lavatelli F, Romeo M, Del Favero E, Cantu L, et al. A Caenorhabditis elegans-based assay recognizes immunoglobulin light chains causing heart amyloidosis. Blood. 2014;123:3543–52.
15. Martinez-Rivas G, Ayala M, Bender S, Roussel M, Jaccard A, Bridoux F, et al. A transgenic mouse model of cardiac AL amyloidosis. Blood. 2021;138(Suppl. 1):1592.
16. Slamova I, Adib R, Ellmerich S, Golos MR, Gilbertson JA, Botcher N, et al. Plasmin activity promotes amyloid deposition in a transgenic model of human transthyretin amyloidosis. Nat Commun. 2021;12:7112.
17. Merlini G, Lousada I, Ando Y, Dispenzieri A, Gertz MA, Grogan M, et al. Rationale, application and clinical qualification for NT-proBNP as a surrogate end point in pivotal clinical trials in patients with AL amyloidosis. Leukemia. 2016;30:1979–86.
18. Palladini G, Paiva B, Wechalekar A, Massa M, Milani P, Lasa M, et al. Minimal residual disease negativity by next-generation flow cytometry is associated with improved organ response in AL amyloidosis. Blood Cancer J. 2021;11:34.
19. Muchtar E, Dispenzieri A, Wisniowski B, Palladini G, Milani P, Merlini G, et al. Graded cardiac response criteria for patients with systemic light chain amyloidosis. J Clin Oncol. 2023;41:1393–403.
20. Minamisawa M, Claggett B, Adams D, Kristen AV, Merlini G, Slama MS, et al. Association of patisiran, an RNA interference therapeutic, with regional left ventricular myocardial strain in hereditary transthyretin amyloidosis: the APOLLO study. JAMA Cardiol. 2019;4:466–72.
21. Solomon SD, Adams D, Kristen A, Grogan M, Gonzalez-Duarte A, Maurer MS, et al. Effects of patisiran, an RNA interference therapeutic, on cardiac parameters in patients with hereditary transthyretin-mediated amyloidosis. Circulation. 2019;139:431–43.
22. Genovesi D, Vergaro G, Giorgetti A, Marzullo P, Scipioni M, Santarelli MF, et al. [18F]-florbetaben PET/CT for differential diagnosis among cardiac immunoglobulin light chain, transthyretin amyloidosis, and mimicking conditions. JACC Cardiovasc Imag. 2021;14:246–55.
23. Palladini G, Schonland S, Merlini G, Milani P, Jaccard A, Bridoux F, et al. The management of light chain (AL) amyloidosis in Europe: clinical characteristics, treatment patterns, and efficacy outcomes between 2004 and 2018. Blood Cancer J. 2023;13:19.
24. Merlini G. AL amyloidosis: from molecular mechanisms to targeted therapies. Hematology Am Soc Hematol Educ Program. 2017;2017:1–12.
25. Khor YM, Cuddy S, Falk RH, Dorbala S. Multimodality imaging in the evaluation and management of cardiac amyloidosis. Semin Nucl Med. 2020;50:295–310.
26. Manwani R, Foard D, Mahmood S, Sachchithanantham S, Lane T, Quarta C, et al. Rapid hematologic responses improve outcomes in patients with very advanced (stage IIIb) cardiac immunoglobulin light chain amyloidosis. Haematologica. 2018;103:e165–e8.
27. Theodorakakou F, Briasoulis A, Fotiou D, Petropoulos I, Georgiopoulos G, Lama N, et al. Outcomes for patients with systemic light chain amyloidosis and Mayo stage 3B disease. Hematol Oncol. 2023;41(4):725–32.
28. Basset M, Milani P, Foli A, Nuvolone M, Benvenuti P, Nanci M, et al. Early cardiac response is possible in stage IIIb cardiac AL amyloidosis and is associated with prolonged survival. Blood. 2022;140:1964–71.
29. Edwards CV, Rao N, Bhutani D, Mapara M, Radhakrishnan J, Shames S, et al. Phase 1a/b study of monoclonal antibody CAEL-101 (11-1F4) in patients with AL amyloidosis. Blood. 2021;138:2632–41.
30. Liedtke M, Palladini G, Molina MA, Kastritis E, Ianus J, Catini J, et al. Enrolling patients in Cardiac Amyloid Reaching for Extended Survival (CARES) trials: two placebo-controlled, double-blind, randomized, international phase 3 trials assessing CAEL-101 in patients with Mayo stage IIIa or stage IIIb AL amyloidosis. J Clin Oncol. 2023;41:TPS8071-TPS.

31. Ioannou A, Patel RK, Razvi Y, Porcari A, Sinagra G, Venneri L, et al. Impact of earlier diagnosis in cardiac ATTR amyloidosis over the course of 20 years. Circulation. 2022;146:1657–70.
32. Maurer MS, Schwartz JH, Gundapaneni B, Elliott PM, Merlini G, Waddington-Cruz M, et al. Tafamidis treatment for patients with transthyretin amyloid cardiomyopathy. N Engl J Med. 2018;379:1007–16.
33. Adams D, Gonzalez-Duarte A, O'Riordan WD, Yang CC, Ueda M, Kristen AV, et al. Patisiran, an RNAi therapeutic, for hereditary transthyretin amyloidosis. N Engl J Med. 2018;379:11–21.
34. Fontana M, Martinez-Naharro A, Chacko L, Rowczenio D, Gilbertson JA, Whelan CJ, et al. Reduction in CMR derived extracellular volume with patisiran indicates cardiac amyloid regression. JACC Cardiovasc Imag. 2021;14:189–99.
35. Adams D, Tournev IL, Taylor MS, Coelho T, Planté-Bordeneuve V, Berk JL, et al. Efficacy and safety of vutrisiran for patients with hereditary transthyretin-mediated amyloidosis with polyneuropathy: a randomized clinical trial. Amyloid. 2023;30:1–9.
36. Keam SJ. Vutrisiran: first approval. Drugs. 2022;82:1419–25.
37. Benson MD, Waddington-Cruz M, Berk JL, Polydefkis M, Dyck PJ, Wang AK, et al. Inotersen treatment for patients with hereditary transthyretin amyloidosis. N Engl J Med. 2018;379:22–31.
38. Viney NJ, Guo S, Tai LJ, Baker BF, Aghajan M, Jung SW, et al. Ligand conjugated antisense oligonucleotide for the treatment of transthyretin amyloidosis: preclinical and phase 1 data. ESC Heart Fail. 2021;8:652–61.
39. Gillmore JD, Gane E, Taubel J, Kao J, Fontana M, Maitland ML, et al. CRISPR-Cas9 in vivo gene editing for transthyretin amyloidosis. N Engl J Med. 2021;385:493–502.
40. Garcia-Pavia P, Aus dem Siepen F, Donal E, Lairez O, van der Meer P, Kristen AV, et al. Phase 1 trial of antibody NI006 for depletion of cardiac transthyretin amyloid. N Engl J Med. 2023;389(3):239–50.
41. Palladini G, Dispenzieri A, Gertz MA, Kumar S, Wechalekar A, Hawkins PN, et al. New criteria for response to treatment in immunoglobulin light chain amyloidosis based on free light chain measurement and cardiac biomarkers: impact on survival outcomes. J Clin Oncol. 2012;30:4541–9.
42. Banypersad SM, Sado DM, Flett AS, Gibbs SD, Pinney JH, Maestrini V, et al. Quantification of myocardial extracellular volume fraction in systemic AL amyloidosis: an equilibrium contrast cardiovascular magnetic resonance study. Circ Cardiovasc Imaging. 2013;6:34–9.
43. Passino C, Aimo A, Masotti S, Musetti V, Prontera C, Emdin M, et al. Cardiac troponins as biomarkers for cardiac disease. Biomark Med. 2019;13:325–30.
44. Dispenzieri A, Gertz MA, Kumar SK, Lacy MQ, Kyle RA, Saenger AK, et al. High sensitivity cardiac troponin T in patients with immunoglobulin light chain amyloidosis. Heart. 2014;100:383–8.
45. Kim D, Choi JO, Kim K, Kim SJ, Kim JS, Jeon ES. Association of left ventricular global longitudinal strain with cardiac amyloid load in light chain amyloidosis. JACC Cardiovasc Imag. 2021;14:1283–5.
46. Cohen OC, Ismael A, Pawarova B, Manwani R, Ravichandran S, Law S, et al. Longitudinal strain is an independent predictor of survival and response to therapy in patients with systemic AL amyloidosis. Eur Heart J. 2022;43:333–41.
47. Lohrmann G, Pipilas A, Mussinelli R, Gopal DM, Berk JL, Connors LH, et al. Stabilization of cardiac function with diflunisal in transthyretin (ATTR) cardiac amyloidosis. J Card Fail. 2020;26:753–9.
48. Chacko L, Karia N, Venneri L, Bandera F, Passo BD, Buonamici L, et al. Progression of echocardiographic parameters and prognosis in transthyretin cardiac amyloidosis. Eur J Heart Fail. 2022;24:1700–12.
49. Ioannou A, Patel R, Gillmore JD, Fontana M. Imaging-guided treatment for cardiac amyloidosis. Curr Cardiol Rep. 2022;24:839–50.
50. Dey D, Slomka PJ, Leeson P, Comaniciu D, Shrestha S, Sengupta PP, et al. Artificial intelligence in cardiovascular imaging: JACC state-of-the-art review. J Am Coll Cardiol. 2019;73:1317–35.

51. Tromp J, Seekings PJ, Hung CL, Iversen MB, Frost MJ, Ouwerkerk W, et al. Automated interpretation of systolic and diastolic function on the echocardiogram: a multicohort study. Lancet Dig Health. 2022;4:e46–54.
52. Howard JP, Francis DP. Machine learning with convolutional neural networks for clinical cardiologists. Heart. 2022;108:973–81.
53. Fontana M, Pica S, Reant P, Abdel-Gadir A, Treibel TA, Banypersad SM, et al. Prognostic value of late gadolinium enhancement cardiovascular magnetic resonance in cardiac amyloidosis. Circulation. 2015;132:1570–9.
54. Fontana M, Ćorović A, Scully P, Moon JC. Myocardial amyloidosis: the exemplar interstitial disease. JACC Cardiovasc Imag. 2019;12:2345–56.
55. Fontana M, Banypersad SM, Treibel TA, Maestrini V, Sado DM, White SK, et al. Native T1 mapping in transthyretin amyloidosis. JACC Cardiovasc Imag. 2014;7:157–65.
56. Karamitsos TD, Piechnik SK, Banypersad SM, Fontana M, Ntusi NB, Ferreira VM, et al. Noncontrast T1 mapping for the diagnosis of cardiac amyloidosis. JACC Cardiovasc Imag. 2013;6:488–97.
57. Banypersad SM, Fontana M, Maestrini V, Sado DM, Captur G, Petrie A, et al. T1 mapping and survival in systemic light-chain amyloidosis. Eur Heart J. 2015;36:244–51.
58. Martinez-Naharro A, Patel R, Kotecha T, Karia N, Ioannou A, Petrie A, et al. Cardiovascular magnetic resonance in light-chain amyloidosis to guide treatment. Eur Heart J. 2022;43:4722–35.
59. Fontana M, Gilbertson J, Verona G, Riefolo M, Slamova I, Leone O, et al. Antibody-associated reversal of ATTR amyloidosis-related cardiomyopathy. N Engl J Med. 2023;388:2199–201.
60. Wang A, Mahmood U, Tang X, Jain D, Pan S. A case of disappearing amyloid on technetium pyrophosphate scan. J Nucl Cardiol. 2023;30(5):1986–91.
61. Smiley DA, Einstein AJ, Mintz A, Shetty M, Chan N, Helmke ST, et al. Gene silencing therapy in hereditary (variant) transthyretin cardiac amyloidosis: a puzzling case of decreasing pyrophosphate uptake on scintigraphy. Circ Cardiovasc Imaging. 2023;16(8):e015243.
62. Dorbala S, Vangala D, Semer J, Strader C, Bruyere JR Jr, Di Carli MF, et al. Imaging cardiac amyloidosis: a pilot study using ^{18}F-florbetapir positron emission tomography. Eur J Nucl Med Mol Imaging. 2014;41:1652–62.
63. Dietemann S, Nkoulou R. Amyloid PET imaging in cardiac amyloidosis: a pilot study using (18)F-flutemetamol positron emission tomography. Ann Nucl Med. 2019;33:624–8.
64. Antoni G, Lubberink M, Estrada S, Axelsson J, Carlson K, Lindsjö L, et al. In vivo visualization of amyloid deposits in the heart with 11C-PIB and PET. J Nucl Med. 2013;54:213–20.
65. Kircher M, Ihne S, Brumberg J, Morbach C, Knop S, Kortüm KM, et al. Detection of cardiac amyloidosis with (18)F-Florbetaben-PET/CT in comparison to echocardiography, cardiac MRI and DPD-scintigraphy. Eur J Nucl Med Mol Imaging. 2019;46:1407–16.
66. Lee SP, Suh HY, Park S, Oh S, Kwak SG, Kim HM, et al. Pittsburgh B compound positron emission tomography in patients with AL cardiac amyloidosis. J Am Coll Cardiol. 2020;75:380–90.
67. Kim YJ, Ha S, Kim YI. Cardiac amyloidosis imaging with amyloid positron emission tomography: a systematic review and meta-analysis. J Nucl Cardiol. 2020;27:123–32.
68. Maurer MS. Gene editing—a cure for transthyretin amyloidosis? N Engl J Med. 2021;385:558–9.
69. Sousa JC, Marques F, Dias-Ferreira E, Cerqueira JJ, Sousa N, Palha JA. Transthyretin influences spatial reference memory. Neurobiol Learn Mem. 2007;88:381–5.
70. Brouillette J, Quirion R. Transthyretin: a key gene involved in the maintenance of memory capacities during aging. Neurobiol Aging. 2008;29:1721–32.
71. Zheng F, Kim YJ, Moran TH, Li H, Bi S. Central transthyretin acts to decrease food intake and body weight. Sci Rep. 2016;6:24238.
72. Kotnik P, Fischer-Posovszky P, Wabitsch M. RBP4: a controversial adipokine. Eur J Endocrinol. 2011;165:703–11.
73. Zemany L, Bhanot S, Peroni OD, Murray SF, Moraes-Vieira PM, Castoldi A, et al. Transthyretin antisense oligonucleotides lower circulating rbp4 levels and improve insulin sensitivity in obese mice. Diabetes. 2015;64:1603–14.

74. Haapaniemi E, Botla S, Persson J, Schmierer B, Taipale J. CRISPR-Cas9 genome editing induces a p53-mediated DNA damage response. Nat Med. 2018;24:927–30.
75. Enache OM, Rendo V, Abdusamad M, Lam D, Davison D, Pal S, et al. Cas9 activates the p53 pathway and selects for p53-inactivating mutations. Nat Genet. 2020;52:662–8.
76. Vergaro G, Aimo A, Barison A, Genovesi D, Buda G, Passino C, et al. Keys to early diagnosis of cardiac amyloidosis: red flags from clinical, laboratory and imaging findings. Eur J Prev Cardiol. 2020;27(17):1806–15.
77. Writing C, Kittleson MM, Ruberg FL, Ambardekar AV, Brannagan TH, Cheng RK, et al. 2023 ACC expert consensus decision pathway on comprehensive multidisciplinary care for the patient with cardiac amyloidosis: a report of the American College of Cardiology Solution Set Oversight Committee. J Am Coll Cardiol. 2023;81:1076–126.
78. Hagenbeek A, Gribben J, Jager U, Kapitein P, Merlini G, Piggin M, et al. Fair pricing of innovative medicines: an EHA Position Paper. Hema. 2020;4:e488.
79. Merlini G, Gribben J, Macintyre E, Piggin M, Doeswijk R. Access to affordable orphan medicines in europe: an EHA Position Paper. Hema. 2020;4:e477.
80. Luzzatto L, Hyry HI, Schieppati A, Costa E, Simoens S, Schaefer F, et al. Outrageous prices of orphan drugs: a call for collaboration. Lancet. 2018;392:791–4.
81. Gurwitz JH, Maurer MS. Tafamidis-a pricey therapy for a not-so-rare condition. JAMA Cardiol. 2020;5:247–8.